'COVID-19 has triggered an avalanche of books and articles examining the public policy responses to the pandemic. However, *Federalism and the Response to COVID-19* is one of the very few books that examines and compares the effectiveness of these responses in federal and quasi-federal countries. As the authors show, the pandemic challenged federal structures and processes everywhere but in this crisis was also an opportunity. This volume showed me which federal countries used the pandemic to make innovations in both the practices and structures of federalism and which were incapable of rising to the challenge.'

Dr Greg Marchildon, *Ontario Research Chair in Health Policy and System Design with the Institute of Health Policy, Management, and Evaluation, University of Toronto, Canada*

'*Federalism and the Response to COVID-19* provides an interesting analysis of the strategies adopted by 23 federal and decentralized countries (as well as the European Union) to deal with the COVID-19 pandemic. The volume provides important insights in how the first wave of the pandemic was handled, exploring the different roles and responsibilities discharged by different levels of government, variations in the success of intergovernmental coordination and interesting innovations in dealing with the health crisis. This volume is a must-read for all those who wish to understand what succeeds and what does not when federal and decentralized administrations respond to emergencies.'

Dr Sandeep Shastri, *Vice Chancellor, Jagran Lakecity University, Bhopal, India*

T0256282

Federalism and the Response to COVID-19

The COVID-19 pandemic bared the inadequacies in existing structures of public health and governance in most countries. This book provides a comparative analysis of policy approaches and planning adopted by federal governments across the globe to battle and adequately respond to the health emergency as well as the socio-economic fallouts of the pandemic.

With twenty-four case studies from across the globe, the book critically analyzes responses to the public health crisis, its fiscal impact and management, as well as decision-making and collaboration between different levels of government of countries worldwide. It explores the measures taken to contain the pandemic and to responsibly regulate and manage the health, socio-economic welfare, employment, and education of its people. The authors highlight the deficiencies in planning, tensions between state and local governments, politicization of the crisis, and the challenges of generating political consensus. They also examine effective approaches used to foster greater cooperation and learning for multi-level, polycentric innovation in pandemic governance.

One of the first books on federalism and approaches to the COVID-19 pandemic, this volume is an indispensable reference for scholars and researchers of comparative federalism, comparative politics, development studies, political science, public policy and governance, health and wellbeing, and political sociology.

The Open Access version of this book, available at: http://www.taylorfrancis.com/books/e/9781003251217, has been made available under a Creative Commons Attribution-Non Commercial-No Derivatives 4.0 license.

Rupak Chattopadhyay is President and CEO of the Forum of Federations, Canada.

Felix Knüpling is Vice President of the Forum of Federations, Canada.

Diana Chebenova is Senior Director at the Forum of Federations, Canada.

Liam Whittington is Program Manager at the Forum of Federations, Canada.

Phillip Gonzalez is Regional Director of Programs for Asia and Australia at the Forum of Federations, Canada.

Routledge Series on the Humanities and the Social Sciences in a Post-COVID-19 World

The COVID-19 Pandemic has changed our lives economically, politically, socially, and emotionally.

The pandemic has impacted around the world in terms of health and wellbeing and brought into sharp focus fault lines and continuities in our lives and societies which are likely to outlive the pandemic. In this light, the humanities and the social sciences will have a crucial role to play as we reimagine and reshape everything we know in the post-pandemic years.

This Routledge series aims to bring forward cutting edge interdisciplinary research on various facets of politics, society, economy, environment, culture, psychology, and wellbeing in the post-COVID world. The books in this series will engage with a range of topical issues that have surfaced in the wake of the pandemic, and study how these emerging trends and critical developments are likely to impact the way in which humanities and social sciences are taught, researched, and understood in the years to come.

Books in this series

Democracy and Public Policy in the Post-COVID-19 World
Choices and Outcomes
Edited by Rumki Basu

Pandemic, Governance and Communication
The Curious Case of COVID-19
Dipankar Sinha

Federalism and the Response to COVID-19
A Comparative Analysis
Edited by Rupak Chattopadhyay, Felix Knüpling, Diana Chebenova,
Liam Whittington and Phillip Gonzalez

For more information about this series, please visit: https://www.routledge.com/Routledge-Series-on-the-Humanities-and-the-Social-Sciences-in-a-Post-COVID-19/book-series/HSSPCW

Federalism and the Response to COVID-19

A Comparative Analysis

Edited by
Rupak Chattopadhyay, Felix Knüpling,
Diana Chebenova, Liam Whittington and
Phillip Gonzalez

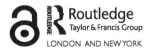

Routledge
Taylor & Francis Group

LONDON AND NEW YORK

Cover image: Getty Images

First published 2022
by Routledge
2 Park Square, Milton Park, Abingdon, Oxon OX14 4RN

and by Routledge
605 Third Avenue, New York, NY 10158

Routledge is an imprint of the Taylor & Francis Group, an informa business

British Library Cataloguing-in-Publication Data
A catalogue record for this book is available from the British Library

Library of Congress Cataloging-in-Publication Data
A catalog record has been requested for this book

ISBN: 978-1-032-07790-1 (hbk)
ISBN: 978-1-032-16987-3 (pbk)
ISBN: 978-1-003-25121-7 (ebk)

DOI: 10.4324/9781003251217

Typeset in Sabon
by codeMantra

Contents

Figures

Tables

Contributors

Zemelak Ayitenew Ayele is Associate Professor and Director at the Centre for Federalism and Governance Studies, Addis Ababa University, Ethiopia.

Rodrigo Ribeiro Bedritichuk is Commission Secretary in the Brazilian Federal Senate.

Daniel Béland is Professor at the School of Political Studies at the University of Ottawa, Canada.

Matías Bianchi is the Founder and Director of the think tank Asuntos del Sur, Argentina, and Adjunct Professor at the University of Arizona, United States.

Peter Bursens is Professor at Universiteit Antwerpen, GOVTRUST Centre of Excellence, Belgium.

Peter Bußjäger is Chairman of the Institute of Federalism in Innsbruck and Professor at the University of Innsbruck, Austria.

David Cameron is Fellow of the Royal Society of Canada and Professor at the University of Toronto, Canada.

Cristina Ares Castro-Conde is Professor at the University of Santiago de Compostela, Spain.

Rupak Chattopadhyay is President and CEO of the Forum of Federations, Canada, and Research Fellow at the Centre for Federal Studies at the University of Kent, United Kingdom.

Diana Chebenova is Senior Director at the Forum of Federations, Canada.

Eduardo Henrique Corrêa da S.P. Néris is Director of Intergovernmental Management for Federative Affairs in the Brazilian Presidency.

Jaap De Visser is Director of the Dullah Omar Institute and Professor at the University of the Western Cape, South Africa.

Mathias Eller is Assistant Professor at the Institute of Federalism in Innsbruck, Austria.

Alan Fenna is Professor at the John Curtin Institute of Public Policy, Curtin University, Western Australia.

Rahel Freiburghaus is a PhD candidate at the University of Bern, Switzerland.

Nataliya Golovanova is Senior Researcher at the Center for Intergovernmental Relations at the Financial Research Institute of the Ministry of Finance of the Russian Federation, Moscow, Russia.

Laura Flamand is Professor at the El Colegio de Mexico.

Phillip Gonzalez is Regional Director of Programs for Asia and Australia at the Forum of Federations, Canada.

Clive Grace O.B.E is Honorary Research Fellow at the Cardiff Business School, Wales.

Monica Naime is a doctoral researcher at the University of Bergen, Norway.

Julius O. Ihonvbere is a member of the National Assembly of the Federal Republic of Nigeria.

Puspa Raj Kadel is Vice Chair of the National Planning Commission, Nepal.

John Kincaid is Director of the Meyner Center for the Study of State and Local Government at Lafayette College, Pennsylvania, United States.

Felix Knüpling is Vice President of the Forum of Federations, Canada.

Mario Kölling is Professor at the Spanish National Distance University (UNED), Spain.

Sabine Kropp is Professor at Freie Universität Berlin, Germany.

J. Wesley Leckrone is Professor and Chair of Widener University, Pennsylvania, United States.

André Lecours is Professor at the School of Political Studies at the University of Ottawa, Canada.

Petra Meier is Professor at Universiteit Antwerpen, GOVTRUST Centre of Excellence, Belgium.

Sameen A. Mohsin Ali is Assistant Professor at the Mushtaq Gurmani School of Humanities and Social Sciences (MGSHSS), Lahore University of Management Sciences, Pakistan.

Sean Mueller is Assistant Professor at the University of Lausanne, Switzerland.

Juan C. Olmeda is Professor at the El Colegio de Mexico.

Rose B. Osoro is Fellow of the Chartered Professional Accountants (FCPA), Kenya.

Francesco Palermo is Professor of Comparative Constitutional Law at the University of Verona and Director of the Institute for Comparative Federalism at Eurac Research in Bolzano/Bozen, Italy.

Patricia Popelier is Professor at Universiteit Antwerpen, GOVTRUST Centre of Excellence, Belgium.

Nina Sajic is a foreign policy advisor to the Presidency of Bosnia and Herzegovina.

Rekha Saxena is Honorary Vice-chairperson, Centre for Multilevel Federalism, India and Professor at the University of Delhi, India.

Johanna Schnabel is Lecturer and Chair of German Politics at the Otto Suhr Institute for Political Science at Freie Universität Berlin, Germany.

Nico Steytler is the South African Research Chair at the Dullah Omar Institute of the University of the Western Cape, South Africa.

Adrian Vatter is Professor at the University of Bern, Switzerland.

Jennifer Wallner is Professor at the School of Political Studies at the University of Ottawa, Canada.

Liam Whittington is Program Manager at the Forum of Federations, Canada, and Research Fellow at the Centre for Federal Studies at the University of Kent, United Kingdom.

Tricia Yeoh is CEO of the Institute for Democracy and Economic Affairs (IDEAS), Malaysia.

Foreword

The COVID-19 pandemic of 2020 is a pivotal event in human history. It has upended societies and economies all over the world. As we enter a period in which governments are rolling out vaccines in their fight against the pandemic, this volume is an effort to pause and take stock of how federations worldwide responded to this crisis. Comprising over 40 percent of the global population and some of the world's largest economies, federal countries cover a considerable part of the world and much of the global economic output.

In the summer of 2020, the Forum of Federations produced a critical series of concise comparative papers that explored how federal and devolved countries initially reacted to the global pandemic. These papers represented a snapshot of a quickly unfolding situation. This series, "Dealing with the COVID-19 crisis in Federal and Devolved Countries," captured the interest of many governance practitioners who used the knowledge while developing and analyzing their own governance responses.

The broad interest in these short papers inspired the Forum of Federations to comprehensively examine how these countries managed the pandemic in the first year. The time period covered by this publication starts from the onset of the COVID-19 virus (as the world understood it to be a threat) until right before vaccine delivery. The first phase of this pandemic covered most of the 2020 calendar year. The volume aims to understand the impact that federalism had in shaping public policy responses to the pandemic and also considers how the crisis has changed the practice of federalism.

In this volume, experiences from 23 federal and devolved countries, plus the EU, are examined. At the time of writing, the pandemic was still raging. Consequently, our observations can only be treated as preliminary. To produce this publication, the Forum of Federations leveraged its global network of experts to commission different country-expert authors for each chapter. Quite apart from colleagues who are editors of this volume, I take this opportunity to thank and recognize others who contributed to the publication by editing, formatting, collecting data, managing author contributions, and gathering permissions: Notably, George Stairs (Project Officer), Carl Stieren, Max Lapointe-Rohde, Asma Zribi (Project Officer), and Deanna Senko.

The Forum team also wants to express our appreciation to the many illustrious authors who contributed numerous research hours to producing their chapters. This manuscript would not have been possible without their insightful and enriching contributions.

A grand thank you as well to our publishers at the Routledge Taylor & Francis Group for their expertise in preparing our manuscript to be presented to the public.

Since its founding, the Forum's mission has been based around the core principle of "Learning From Each Other," an institutional axiom which guides our comparative research. The Forum hopes that this volume represents accessible and valuable contribution to research on federalism and the pandemic.

John Light, Senior Director of Communications

Acronyms and abbreviations

AC	Autonomous Community
ADF	Australian Border Force or the Australian Defense Force
AMBA	Metropolitan Area of Buenos Aires
ASHA	Accredited Social Health Activist
ATP	Work and Production Assistance
BFI	Bank and Financial Institutions
BGP	Basic Guarantee Program
BJP	Bharatiya Janata Party
B-VG	Austrian Federal Constitution (*Bundes-Verfassungsgesetz*)
CAF	Council for the Australian Federation
CARES Act	Coronavirus Aid, Relief, and Economic Security Act
CCC	Coordination and Crisis Centre
CCI	Council of Common Interests
CCMC	COVID-19 Crisis Management Centre
CCOP	COVID-19 Crisis Combat Operations Center
CCSERS	COVID-19 County Socio-Economic Re-Engineering and Recovery Strategy
CDC	US Centers for Disease Control and Prevention
CDU	Christian Democratic Union of Germany
CELEVAL	Belgian National Evaluation Unit (*Cellule d'Évaluation*)
CERB	Canada Emergency Response Benefits
CESB	Canada Emergency Student Benefit
CEWS	Canada Emergency Wage Subsidy
CHF	Swiss Franc
CHT	Canada Health Transfer
CIS	Commonwealth of Independent States
CMCO	Controlled Movement Control Order
COAG	Council of Australia Governments
COBRA	Cabinet Office Briefing Rooms
COF	Council of the Federation
COFESA	Federal Council for Healthcare (*Consejo Federal de Salud*)
CoG	Council of Governors
CoM	Council of Ministers
CPM	Civil Protection Mechanism
CST	Canada Social Transfer
Cst	Federal Constitution of the Swiss Confederation

CSU	Christian Social Union
DIY	Do-It-Yourself
ECMO	Extracorporeal membrane oxygenation
EDP	Ethiopian Democratic Party
EFDCA	Ethiopian Food and Drug Control Authority
EpidA	Federal Act on the Control of Communicable Human Diseases
ESP	Economic Stimulus Programme
EU	European Union
F&B	Food and Beverage
FATA	Federally Administered Tribal Areas
FB&H	Federation of Bosnia and Herzegovina
FCT	Federal Capital Territory
FMMIF	Federal Mandatory Medical Insurance Fund
FPE	State Participation Fund
FPM	Municipality Participation Fund
FRSC	Federal Road Safety Commission
FY	Fiscal Year
GDK	Conference of Cantonal Directors for Health (*Schweizerische Gesundheitsdirektorenkonferenz*)
GDP	Gross Domestic Product
GEES	Group of Experts in charge of the Exit Strategy
GFC	Global Financial Crisis
GNI	Gross National Income
GST	Goods and Services Tax
HDI	Human Development Index
HLCC	High Level Coordination Committee
HoF	House of Federation
ICT	Islamabad Capital Territory
ICU	Intensive Care Unit
IFE	Emergency Family Income (*Ingreso Familiar de Emergencia*)
IfSG	German Infection Protection Act (*Infektionsschutzgesetz*)
IGR	Inter-governmental Relations
IMF	International Monetary Fund
INEC	Independent Electoral Commission
INSABI	National Institute of Health for Wellness (*Instituto de Salud para el Bienestar*)
ISI	Inter-Services Intelligence
JEE	Joint Entrance Exam
JOC	Joint Operating Centers
KdK	Conference of Cantonal Governments (*Konferenz der Kantonsregierungen*)
KNBS	National Bureau of Statistics
LGAs	Local Government Areas
MCO	Movement Control Order
MFF	Multiannual Financial Framework
MinMECS	Ministers and Members of Executive Councils
MITI	Ministry of International Trade and Industry
MoH	Ministry of Health

MoNHSCR	Ministry of National Health Service Coordination and Regulation
MoP	Ministry of Peace
MPI	Multidimensional Poverty Index
MPK	Prime Minister's Conference (*Ministerpräsidentenkonferenz*)
MSME	Micro, Small, and Medium Enterprises
MySED	Malaysia Strategy for Emerging Diseases and Public Health Emergencies
NCC	National Coordination Committee
NCCC	National Coronavirus Command Council
NCCRCP	National Coordination Committee on the Response to the Corona Virus Pandemic
NCDC	National Centre for Disease Control
NCLG	National Council on Local Governments
NCOC	National Command and Operations Centre
NDMA	National Disaster Management Authority
NDRMC	National Disaster and Risk Management Commission
NEBE	National Elections Board of Ethiopia
NEBR	National Economic and Business Response
NECC	National Emergency Coordination Centre
NEET	National Eligibility Cum Entrance Test
NGOs	Non-Governmental Organizations
NHS	National Health System
NIH	National Institute of Health
NIMC	National Identity Management Commission
NIN	National Identity Numbers
NMS	Nairobi Management Service
NOA	National Orientation Agency
NPR	Nepal Rupees
NSC	National Security Council
NSW	New South Wales
NT	National Treasury
NTA	National Testing Agency
OECD	Organization for Economic Co-operation and Development
OFC	Oromo Federalist Congress
PCC	President's Coordinating Council
PCR	Polymerase Chain Reaction
PHCC	Primary Health Care Centers
PHI	Public Health Institute
PKR	Pakistani Rupee
PN	Perikatan Nasional
PNV	Basque Nationalist Party (*Partido Nacionalista Vasco*)
PP	Popular Party (*Partido Popular*)
PPE	Protective Personal Equipment
PPP	Pakistan People's Party
PSOE	Spanish Socialist Workers' Party (*Partido Socialista Obrero Español*)
PTF	Presidential Task Force
PTI	Pakistan Tehreek-e-Insaf

PWD	Persons with Disabilities
R&D	Research and Development
RDT	Rapid Diagnostic Tests
RF	Russian Federation
RGP	Regional Guarantee Program
RKI	Robert Koch Institute
RMCO	Recovery Movement Control Order
RMG	Risk Management Group
RS	Republika Srpska
RT-PCR	Reverse Transcription – Polymerase Chain Reaction
SAARC	South Asian Association for Regional Cooperation
SAHOs	Stay-At-Home Orders
SC	Spanish Constitution
SEAF	Special Secretariat for Federative Affairs
SEDCs	State Economic Development Corporations
SIAPR	National Early Warning and Rapid Response System (*El Sistema Nacional de Alerta Precoz y Respuesta Rápida*)
SISA	Argentine Integrated Health Information System (*Sistema Integrado de Información Sanitaria Argentino*)
SMEs	Small and Medium Enterprises
SoE	State of Emergency
SOPs	Standard Operative Procedures
SURE	The temporary Support to mitigate Unemployment Risks in an Emergency
TEMCOs	Targeted Enhanced Movement Control Orders
TEU	Treaty of the European Union
TFC	Tourism Finance Corporation
TPLF	Tigray People's Liberation Front
UC	Unemployment Compensation
UCR	Radical Civic Union (*Unión Cívica Radical*)
UGC	University Grants Commission
UNICEF	United Nations International Children's Emergency Fund
UTs	Union Territories
VAT	Value-Added Tax
WHO	World Health Organization

1 An introduction to COVID-19 and federalism

Rupak Chattopadhyay, Felix Knüpling and Liam Whittington

The COVID-19 pandemic is an unprecedented international event. The spread of the coronavirus – the biggest public health crisis in a century and the first of this scale in the globalized modern world – has prompted unparalleled responses by national governments. The proliferation of 24-hour news coverage and social media has allowed people across the world to follow, in real time, the unfolding and visible impacts of the pandemic.

This book is about the impact of the crisis on federal and multilevel systems, which account for approximately 40 percent of the world population.[1] In 2020, as governments grappled with fluctuating waves of the COVID-19 pandemic, the effectiveness of public policy varied among federal nations. Federal countries such as Australia and Canada managed to keep mortality low, whereas others such as Brazil, Spain, and the United States suffered some of the highest numbers of fatalities anywhere around the world, both in absolute and relative terms (Brunner et al. 2020; Ionova 2020; Kontis et al. 2020, pp. 1919–1928; Ritchie et al. 2021).

A 2015 Forum of Federations workshop on "Emergency Management in Federal Countries," which brought together emergency management professionals from half a dozen nations, did not even consider the question of transnational pandemics (Forum of Federations 2015). Focusing primarily on natural disasters such as fires, earthquakes, floods, and climate adaptation, the subsequent report reflected the recurring issues that routinely demand the attention of emergency management departments in all countries. Perhaps because recent pandemics such as SARS-CoV and H1N1 had a relatively limited geographic footprint, the COVID-19 tsunami took policy makers everywhere by surprise (Relman, Chofness and Mack 2010; World Health Organization 2003). The novelty of the virus, and a lack of information on its origin and effects in the early phases of the outbreak, enabled it to spread unchecked for several months before controls were subsequently introduced (World Health Organization 2020; Wu et al. 2020).

While, in most federal countries, the constitutional power to deal with national disasters or emergencies resides with the federal government, the delivery of health services is often the remit of constituent units, such as states, provinces, and cantons, as well as local governments.[2] Thus, responding to the public health and economic crisis brought on by the pandemic has required policy interventions at the level of federal governments as well as constituent units (OECD 2020). This has necessitated unprecedented levels of intergovernmental interaction and coordination between all orders[3] in a federation.

DOI: 10.4324/9781003251217-1

The pandemic has clearly raised questions about the effectiveness of the governance response to the crisis in federal (and devolved) countries. This touches on issues such as the roles and responsibilities of various orders of government and the adequacy of existing institutions and processes of intergovernmental relations. Furthermore, whether the pandemic has led to innovations in the practice of federalism, and thus whether federal countries now are better prepared to handle future pandemics, is a topic of substantial importance.

Following Oates' (1999) notion of "laboratory federalism," innovation in public policy through experimentation and mutual learning can be considered as one of the important advantages of federal systems. Accordingly, federal countries may be uniquely suited to grappling with the complexity and uncertainty of emergencies such as pandemics (Ferejohn, Eskridge and Bednar 2001; Greer et al. 2020). Federal models, so the theory purports, provide policy makers with opportunities to develop solutions tailored to different scales and circumstances, experiment with innovative policy measures, and engender policy learning and convergence over time. Conversely, political scientists argue that regulatory overlaps and coordination deficits are inherent in many federal systems, which may hinder the pursuit of effective responses to an emergency such as the COVID pandemic (*ibid.*).

The complex mosaic of actions adopted within many federal and multilevel systems prompts this comparative publication toward enhancing understanding on how different institutional frameworks, governance mechanisms, and political dynamics interact to shape emergency response. Of particular interest is the extent of cooperation between different orders of government, as well as effective and ineffective practice in pandemic management in federal and multilevel systems.

This volume provides a comparative overview of the policy response of 23 federal or federal-type countries, and one supra-national organization, to the pandemic: Australia, Austria, Argentina, Belgium, Bosnia and Herzegovina, Brazil, Canada, Ethiopia, Germany, India, Italy, Kenya, Malaysia, Mexico, Nepal, Nigeria, Pakistan, Russia, South Africa, Spain, Switzerland, the United Kingdom, the United States, and the European Union. By federalism, we understand a system of governance which has at least two orders of government (one for the whole country and one for the constituent units) whose spheres of decision-making authority are protected constitutionally[4] (Anderson 2008).

We recognize that the case studies covered in this volume include countries which do not strictly fall under the category of federalism. This includes the devolved multinational United Kingdom, Italy, which alongside to its federal features also exhibits strong elements of a unitary system of governance, and the supra-national case study of the European Union. Case studies of countries which do not refer to themselves as federal, such as Spain and South Africa, are also included.

The cases cover the majority of federal or federal-type countries from both the Global North and the Global South, with great institutional variation, differing levels of economic development, and diverse demographic profiles. While we acknowledge the challenges of comparative analysis of 24 very different case studies, we believe that there is significant value in this endeavor. Despite the uniqueness of each case and the many differences between the nations analyzed – in terms of their history, constitutional and institutional structures, and political and economic development – they do have common features and face the challenge of coordination and collaboration (Hueglin and Fenna 2015).

The issue of coordination and collaboration between orders of government also guides our categorization of case studies. Comparing the response to the pandemic from a governance perspective, we identify three categories:

• National Government Dominated Responses;
• Strong Collaboration and Coordination between Jurisdictions;
• Weak Collaboration between Jurisdictions.

The categorization of the case studies is elaborated in greater detail in the comparative chapter, accompanied by identification of key trends across the countries analyzed.

At the time of writing in early 2021, globally the COVID-19 crisis is still very much ongoing and unlikely to abate in the short term. This volume focuses on examining the response to (as well as the impact of) the pandemic in the year 2020. During this period, many countries around the world experienced multiple waves of COVID-19 infections, some more or less severe than others. It is important to note that the phrase "first wave" (or indeed second or third wave) does not refer to a universal period of time globally. This is because COVID-19 peaked at different points in time in different countries. For example, the first wave peaked in Germany in late March 2020, in Canada in April 2020, and in India only in October 2020 (Ritchie et al. 2020). The country case studies therefore focus on the impacts of COVID-19 as the pandemic ebbed and flowed in the respective country over the course of 2020.

The chapters in this book consider how the pandemic has tested not just systems of government but also the robustness of existing governing arrangements in a range of areas. In many federations, emergency management is a federal responsibility, and the federal government tends to have some regulatory or oversight power over health care systems. However, the delivery of health care services is typically either a constituent unit or concurrent responsibility (Marchildon and Bossert 2018). Given the clustering of infection in urban areas, local governments have become essential components of the COVID-19 management strategy, particularly in delivering sanitation services, managing public spaces, and enforcing quarantine/lockdown restrictions (OECD 2020). Consequently, effective pandemic management has required closer coordination between the various orders of government.

In this volume, chapter authors will help readers understand the institutional and policy context in which countries have responded to COVID-19, and how these conditions shaped the response. The political scientists, serving government officials, and senior governance practitioners who comprise the authors of this book bring a wealth of academic and practical experience to their analysis. We believe, therefore, that the case studies will be of value to both researchers and governance practitioners, as well as anyone with an interest in the field of emergency management.

In the first section of each chapter, authors provide an analysis of how the institutional architecture of each country shaped their responses to the health and economic crisis brought on by the pandemic. They consider how effective intergovernmental coordination has been in each country and whether existing intergovernmental institutions and processes were fit for purpose. The extent to which constituent unit governments were able to effectively deliver health care services is also assessed.

In the second section, the analysis focuses on lessons learnt as a consequence of the first year of the pandemic. Many countries emerged from 2020 having suffered at least one wave of infections, and face the challenge of "living with the virus" as well as tackling subsequent resurgences in cases. During peaks in cases, governments have, in a context of great uncertainty, been forced to make unenviable decisions to protect the lives of citizens. The unprecedented imposition of lockdowns, school closures, and stay at home orders as a last resort underscores the challenge of balancing the health dimension of the pandemic with the potentially severe economic, social, and psychological consequences of the pandemic response. The effects of both COVID-19 and the policies employed to control it will most likely keep governments occupied for years to come. Are there lessons learnt to date that can produce improvements in how governments deal with future outbreaks?

Finally, each chapter offers reflections on how COVID-19 is likely to transform the nature of the federation (or governance system in federal-type nations). Does the pandemic change everything or nothing? Or only some things? The questions of economic recovery, the precariousness of constituent unit finances, and the importance of the graduated bespoke responses that constituent unit governments can provide are particularly germane to our understanding of how federal relations are rebalanced in post COVID-19 world.

Notes

1 The analysis focuses on countries that are explicitly and constitutionally federal, and countries with governance systems in which governance powers and responsibilities are devolved from the central level to the subnational level. For a definition of federal and multilevel systems, see Anderson (2008, pp. 1–6).
2 In this book, we refer to the government with national powers as either "federal" or "central" government, recognizing that, in some federations, this order of government has a different title, such as "Union government" (in India), "central government" (in Spain), or "Commonwealth government" (in Australia). By "constituent units," we refer to the federal entities that make up the federation, such as provinces (Canada), states (Brazil, India, USA), cantons (Switzerland), *Länder* (Austria and Germany), or Autonomous Communities (Spain). See Anderson (2008, p. 2).
3 "Orders" of government refers to all constitutionally recognized layers of government in a federation. The authors of this book sometimes also refer to "levels" of government.
4 In some federations, local government is also recognized as a (third) distinct order of government.

Bibliography

Anderson, G., 2008. *Federalism: An Introduction*. Toronto: Oxford University Press.
Brunner, J.H., Sigurdsson, F.S., Svennebye, L. and Täube, V., 2020. *COVID-19: Excess Mortality in Select European Countries*. Luxembourg: European Free Trade Association Statistical Office. Ferejohn, J., Eskridge, W. and Bednar, J., 2001. A Political Theory of Federalism. *In*: Ferejohn, J., Rakove, J. and Riley, J., eds. *Constitutional and Democratic Rule*. New York: Cambridge University Press,5–8.
Forum of Federations, 2015. Emergency Management in Federal Countries. Ottawa: Forum of Federations. Available from: http://www.forumfed.org/publications/report-emergency-management-in-federal-countries/ [Accessed 8 April 2021].
Greer, S., Rozenblum, S., Wismar, M. and Jarman, H., 2020. How Have Federal Countries Organized Their Covid Response? COVID-19 Health System Monitor. *World Health Organization*, 16 July. Available from: https://analysis.covid19healthsystem.org/index.php/2020/07/16/how-have-federal-countries-organized-their-covid-19-response/ [Accessed 8 April 2021].

Hueglin, T.O. and Fenna, A., 2015. *Comparative Federalism: A Systematic Enquiry*. Toronto: University of Toronto Press.

Ionova, A., 2020. Brazil's First Wave Isn't Over Yet. ForeignPolicy.com. Foreign Policy, 29 October. Available from: https://foreignpolicy.com/2020/10/29/brazils-first-wave-not-over-yet-coronavirus-pandemic-manaus-bolsonaro/ [Accessed 8 April 2021].

Kontis, V., Bennett, J.E., Rashid, T., Parks, R.M., Pearson-Stuttard, J., Guillot, M., Asaria, P., Zhou, B., Battaglini, M., Corsetti, G., McKee, M., Di Cesare, M., Mathers, C.D. and Ezzati, M., 2020. Magnitude, Demographics and Dynamics of the Effect of the First Wave of the COVID-19 Pandemic on All-Cause Mortality in 21 Industrialized Countries. *Nature Medicine*, 26, 1919–1928. Available from: https://doi.org/10.1038/s41591-020-1112-0 [Accessed 8 April 2021].

Marchildon, G.P. and Bossert, T.J., 2018. *Federalism and Decentralization in Health Care: A Decision Space Approach*. Toronto: University of Toronto Press.

Oates, W.E., 1999. An Essay on Fiscal Federalism. *Journal of Economic Literature*, 37 (3), 1120–1149.

OECD, 2020. *The Territorial Impact of COVID-19: Managing the Crisis Across Levels of Government*. Paris: Organisation for Economic Cooperation and Development.

Relman, D.A., Choffnes, E.R. and Mack, A., Rapporteurs, 2010. *The Domestic and International Impacts of the 2009-H1N1 Influenza A Pandemic: Global Challenges, Global Solutions: Workshop Summary*. Washington, DC: Institute of Medicine.

Ritchie, H., Ortiz-Ospina, E., Beltekian, D., Mathieu, E., Hasell, J., Macdonald, B., Giattino, C. and Roser, M., 2021. Coronavirus (COVID-19) Deaths. Oxford: Our World in Data. Available from: https://ourworldindata.org/covid-deaths [Accessed 8 April 2021].

World Health Organization, 2020. *Report of the WHO-China Joint Mission on Coronavirus Disease 2019 (COVID-19)*. Geneva: World Health Organization.

World Health Organization Department of Communicable Disease Surveillance and Response, 2003. *Consensus Document on the Epidemiology of Severe Acute Respiratory Syndrome (SARS)*. Geneva: World Health Organization.

Wu, J., Cai, W., Watkins, D. and Glanz, J. How the Virus Got Out [online]. *The New York Times*, 22 March. Available from: https://www.nytimes.com/interactive/2020/03/22/world/coronavirus-spread.html [Accessed 8 April 2021].

2 Federalism and the COVID-19 crisis in Argentina

Matías Bianchi

2.1 Introduction

Argentina is a country of extremes, and its experience in managing the COVID-19 pandemic is no exception. It went from being a poster child for best responses to COVID-19 to joining the list of the top ten countries with the most infections per day in the world at the time of writing.

Argentina's initial approach to the pandemic was promising, with President Alberto Fernandez taking rapid and strong measures to limit social interaction and mixing, strengthening the public healthcare system, and providing economic relief to the population.

By mid-June 2020, the country had a death rate of 25 per million inhabitants, ten times less than the other federal counties in the Western Hemisphere (the United States had 322, Mexico 197, Brazil 220, and Canada 224). A key aspect of that relative success was the national consensus and political collaboration the government managed to achieve. Right from the beginning of the pandemic, the government activated federal institutions seeking intergovernmental collaboration.

Measures against COVID-19 included the following:

- Strengthening the Federal Council for Healthcare (COFESA);
- Inviting governors to help the federal government decide the limits and extent of the social distancing phases; and
- Setting up of a coordination space for the metropolitan area of Buenos Aires.

In April 2020, the president enjoyed an astonishing 90 percent approval rate, and despite the dire economic crisis, 60 percent of Argentines agreed that the country was heading in the right direction (Zubán Córdoba 2021).

Yet, by the beginning of 2021, Argentina had one of the fastest rates of infections in the world and reached 1,049 deaths per million, catching up to the United States (1,286), Brazil (1,035), and Mexico (1,191) and doubling that of Canada (517). At this moment, it is difficult to find a clear explanation for that changing trend of the pandemic.

One contributing factor, undoubtedly, was the weakening of the political consensus over COVID-19 policies. In Argentina, large portions of the population stopped complying with the social distancing measures because of fatigue, the economic crisis, and the aggressive position against the government by some of the political opposition and the mainstream media. Despite these challenges, the situation at the time

DOI: 10.4324/9781003251217-2

Table 2.1 Cases of COVID-19 in Argentina

Argentina	
Total Cases – 14 February 2021[a]	2,025,798
New Cases – 15 February 2021[a]	4,245
Seven-day avg New Cases – 22 October 2021[b]	14,941

a Total cases and new cases source: https://coronavirus.jhu.edu/map.html
b Seven-day avg new cases source: https://www.google.com/search?client=firefox-b-d&q=world+coronavirus+statistics+data

Table 2.2 Key Statistics on COVID-19 in Argentina as of 10 January 2021

Cumulative Cases	Cumulative Cases per 100,000 Population	Cumulative Deaths	Cumulative Deaths per 100,000 Population	Case Fatality Percentage
1,703,352	3,768.8	44,273	98.0	2.6

Source: World Health Organization Weekly epidemiological update – 12 January 2021. Geneva: WHO, 2021. Available from https://www.who.int/publications/m/item/weekly-epidemiological-update

of this writing was still under control, and the healthcare system had not collapsed. The government's success in flattening the curve during the first four months gave it time to build 12 new hospitals, double the number of ICU beds, and take advantage of new treatments.

By 14 February 2021, Argentina, the 32nd largest country in the world by population (World meters 2021), had the 12th highest number of COVID-19 cases: 2,025,798. The highest seven-day average of new cases per day was 14,941 on 22 October 2020, which was on a downward slope to 4,245 on 15 February 2021 (Tables 2.1 and 2.2).

2.2 COVID-19 in Argentina

When the COVID-19 pandemic arrived in Argentina, the country was in the middle of a two-year long economic recession. Its economy had contracted by 4 percent during this period; unemployment reached 9.8 percent (8.4 percent in 2017); and 35.5 percent of the population was below the poverty line (27.2 percent in 2017; Manzanelli et al. 2020). President Fernández, who had taken office only three months before the pandemic hit, was focused on renegotiating the foreign debt, which represented 90 percent of the GDP and was at a serious risk of default. The pandemic added fuel to an already smoldering fire.

The provinces in Argentina are responsible for delivering public healthcare. The federal government is responsible for healthcare system co-ordination. The country's response to the COVID-19 pandemic took place in two phases.

The first phase was by and large a success story. The federal government reacted quickly and decisively to the crisis. On March 19, with only 97 registered cases in the country and two deaths, the President declared a total lockdown. This early strict social distancing measure helped to flatten the curve and allowed the government to gain much needed time. During this time, research and experimental treatments with anti-inflammatories progressed, such as the use of convalescent plasma, among other treatments.

The first phase also allowed the government to do the following:

- Build 12 modular hospitals;
- More than double the number of ICU beds and available ventilators;
- Dramatically increase testing capabilities, train personnel on emergentology;
- Implement protocols for workers in essential areas such as pharmacies, supermarkets, and others.

Moreover, despite its fiscal and financial fragility, the federal government reacted with a series of economic measures that represented roughly 5 percent of the GDP, aiming at providing relief to people and private companies (Manzanelli et al. 2020). The most important ones thus far have been the following:

- Credits at subsidized rates. By September 2020, 102,000 private companies received 410b pesos ($5.5b USD);
- An Emergency Family Income (IFE in Spanish), which provides 10,000 pesos ($120 USD) to lowest income households, informal workers, and domestic workers. As of December, this program had issued three rounds of payments benefiting 9 million people for an amount of 265b pesos ($3.5b USD);
- Work and Production Assistance (ATP in Spanish), which focuses on benefits to employers and independent formal employees who are not included in IFE. The ATP covers a portion of their salary and reduces employer contributions. As of December, there had been seven rounds of payments benefiting at least 420,000 companies and 2.3 million workers for a total of 370b pesos ($4b USD).

Other important monetary transfers to households – all provided by the federal government – have amounted to roughly 1 percent of the GDP (Díaz Laingou et al. 2020). For example, the government issued an extra payment to beneficiaries of social programs such as *Asignación Universal por Hijo* (Universal Child Allowance) and *Asignación Universal por Embarazo* (Universal Pregnancy Allowance). They also provided additional funds to a food stamps program, called *Alimentar* – 1.5 million cards estimated at $90b pesos ($1b dollars) and a program designed to boost jobs (Potenciar el trabajo) – 65b pesos ($0.8b dollars), an 150 percent increase from what was originally planned. Finally, they issued additional subsidies for senior citizens.

Early results were very promising. By mid-June 2020, the country had "only" 35,000 confirmed cases and a low death rate. The incidence was concentrated with nine out of ten cases registered in the metropolitan area of Buenos Aires (AMBA). This is the third largest metropolitan area in Latin America, and even though it occupies only 1 percent of the national territory, this region holds 37 percent of Argentines. It also concentrates most of the wealth of the country and most of its vulnerable populations. The poorer areas of Greater Buenos Aires contain more than 1,400 slums. One out of four households lack fresh water, and 40 percent have no sewage. In these areas, children have limited access to computers and internet for education, and fewer parks for recreation.[1]

Outside of AMBA, most provinces had low levels or no detected cases. The overall results during the first four months of the pandemic were considerably better than in most countries in the Western Hemisphere (see Figure 2.1). In mid-June, *Time Magazine* and the Eurasia Group included Argentina among the top performing countries

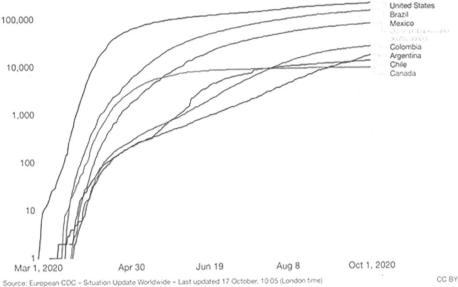

Figure 2.1 Cumulative Confirmed COVID-19 Deaths.

in the world and the only one from Latin America, in terms of their pandemic response. The report highlighted competent management of the health crisis, strong economic measures, and the country's political leadership.

The economic impact of the pandemic has been dire. Economic activity declined by 12.9 percent between February and June (CEP XXI 2020, p. 10). Even though the economy has been recovering since then, it is estimated that the country's total economic activity will have declined by 10.5 percent of GDP in 2020. Adding to this drop is the accumulated 4 percent decline since 2018, placing Argentina among the worst economic performers in the region (ECLAC 2020). Also, a full 40.9 percent of the population currently live in poverty, which means that there are 2.5 million newly impoverished citizens. UNICEF estimates that the number of children below the poverty line will reach 63 percent by the end of 2020, an increase from 7 million to 8.3 million (Télam 2020b).

Nevertheless, without the economic relief policies, it was estimated that poverty would have increased 2.6 percent more, affecting 43.5 percent of the population (Díaz Langlou et al. 2020). The early government measures, therefore, saved 1.2 million Argentines from falling below the poverty line. Moreover, with the resumption of some productive activity in May, economic indicators have slowly started to grow once again. By September 2020, industrial and construction indicators showed similar pre-pandemic levels of activity and have continued to increase (CEP XXI 2020).

The measures that worked to contain the spread of COVID-19 at the beginning of the outbreak seem to have lost steam. The infection rate has dramatically risen since July. Whereas AMBA's infection curve has begun to flatten, we are now starting to see worrying trends in the provinces of Santa Fe, Córdoba, Jujuy, and Neuquén. From August and into September, Argentina joined the top ten countries in the world in terms of infection rates and currently ranks 12th in the total number of deaths. Paradoxically, while health conditions worsened, the government started to loosen measures. In a first move toward reopening, the government announced a new phase in June that eased quarantine restrictions for large portions of the national territory with low levels of contagion. On that date, social and economic activity restarted but had to follow strict health guidelines, including restricting social gatherings to ten people or fewer and maintaining 2 meters from each other while using face masks in public spaces.

While the situation becomes very delicate, the health care system has not collapsed. ICU beds never surpassed manageable capacity of 65 percent at the national level and none of the district health systems collapsed.

2.3 COVID-19 and federalism in Argentina

Argentina is a federal country divided into two levels of government: a central government and 23 provinces plus the City of Buenos Aires, which has the autonomy of a province. The country's federal structure has created a unique set of dynamics that deeply affects governance in the country.

On the one hand, Argentine provinces hold important institutional powers. They have the right to write their own constitutions and legal frameworks. Also, because of unequal apportionment in Congress and the federal structure of the party system, provinces are rather influential in the national political arena. Moreover, they enjoy important autonomy from national politics. Additionally, a 1994 constitutional reform established that provinces were responsible for the provision of key aspects of public policy, including most education, healthcare, justice, and security.

On the other hand, most Argentine provinces are fiscally very weak. On average, provinces collect only 20 percent of total fiscal revenues even as they execute roughly half of total expenditures. There is much variation in revenue collection across the provinces. The City of Buenos Aires, for example, collects 90 percent of its own fiscal needs, while a group of seven provinces collect less than 10 percent. This important vertical fiscal imbalance is covered by transfers from the national government. The main distribution, three quarters of the total fiscal pie, is provided by a formula-based tax sharing scheme ("*Ley de Coparticipación Federal*") that automatically transfers to provinces a percentage of funds of the total collected. The rest are oil and mineral royalties that accrue directly to the provinces of origin, and other funds that the national government redistributes on a discretionary basis.

A third outstanding feature of Argentina is the dramatically uneven levels of development within the national territory. The Metropolitan area of Buenos Aires, which represents 1 percent of the national territory, is home to 37 percent of the population and produces more than 50 percent of the gross domestic product. This area, along with Santa Fe, Córdoba, and Mendoza, concentrate a full two thirds of the national population, 75 percent of the national economy, and 85 percent of industrial production. At the other extreme, the country's poorest eight provinces, only 16 percent of the population, produce less than 1 percent of the national economy and have only marginal participation in exports and investment (Bianchi 2016).

This unique scheme of politically powerful but fiscally highly dependent provinces in a very heterogeneous country has created paradoxical dynamics of governance.

The federal government can be overseen by either powerful or extremely weak presidents, depending on their fiscal strength and their territorial political coalition. The power of the chief executive affects decision-making about public policy at the national level. The president's strength – or weakness – can also impact local or provincial governments that try to address local policy challenges.

2.3.1 Healthcare

Argentina spends 10 percent of its GDP on healthcare, making it the highest in Latin America and equivalent to OECD levels (PAHO 2020). At the time of the outbreak, Argentina had double the average number of beds and doctors per inhabitant in Latin America (ECLAC 2020). This strength has been crucial for avoiding a collapse of the system during the pandemic so far.

Provinces are in charge of healthcare in their own territories, and their spending represents 70 percent of the total. Also, during the decentralization process in the 1990s, hospitals were transferred from the national sphere to the provinces, and provincial policy autonomy over healthcare, in general, grew. Still, some municipal governments are also in charge of primary and/or secondary care, and the national government holds some general and limited authority. Overall, given the level of decentralization, the healthcare system replicates the unequal and heterogenous profile of the country. The public system only represents less than a half of the total healthcare spending, while the rest is covered by private and pre-paid insurance. One third of the population is covered by the public sector and over 50 percent by pre-paid health services (PAHO 2020).

2.3.2 Intergovernmental coordination

Responses to the COVID-19 pandemic require cooperation among different levels of government. Different federal constituent units need to collaborate to provide healthcare, social subsidies, and sharing infrastructure or data. President Fernández relied on intergovernmental cooperation from the beginning. He activated existing federal institutions and created other *ad hoc* institutions to address key policy challenges emerging from the pandemic.

The President consulted with governors to define the duration and scope of early social distancing measures. Ultimately, he decided to delegate to them the task of defining social distancing measures and the openings or lockdowns of activities in their territories.

Several other measures were adopted with the goal of coordinating initiatives, regardless of political stripes. The national government and the province of Córdoba negotiated with the most important producer of ventilators in the country, located in that province, so that ventilators would not be exported. Moreover, to avoid competition among provinces over equipment, the distribution of ventilators would be made by a series of criteria defined by the provinces (*La Nueva Mañana* 2020).

The Carlos Malbrán Health Institute was the only institution in the country at that time with the technical capacity to make the COVID-19 tests. The National Administration of Laboratories worked with them to decentralize testing capabilities along the national territory (Télam 2020a). Local governments have also played a role in supervising compliance over price controls or the distribution of foodstuffs and other supplies.

The most outstanding example of vertical coordination was done by the Federal Council for Healthcare (COFESA in Spanish). Created in 1981, COFESA is the formal space designated for coordination between the national and provincial ministries of health. The most important health measures for the pandemic were decided and put together in this space.

These important health measures included the following:

- Tracing of the epidemiology in each district;
- Acquisition and distribution of medicines and devices;
- creation of the "DetectAr" program (aimed at identification, detection, and tracing COVID-19 cases); and
- The coordination of the integrated database system (SISA in Spanish).

At the same time, important levels of horizontal cooperation across provinces have been observed. For example, the governments of the City and the Province of Buenos Aires, which are led by opposing political parties, have established a special board to coordinate measures.

These measures of cooperation by the "two Buenos Aireses" include the following:

- Monitoring healthcare structure;
- Monitoring information on public transportation; and
- Supervising of the social compliance of the social distancing policies (Perfil 2020).

Other examples of intergovernmental collaboration include the government of Córdoba sending emergency room-doctors to Jujuy (Somos Jujuy 2020) or the governments of San Luis and La Pampa allowing bilateral unrestricted circulation of traffic (Télam 2020c).

The scenario has not been completely bright. Most of these initiatives lack institutionalization and rely primarily on the political will of leaders. Moreover, certain measures have been implemented in violation of the federal constitution. For example, a dozen provinces breached the constitution by unilaterally closing their borders. One governor expelled foreign citizens from their province. Despite these complications, cooperation among the different levels of government has been predominant.

2.3.3 A changing scenario

Vertical and horizontal solidarity, plus collaboration, emerged in Argentina during the first months of the pandemic. This cooperation was promising, especially when compared to other federal countries such as Mexico, the United States, and Brazil. Thanks to his approach to governing during the pandemic, President Fernandez managed to obtain a multiparty cooperation of governors and congressional figures[2] as well as an impressive support from society. Despite the looming threat of debt default and the dire economic crisis, the president managed to retain an approval rating at or above 75 percent for three months (see Figure 2.2), and a majority of the population believed the country was heading in the right direction through June (Zubán Córdoba 2020).

Things started to change in late June. The most important change was that Fernández's coalition of support faltered. Openly violating the mandatory social distancing policy, the opposition organized a national protest on 20 June 2020 – the first of many – holding slogans that declared "Save the Republic," "Save democracy," and "No to Argenzuela"[3] (*La Nación* 2020). Later that week, Alfredo Cornejo, president of the opposition party, UCR, and former governor of Mendoza, declared that the province should become an independent country (*La Nación* 2020). These expressions by the opposition were covered amply by mainstream media outlets. Moreover, given the generalized fatigue of the population over the strict social distancing measures and the economic crisis, it is perhaps not surprising that the political support of the president started to decline. By September 2020, the support for the president dropped by 30 percent, and a majority of Argentines felt that the country was heading in the wrong direction (see Figure 2.3). Due to this loss of support, the government started to loosen measures. Additionally, many citizens stopped complying with the social distancing measures.

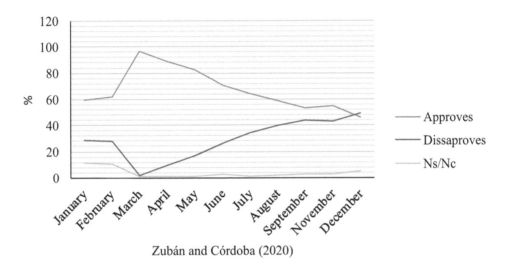

Zubán and Córdoba (2020)

Figure 2.2 The Fernández Administration's Approval Rating.

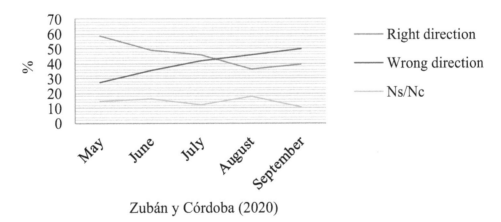

Zubán y Córdoba (2020)

Figure 2.3 Argentinians' Views on Whether the Country is Heading in the Right Direction During COVID-19.

Table 2.3 Case-fatality Ratio and Total Deaths in Argentina

Argentina	
Case-fatality ratio – 14 February 2021[a]	2.5%
Total deaths – 14 February 2021[b]	50,236

a   Case-fatality ratio source: https://coronavirus.jhu.edu/data/mortality
b   Total deaths source: https://coronavirus.jhu.edu/map.html

Consequently, the rate of contagion and deaths grew. In the second half of the year, Argentina's infection rates dramatically increased and became one of the fastest rates in the world.

The number of deaths in Argentina from COVID-19 was 50.236 on 14 February 2021, 11th highest in the world (Johns Hopkins Coronavirus Resource Center data 2021). The case-fatality rate on that same date was 2.5 percent, the sixth highest in the world (Table 2.3).

2.4 Towards Argentina's federalism for the 21st century

So far, there are two important lessons learned from the COVID-19 pandemic, and in the case of Argentina, both are intimately related to the federal organization of the country.

The first one is that the pandemic disproportionately affects the most vulnerable populations. Argentina is geographically the most unequal federal country in the world.[4] The pandemic has revealed its monocephalic nature. During the first wave, 90 percent of the cases occurred in the Metropolitan Area of Buenos Aires, where most of the wealth and vulnerabilities are concentrated. Only months later, when the disease impacted the more peripheral provinces, did it become clear that much of the country was too weak fiscally and administratively to respond to it.

A second lesson learned is the weak institutionalization of coordination mechanism of federalism in Argentina. Most of the coordination and collaboration depended on the political capital and drive of the President. When the latter weakened, also the cooperation and coordination did.

The COVID-19 pandemic is a global challenge, and thus, it is not enough to address the crisis solely from the national, provincial, or local level. Federalism is a political system that seeks "unity in diversity," aiming at cooperation and solidarity among its parts. Therefore, more than ever, institutional arrangements like federalism have the potential to provide the infrastructure to develop common solutions for complex and global challenges such as the COVID-19 pandemic. In Argentina, the provinces control crucial areas such as healthcare, education, and security; the national government concentrates the financial resources for social plans, infrastructure, and sciences; and the local governments manage local utilities, food provision, and social circulation. Cooperation among different levels of government is crucial to slow down the disease and, eventually, to contain it.

Comparatively, the initial scenario in Argentina was promising, with President Fernández activating federal institutions and creating other multilevel horizontal and vertical policy coordination schemes. That governance profile helped to flatten the curve and gave the government time to acquire equipment, to build new hospitals, to adopt protocols, and to train personnel.

Yet, those measures also revealed the country's weaknesses. Most of these initiatives lacked institutionalization and relied primarily on the political leadership of the President. For example, the regulation of COFESA is overly general in its functions and structure (as are most federal councils), and it lacks financial autonomy. Rodriguez and Tobar (2003) point out that, since its creation, COFESA has had scarce influence in the decision-making process on healthcare policies, and its activity has been highly dependent on the corresponding political will of the leaders.

Due to these reasons, Argentina desperately needs a "Federal Pact" that could strengthen the mechanisms of solidarity and cooperation. This pact should include the fiscal resources, administrative capabilities, and productive policies that could guarantee an equivalent level of opportunities to Argentines regardless of where they live, as the Federal Constitution mandates. To achieve this, it is crucial that fiscal equalization schemes, investment in infrastructure, and other measures follow standards and benchmarks based on development indicators and policy priorities.

This pact should also include a strengthening and institutionalization of the coordination schemes such as the Federal Councils. They require more clarity and uniformity in their legal frameworks, an increase in financial autonomy, decision-making power, and better clarification of their roles and functions.

We can hope that the political impetus achieved during the pandemic sets a positive precedent for the country, generating the inertia needed to strengthen a more solidary and collaborative federal system that the country so desperately needs.

Notes

1 In Greater Buenos Aires, 44 percent of the population has no access to computers, 20 percent has no access to the internet, while, in the City of Buenos Aires, those figures are 20 percent and 8 percent, respectively (Observatorio del Conurbano Bonaerense 2020).
2 "President, you are our commander" declared Mario Negri, head of the most important opposition party in Congress (Infobae 2020).
3 This is a common reference on Venezuala.
4 The income of the wealthiest region is nine times higher than the poorest. That figure is seven times, Mexico 6 and 1.7 in Canada (Cetrángolo and Gómez Sabaini 2007, cited in Bianchi 2016).

Bibliography

Bianchi, M., 2016. Territorio, poder y desarrollo: la articulación de políticas industriales en San Luis y Rafaela. *In*: Mauro, S., Ortiz de Rozas, V. and Narvaja, M., eds. In *Política Subnacional en Argentina. Enfoques y Problemas*. Buenos Aires: CEAP-UBA Sociales, 337–362.

CEP XXI, 2020. Informe de Panorama Productivo, Septembre 2020, Ministerio de Desarrollo Productivo. Available from: https://www.argentina.gob.ar/sites/default/files/informe_de_panorama_productivo_-_septiembre_2020.pdf [Accessed 16 February 2021].

Díaz Laingou, G., Kessler, G., della Paolera, C. and Karczmarczy, M. Septiembre 2020. *Impacto social del COVID-19 en Argentina*, Documento e trabajo #197, CIPPEC Available from: https://www.cippec.org/wp-content/uploads/2020/10/197-DT-PS-Impacto-social-del-COVID-19-en-Argentina.-D%C3%ADaz-Langou-Kessler...-1.pdf [Accessed 16 February 2021].

ECLAC, 2020. La pandemia del COVID-19 y su efecto en las tendencias de los mercados laborales, julio 2020. Comisión Económica para América Latina y el Caribe (CEPAL). Weller, Jurgen, author. Available from: https://www.cepal.org/es/publicaciones/45759-la-pandemia-covid-19-su-efecto-tendencias-mercados-laborales [Accessed 16 February 2021].

Infobae, 2020. *"Presidente, usted es el comandante": el mensaje anti grieta de la oposición para respaldar a Alberto Fernández.* Available from: https://www.infobae.com/coronavirus/2020/03/19/presidente-usted-es-el-comandante-el-mensaje-anti-grieta-de-la-oposicion-para-respaldar-a-alberto-fernandez/ [Accessed 16 February 2021].

Johns Hopkins Coronavirus Resource Center, 2021. The Johns Hopkins University & Medicine. Available from: https://coronavirus.jhu.edu/map.html [Accessed 10 February 2021].

La Nación, 2020. Alfredo *Cornejo, sobre la independencia de Mendoza: "Debemos pensarlo seriamente"*, 30 June 2020. Available from: https://www.lanacion.com.ar/politica/alfredo-cornejo-independencia-mendoza-debemos-pensarlo-seriamente-nid2388507 [Accessed 16 February 2021].

La Nueva mañana, 2020. "En Córdoba, se pasó de fabricar 30 respiradores a 110 al mes." Available from: https://lmdiario.com.ar/contenido/230020/cordoba-el-pulmon-del-pais [Accessed 16 February 2021].

Manzanelli, Pablo, Daniela Calvo and Eduardo Basualdo, 2020. Un Balance Preliminar de la Crisis Economíca Argentina en el Marco del Coronavirus, Documento de Trabajo 17, CIFRA-CTA/FLACSO. Available from: https://www.flacso.org.ar/wp-content/uploads/2020/06/Crisis-coronavirus_DT-FLACSO_AEyT-CIFRA_junio2020.pdf [Accessed 16 February 2021].

Observatorio del Conurbano Bonaerense, 2020. *2da serie Especial COVID-19: AMBA resiste: Actores territoriales y políticas públicas.* Buenos Aires, Argentina: Universidad Nacional General Sarmiento. Available from: https://www.ungs.edu.ar/new/2da-serie-especial-covid-19-amba-resiste-actores-territoriales-y-politicas-publicas [Accessed 16 February 2021].

PAHO, Cuánto Gasta Argentina en Salud, 2020. Available from: https://www.paho.org/arg/index.php?option=com_content&view=article&id=10420:cuanto-gasta-argentina-en-salud-un-analisis-de-las-cuentas-cn-el-sector-publico-privado-y-de-la-seguridad-social&Itemid=225 [Accessed 16 February 2021].

Perfil, 2020. Larreta y Kicillof definen cómo seguirá la cuarentena en el AMBA. Available from: https://www.perfil.com/noticias/politica/horacio-rodriguez-larreta-axel-kicillof-coordinaron-como-sigue-cuarentena-amba.phtml [Accessed 16 February 2021].

Rodrigáñez Riccheri, Pilar and Federico Tobar, 2003. El Consejo Federal de Salud Argentino (CO. FE. SA): Actor clave en la construcción de un federalismo sanitario efectivo, Ministerio de Salud, 2003. Available from: https://www.academia.edu/39998014/Tobar_F_and_Rodriga%C3%B1ez_P_Hacia_un_federalismo_sanitario_efectivo_2004 [Accessed 16 February 2021].

Somos Jujuy, 2020. Córdoba enviará médicos terapistas para ayudar a la lucha contra el Covid_19 en Jujuy. 14 July 2020. Available from: https://www.somosjujuy.com.ar/salud/175831-cordoba-enviara-medicos-terapistas-para-ayudar-a-la-lucha-contra-el-covid_19-en-jujuy [Accessed 16 February 2021].

Télam, March 2020a. El Malbrán comenzó el proceso de descentralización del diagnóstico", March 20. Available from: https://www.telam.com.ar/notas/202003/442857-malbran-descentralizacion-diagnostico-coronavirus.html [Accessed 16 February 2021].

Télam, May 2020b. El 2020 finalizará con casi 63% de la infancia en situaciión de pobreza en Argentina. May 8. Available from: https://www.telam.com.ar/notas/202008/498702-el-2020-finalizara-con-casi-63-de-la-infancia-en-situacion-de-pobreza-en-la-argentina.html [Accessed 16 February 2021].

Télam, June 2020c. Habilitan la libre circulación entre San Luis y La Pampa sin cumplir cuarentena", June 19. Available from: https://www.telam.com.ar/notas/202006/478806-la-pampa-flexibilizacion-san-luis-cuarentena.html# [Accessed 16 February 2021].

World Meters 2021. Available from: https://www.worldometers.info/coronavirus/ [Accessed 1 February 2021].

Zubán y Córdoba Asociados, Informe de Opinión, January 2020. Available from: https://zubancordoba.com/portfolio/informe-nacional-enero-2021/ [Accessed 10 February 2021].

3 Australian federalism and the COVID-19 crisis

Alan Fenna

3.1 Introduction

Australia's federal system handled the COVID-19 pandemic throughout 2020 re-markably well — lauded, indeed, for the unusually cooperative manner in which it functioned (e.g., Saunders 2020; Williams 2020). This was reflected in public opinion, with Australians giving their governments full marks (PRC 2020). There was certainly some friction between the Commonwealth and the States, manifestations of the inevitable tension between the necessity and the cost of prophylactic measures; however, it proved of little detriment.

Things might well have been otherwise, with the stresses of the crisis exposing yet again some of the oft-remarked debilities of federal governance in Australia.[1] In terms of pandemic threats, some health experts had earlier warned of the danger of relying on Australia's 'patchwork of legislative measures,' arguing that those would prove 'cumbersome and difficult' in an emergency such as this (Howse 2004; also Brew and Burton 2004). Others have been more sanguine — emphasizing the degree to which the system's complex arrangements provide a desirable level of 'flexibility and choice' as demonstrated in the management of the H1N1 pandemic in 2009 (Bennett, Carney and Bailey 2012).

Meanwhile, the crisis might have elicited another round of heavy-handed unilateralism from the Commonwealth government and a further ratcheting up of the secular process of centralization that has been broadly experienced by the established federations, particularly Australia, over the longer term (Dardanelli et al. 2019; Fenna 2019a). After all, this crisis came immediately on the heels of a catastrophic bushfire season where, in response to some coordination issues, the prime minister immediately called for greater Commonwealth disaster management powers (Benson and Chambers 2020; PM 2020a; RCNNDA 2020). Instead, though, Australia's handling of the pandemic showcased the continuing importance of the States and a surprising degree of popular support for their individual actions. It also demonstrated some of the ways in which divided jurisdiction can be an asset in crises of this nature (Table 3.1).

Table 3.1 Key Statistics on COVID-19 in Australia to 31 December 2020

Cumulative Cases	Cumulative Cases per 100,000 Population	Cumulative Deaths	Cumulative Deaths per 100,000 Population	Case Fatality Percentage
28,405	112.1	909	3.6	3.2

Source: World Health Organization Weekly epidemiological update – 12 January 2021. Geneva: WHO, 2021. Available from https://www.who.int/publications/m/item/weekly-epidemiological-update

DOI: 10.4324/9781003251217-3

3.2 Impact of COVID-19 in Australia

Australia's first case, a passenger arriving from China, was confirmed on 25 January 2020 (McLean and Huf 2020, p. 3). Cases peaked at fewer than 500 per day at the end of March and rapidly subsided to nil through May and June for a total of approximately 7,000 cases. A more severe second outbreak subsequently occurred in Victoria, leading to the declaration of a 'state of disaster' by the State government on 2 August (McLean and Huf 2020, p. 3). That 'second wave' peaked at 700 cases per day in late August and subsided more slowly through September, driving total cases up more than three times what they had been and increased deaths sevenfold. Three quarters of those deaths occurred in aged-care facilities (RCACQS 2020, p. 2). With a population of 25 million, Australia had 28,405 recorded cases of COVID-19 and 909 associated deaths in 2020 — a very modest rate of 35 per million.

Economically and fiscally, the cost of the containment measures was substantial. Three decades of economic good fortune in Australia finally ran out as the lockdowns induced the largest quarterly decline in gross domestic product (GDP) on record — falling 7 percent in the April–June period — and ushering in the country's first recession since 1990–1991. On the fiscal side, 2020 was to have been a year of celebration for the conservative 'Coalition' parties holding office in Canberra, with the Commonwealth budget scheduled to return to surplus for the first time since the Global Financial Crisis (GFC) of 2008–2009. Instead, the budget went from a projected surplus of $8bn to a deficit of $92bn over the 2019–2020 financial year (Frydenberg and Cormann 2020), and the deficit for 2020–2021 was budgeted at $214bn (Treasury 2020a). At 11 percent of GDP, that is more than twice the size of the deficits run during the GFC by an avowedly Keynesian Labor government in Australia (Fenna 2010; Treasury 2009). Continuing deficits for the foreseeable future were projected to drive Commonwealth net debt from 25 percent to 44 percent of GDP and budgets in the worst-hit States were also thrown into deficit.

3.3 Emergency management in the federation

Australia is famously a 'land ... Of droughts and flooding rains' (Mackellar 1911), not to mention other natural disasters such as bushfires and cyclones. While responsibility for emergency management lies with the States, resource limitations, spillovers, national dimensions, and external border issues create a role for the Commonwealth.

3.3.1 The constitutional structure

In design, Australia is a classic 'dual' federation made up of the six founding States and the Commonwealth. The States were granted the full range of powers and responsibilities they possessed prior to federating other than those expressly denied them (s. 107). The Commonwealth, meanwhile, was assigned a limiting list of specific enumerated powers, mainly concerned with ensuring the common market and managing Australia's border and external relations (ss. 51 and 52). Few of those are exclusive, but for the concurrent ones, the Commonwealth is granted primacy (s. 109). The States shoulder responsibility for most service delivery.

While thus decentralized by design, a century of centralization has greatly expanded the role and influence of the Commonwealth (Fenna 2019a). The Commonwealth's enumerated powers have been given broad interpretation by the High Court, and it has assumed a position of fiscal dominance allowing extensive use of the 'spending power' (Fenna 2008). Controlling the three main tax bases and raising 80 percent of all the tax revenue in Australia, the Commonwealth has financial resources far in excess of its program requirements, while the States are dependent on the Commonwealth for almost half their revenue needs. Reform is periodically mooted, but almost never achieved (Fenna 2017). Under Section 96 of the Constitution, the Commonwealth is at liberty to apply 'such terms and conditions' as it 'thinks fit' to those transfers on which the States depend, and conditional or 'tied' grants make up more than half of the amount the States receive in transfers (Treasury 2020b). This has allowed the Commonwealth to indulge in 'opportunistic' or 'coercive' federalism and has made Australia part of that tendency whereby 'officially dualist regimes are being pragmatically, casuistically, informally, and partially transferred into integrated or hybrid ones' (Poirier and Saunders 2015, p. 492).

There is also a high degree of fiscal equalization, such that each State and Territory enjoys the ability to deliver services of an equivalent standard. These realities reflect the extent to which Australia is a culturally homogeneous federation, and there is broad support for the principle of a common citizenship.

3.3.2 Responsibility for emergency management

The Commonwealth's enumerated powers do not include any explicit authority to legislate for civil emergencies. "Recently, however, the Commonwealth Parliament has passed laws that purport to give it significant control over the management of a certain type of civil emergency, a 'biosecurity emergency'" (Lee et al. 2018, p. 171). Using its assigned authority for quarantine (s. 51.ix) and sundry other provisions, the Commonwealth's recently overhauled statutory framework for dealing with disease threats to plants, animals, and humans, the *Biosecurity Act 2015* asserts sweeping control powers.[2] 'During a human biosecurity emergency period, the Health Minister may determine any requirement' and 'give any direction, to any person, that the Health Minister is satisfied is necessary' for containing the spread of the disease, according to the Act (ss. 477 and 478).

Insofar as the Commonwealth has significant infrastructure for responding to emergencies, that is either the Australian Border Force or the Australian Defence Force (ADF). The Commonwealth's one service delivery responsibility directly relevant to this crisis is aged care (RCACQS 2020, p. 2).

It is the States that operate the public hospitals, the government school systems, and the police and emergency services agencies. They also have primary jurisdiction over public health as well as criminal and civil law; they license and regulate the operation of the thousands of businesses, facilities, and services that are potential sites of contagion, and they provide thousands more public amenities of their own that likewise present risks. The States each have their respective public health and emergency management Acts (McLean and Huf 2020). Reflecting these constitutional and practical realities, the Commonwealth has consistently acknowledged that 'state and territory governments have primary responsibility for the management of communicable disease emergencies' (Health 2018).

3.4 Australian federalism in the crisis

Leaving aside the question of how competently individual governments responded, the issue here is how, and how well, did Australian federalism respond to the crisis?

Was there an effective division of responsibilities? Did governments have capacity commensurate with their responsibilities? Did divided jurisdiction provide any benefits? Were the potential disabilities of divided jurisdiction avoided? On that last point, many commentators have emphasized the importance of *coordination* in federal systems — which may have the dual benefit of reducing policy incoherence and protecting constituent units from coercive unilateralism (Schnabel 2020, p. 49). 'The COVID-19 outbreak is an extraordinary situation that requires this essential intergovernmental framework to function extremely well,' averred the OECD (2020a).

3.4.1 Managing the crisis

Australian border restrictions were implemented in response to emerging signs of the pandemic, beginning with a restriction on foreign nationals from China on 1 February. Further tightening occurred, and with the declaration by the Commonwealth of a 'human biosecurity emergency' under the *Biosecurity Act* on 18 March, the country's borders were closed to non-residents. To minimize the problem of returning travellers, the Commonwealth also moved soon after to impose a ban on residents leaving Australia and quarantining requirements on those returning. All States except New South Wales (NSW) declared a 'state of emergency' (McLean and Huf 2020, p. 8). As discussed further below, four of the six States then closed their domestic borders. In tandem, measures were imposed to limit human contact, including bans on mass gatherings, closure of restaurants and other services, and more contentiously, schools. Aside from external border control, most of the response was initiated and organized by the States — though, as discussed below, in the context of intergovernmental coordination.

3.4.2 The intergovernmental relations context

Like most other federations, Australia has an extensive array of arrangements through which intergovernmental relations in the form of 'executive federalism' are practised. At the apex of these is the first ministers' meeting, which, in 1992, was formalized as the Council of Australia Governments (COAG). COAG was a 'summit meeting' of Australia's heads of government together with the president of the Australian Local Government Association that met infrequently and for brief moments, on terms dictated by the prime minister (Anderson 2008; Phillimore and Fenna 2017). On the next tier down are the portofolio-based ministerial councils, which have a long history in Australia.

While a relatively dense network, Australian intergovernmental relations have a low level of institutionalization. Neither COAG nor the ministerial councils have any statutory basis, and despite the frequent use of intergovernmental agreements in Australia, they have not been formalized via that means either. On various occasions, suggestion has been made that a more defined 'institutional architecture' would enhance the functioning of Australian federalism (e.g., PMC 2015). There is little incentive, though, for the Commonwealth to tie its hands in that way. This reinforces the vertical and Commonwealth-dominated nature of cooperative federalism in Australia (Phillimore and Fenna 2017). Meanwhile, there is virtually nothing by way of horizontal arrangements to provide a counterbalance — the Council for the Australian Federation (CAF) being the main, but only very briefly effectual, exception.

Commonwealth hegemony was reflected in the fluctuating fortunes of COAG: being enlisted energetically when the government of the day needed a high level of cooperation from the States to advance its agenda and neglected when no longer needed. In the mid-1990s, the Commonwealth sought sweeping micro-economic reform in areas of State responsibility and was obliged to adopt a collaborative approach (Fenna 2019b; Painter 1998). Similarly, COAG became the 'engine room' of the federation during the frenetic Rudd government years of the GFC (Fenna and Anderson 2012).

Under the auspices of COAG, Australia's governments established a framework for roles and responsibilities in the event of a threat such as COVID-19, beginning over a decade ago with the *National Health Security Act 2007*, the *National Security Health Agreement*, and model arrangements (COAG 2008b). A range and succession of emergency planning documents followed.[3] In 2018, for instance, State and Territory health ministers and the intergovernmental emergency management committee signed off on the *Emergency Response Plan for Communicable Disease Incidents of National Significance: national arrangements*, the 'National CD Plan.'[4] In 2019, the Commonwealth and the States and Territories signed the *Intergovernmental Agreement on Biosecurity*. In general, these agreements 'reinforce that the States are primarily responsible for exercising special powers in response to civil emergencies, whereas the responsibilities of the Commonwealth generally lie in providing logistical and financial support as required' (Lee et al. 2018, p. 174; also Home Affairs 2019). This was similarly the message of the *Australian Health Sector Emergency Response Plan for Novel Coronavirus (COVID-19)*, released in the early stages of the pandemic. One way in which the Commonwealth plays that supporting role is through its maintenance of the National Medical Stockpile, established for States to draw on in times of emergency (ANAO 2020). The other role consistently identified for the Commonwealth in these planning documents was coordination — though quite what that entails is an open question.

3.4.3 Loose coordination through 'national cabinet'

At its meeting on 13 March 2020, COAG announced the *National Partnership Agreement on COVID-19* (Australia & States and Territories 2020; COAG 2020). This reaffirmed the division of labour laid down in existing framework documents and provided extra Commonwealth funding to support health services. It was immediately followed by the prime minister's (2020d) announcement that a new intergovernmental forum would swing into operation: 'National Cabinet,' a cabinet-style meeting of the first ministers.[5] This innovation attracted particular — and typically very favourable — attention as embodying an elevated spirit of cooperative federalism in Australia.

National Cabinet was not a cabinet in any proper sense of the term; it was executive federalism in a fresh and more dynamic guise. Most importantly, as with other intergovernmental meetings in Australia and elsewhere, decisions cannot be made binding. At the same time, it is more than just COAG re-badged: at the height of the first wave, National Cabinet meetings were held weekly and were apparently characterized by genuine discussion and consensus decision-making — 'co-design,' as the Victorian government (2020) very approvingly expressed it. Reflecting National Cabinet's *raison d'être* here, its main supporting body has been the Australian Health Protection Principal Committee [*sic*], comprising Commonwealth and State chief medical officers. The idea has been that Australia's governments collectively and individually follow the best available expert medical advice from across the federation.

National Cabinet provided *loose coordination*. Collective decisions were made, but the States remained at liberty to implement them as they saw fit. 'Each and every state and territory that is represented here is completely sovereign and autonomous in the decisions that they make,' declared the prime minister (2020d), albeit with some exaggeration. This collegial quality helps explain why the premiers were so enthusiastic. 'The National Cabinet has been effective because it has established national principles that recognize the sovereignty of states and territories to implement policies according to local circumstances' (Victoria 2020). For some commentators, though, this was a lamentable deficiency — with announcements like early May's 'roadmap' out of the pandemic being derided as a mere 'menu' from which the States could choose at whim, the result being no end to the 'confusion' (e.g., Crowe 2020).[6] Such flexibility would seem, though, to be consistent with the OECD's (2020b) advice and indeed with the ethos of federalism more generally: 'Consider adopting a "place based" or territorially sensitive approach to exit-strategy implementation and recovery policies.' It was, after all, a 'roadmap,' not a set of driving instructions.

3.4.4 Coordination on the ground

Quite distinct from the question of peak level political coordination is the practical coordination that may be required at the administrative or service-delivery level. Various mechanisms for that purpose were activated as soon as the nature of the threat became apparent such as the National Coordination Mechanism in the Commonwealth Department of Home Affairs.

While many aspects of this crisis were readily handled by jurisdictions acting autonomously, coordination was necessary at points where the two levels of government intersected. One such intersection was the maritime international border point, where States control the ports and have responsibility for public health, while the Commonwealth has control over customs, immigration, emigration, and quarantine. Passengers disembarking in Sydney from the Ruby Princess cruise ship in March were one of the main vectors of infection in NSW. A NSW commission of inquiry subsequently found, however, that the main issue was not poor coordination between relevant Commonwealth and State services, but rather procedural lapses within the relevant State government agency (SCIRP 2020).

A particularly important point of intersection, given the locus of mortality, was that between Commonwealth responsibility for aged care and State responsibility for public hospitals.[7] This does appear to have been an area where inadequate coordination contributed to the problem (RCACQS 2020, pp. 3, 11 and *passim*). It is also reflective of a broader and oft-noted operational tension in Australian federalism arising from the way responsibility for different aspects of health care and aged care have come to be somewhat promiscuously divided between the Commonwealth and the States (Fenna, Phillimore and Ramamurthy 2021).

Finally, there was the quarantining débâcle in Victoria that sparked the much-more severe second wave and led to imposition of an extended hard lockdown in the State. Having elected not to call on Commonwealth resources in the form of ADF personnel, the State government failed to ensure hermetic quarantine of overseas arrivals into Victoria. On the face of it, that was not a failure of federalism, but the result of poor preparation, decision-making, and management *within* the State government (CHQI 2020). However, several commentators argued that, since quarantine is a Commonwealth enumerated power, the Commonwealth should not be leaving that important responsibility to the States (e.g., Van Onselen 2020). Management of quarantine had been identified in the H1N1 pandemic review as requiring clarification (DHA 2011; also DCSH 1988).

3.4.5 Sources of friction

As always, conflict gets plenty of attention. In this case, the main friction has been between the Commonwealth's desire to minimize the economic disruption and the States' insistence on containing the disease. This manifested itself in ongoing dispute over the stringency of lockdown measures and the closure of borders.

3.4.5.1 Economy and society

Such a conflict is to be expected: while both levels of government suffered financially from the crisis and both spent generously on tiding businesses and individuals through the crisis, it was the Commonwealth that bore the lion's share of both the economic and the fiscal burden. The OECD (2020a, 2020b) raised concerns about the fiscal impact of the crisis on *subnational* governments, but presumably that applies to systems with higher levels of fiscal decentralization. Not only is the Commonwealth the primary fiscal actor, but having responsibility for macroeconomic performance, it was also exposed to the economic fallout in a way the States were not. This was compounded by an ideological tension, where those on the right opposed strict measures on economic grounds (e.g., Wilkie 2020). In office at the Commonwealth level were the centre–right Coalition parties, whose emphasis has been on fiscal prudence.[8] In office in the three States with whom there was the most intergovernmental conflict (Queensland, Victoria, Western Australia) was, meanwhile, the centre–left Labor Party.

Fiscally, the crisis threatened to be a disaster for the Commonwealth. The conservative parties holding office federally had built their economic strategy around restoring the public finances — public finances that were still recovering from Australia's energetic response to the last crisis, the GFC, a decade ago. To shore up the economy through the pandemic, the Commonwealth committed a vast sum to its 'JobKeeper' and 'JobSeeker' programs. The former, 'one of the largest labour market interventions in Australia's history,' was budgeted at $130bn (Bishop and Day 2020, p. 1; Frydenberg and Morrison 2020).[9] The longer the economy was to be kept in hibernation, the more costs would rise. As noted above, hibernation cost the economy and the Commonwealth fisc dearly. The recession also presented a fiscal challenge for a number of the States, and Victoria, the worst-hit, launched its own stimulus program. That drove the State's 2020–2021 budget into substantial deficit. Though large, at 5 percent of gross state product Victoria's deficit was less than half the Commonwealth's 11 percent of GDP (PBO 2020; Treasury 2020a).

The States have been at the frontline of the pandemic and containment was their dominant concern. It was the States who pushed in National Cabinet for stronger measures to contain the spread of the virus, and it was they who led the way. Once it became apparent that the measures were succeeding, the Commonwealth made clear its desire to see them unwound as quickly as possible, but the States were more cautious. The resumption of face-to-face classroom teaching in Australia's schools was a particularly contentious point. In the middle of April, the prime minister (PM 2020c) announced that "National Cabinet agreed with the AHPPC health advice that 'on current evidence, schools can be fully open.'" At one point, the Commonwealth education minister took the dispute public only to be forced into a backdown — going from 'raging bull to mewling kitten,' it was said (Murphy 2020). Despite ongoing rhetorical pressure from the Commonwealth, the States continued to make their own, more circumspect, decisions.

3.4.5.2 Border wars

Another flashpoint was State government border closures, which commenced in March and in several cases continued as other lockdown measures were being eased in May. These were not unprecedented, having occurred in response to the Spanish Flu epidemic a century earlier (Cumpston 1978; Hyslop 1998). However, such action is, on the face of it, in flagrant violation of s. 92 of the Commonwealth Constitution, which stipulates that 'trade, commerce and intercourse among the States ... shall be absolutely free.' As in 1919, though, these have been exceptional times, and the border closures were hugely popular with voters. The closures were deplored by the Commonwealth, which joined a constitutional challenge but withdrew at the 11th hour when the second wave accelerated. On 6 November, the High Court dismissed the challenge, declaring that, under the circumstances, border closures were valid emergency measures consistent with s. 92.[10]

3.4.5.3 An asymmetric power

The *Biosecurity Act* equips the Commonwealth with potentially enormous powers to close things down, but that was not much use in this crisis since the States needed no prompting in that regard. What the Commonwealth so conspicuously lacked is the power to force the States to open things back up. The Commonwealth exercised a modicum of brute power to get its way: using its dominant fiscal position to bribe Australia's extensive array of private schools into reopening (Karp 2020). This was a rather minor invocation of its power, however, because the private schools are *de facto* within Commonwealth jurisdiction. The Commonwealth has not hesitated in the past to use its spending power to coerce the States in regards to schooling more generally, but it refrained in this crisis. In part, this no doubt reflected the high degree of public support enjoyed by the State governments; in part, it reflected the clumsy nature of such an instrument in these circumstances.

3.5 Discussion and conclusion

Australia's federal system proved adept at handling this crisis through 2020 and, if anything, to have been enhanced by it. Federalism demonstrated the advantages of subsidiarity and of what is sometimes pejoratively termed 'balkanization,' with States calibrating their measures to the local severity of the problem and using their borders as a barrier to the spread of the virus. At the same time, collegial national leadership and loose coordination provided collective decision-making where necessary and an overall sense of national direction and purpose.

3.5.1 Loose coordination: a system suited for pandemic

Australia's intergovernmental arrangements had laid the basis for coordinated action when called for — particularly given the investment over the preceding decade or so in establishing emergency *modus operandi*. At the peak level, COAG transitioned effortlessly into National Cabinet, where more rapid, collegial, and informal decision-making could occur. National Cabinet proved such an impressive exercise in collaborative intergovernmentalism because the Commonwealth had little choice but to rely in the main on the States for management of the crisis.

With the exception of some operational areas, tight coordination was not necessary since the approach of State-by-State management and jurisdictional quarantining was well-suited to controlling the spread of infection. This was particularly so given the large geographical size of the Australian States and the limited number of points where population centres are on or near borders. Much more so than the bushfires, a pandemic lends itself to the kind of decentralized and non-coordinated response federalism can provide. Borders, in the form of State regulatory diversity, have been a major target for federalism critics in Australia. This has particularly been the case for business — determined that there be, in COAG's words, a 'seamless national economy' (BCA 2008; COAG 2008a). In 2020, though, borders, were back. Unlike fire, the virus requires human vectors, so can be contained through such simple means. Individual jurisdictions, meanwhile, can calibrate their response to local conditions, and, since the main suppression mechanism is regulatory, resource limitations are not a major factor.[11]

Insofar as adverse spillovers occurred, they primarily took the form of economic ramifications for the rest of the economy in cases where major jurisdictions adopted a full lockdown approach, as Victoria did during the second wave. Finally, if as was frequently alleged, the second wave was the consequence of policy and administrative mis-steps by the Victorian government, then federalism might also be seen as having delivered on its promise of quarantining poor politics or policy to individual jurisdictions. The need for rapid response combined with indeterminacies in the transmission of the virus, however, left little scope for federalism to demonstrate its much-touted potential for policy experimentation and learning — though there was some evidence in the respect of contact-tracing methods where NSW seemed to operate so much more effectively than Victoria (LSIC 2020; Paynter 2020).

3.5.2 National cabinet: a new normal?

Because National Cabinet has been such an unusual case of collaborative leadership and joint decision-making, it has been hailed as unprecedented and as representing a step forward in Australian federalism. Propelled by its success, the prime minister and premiers announced towards the end of the 'first wave' that the new arrangement would be made permanent and the 'COAG model' would be abandoned (PM 2020b).

Superseding COAG was to be an annual meeting bringing together National Cabinet, the Council on Federal Financial Relations, and the president of the Australian Local Government Association. A new label was, in turn, coined for this meeting: the National Federation Reform Council. 'This new model' was touted by the prime minister as 'a congestion busting process that will get things done' (PM 2020b). However, not only does much of the work of intergovernmental relations depend upon bureaucratic processes, but COAG also had its celebrated episodes of energetic 'reformism' when that was the zeitgeist, and it is difficult to avoid the conclusion that National Cabinet should be seen as a crisis mode, rather than a new mode, of intergovernmentalism. The complex and conflictual realities of intergovernmental relations, as well as the top-down nature of Australian federalism outside of such exceptional crisis times, will surely lead the 'new normal' to look awfully similar to the old normal.

3.5.3 *Getting the balance right?*

There was certainly friction, but there is little indication that it was an impediment to effective action and no indication that it escalated into real conflict. Quite possibly, the balance between the Commonwealth's insistence on minimizing fiscal and economic damage and the States' preoccupation with minimizing infection ensured a good compromise. State government prudence was regularly criticized for inflicting excessive economic harm, and if they had more fiscal autonomy in the federation, perhaps the States would have acted differently. However, one cannot readily know whether that would have been for the better. In many ways, as well, their assertiveness was a healthy sign that the States retain some ability to act in defiance of the Commonwealth — a crucial trait of a federal system, particularly one such as Australia's where so much centralization has occurred. Through the first year of the pandemic it would seem that the 'patchwork' that is Australian federalism did not work too badly.

Notes

1 Some of these were canvassed in the abortive Reform of the Federation White Paper process of 2014–2015 (RFWP 2014).
2 It is a motley collection of provisions including everything from the external affairs and trade-and-commerce powers to the "postal power"; see s. 24.
3 Including the *National Catastrophic Natural Disaster Plan, National Health Emergency Response Arrangements*, and the *Australian Government Crisis Management Framework*.
4 The Emergency Management Committee reported to the Ministerial Council for Police and Emergency Management — which, in turn, reported to COAG. That ministerial council was replaced in October 2020 by the National Emergency Management Ministers' Meeting.
5 Minus the ALGA representation that was a feature of COAG.
6 *Roadmap to a COVID-Safe Australia: A Three-Step Pathway for Easing Restrictions* (8 May 2020). https://www.pm.gov.au/sites/default/files/files/covid-safe-australia-roadmap.pdf [Accessed 8 March 2021].
7 It is one of the anomalies of Australian federalism that the Commonwealth has assumed responsibility for aged care — a *de facto* extension of its mandate under s. 51 (xxiii) to provide 'invalid and old-age pensions.'
8 That is the coalition between the Liberal Party and the National Party with Liberal leader Scott Morrison as prime minister.
9 Providing 'the equivalent of around 70 percent of the national median wage' meant that it equated 'to a full median replacement wage' for 'workers in the accommodation, hospitality and retail sectors.' Treasury subsequently revised the estimated cost down substantially. Research by Bishop and Day (2020) suggests that the program was very effective.
10 *Palmer and Anor v. State of Western Australia and Anor*, HCA (2020).
11 Resource limitations were a factor in some important respects — the decision by the Victorian government to employ private contractors to supervise quarantine rather than taking the Commonwealth up on its offer of ADF personnel being a case in point.

Bibliography

ANAO, Australian National Audit Office, 2020. *Planning and Governance of COVID-19 Procurements to Increase the National Medical Stockpile*. Canberra: Commonwealth of Australia.

Anderson, G., 2008. The Council of Australian Governments: A New Institution of Governance for Australia's Conditional federalism. *University of New South Wales Law Journal*, 31 (2), 493–508.

Australia, Commonwealth & States and Territories, 2020. *National Partnership on COVID-19 Response*. Canberra: Council of Australian Governments.

BCA, 2008. *Towards a Seamless Economy: Modernising the Regulation of Australian Business*. Melbourne: Business Council of Australia.

Bennett, B, Carney, T. and Bailey, R., 2012. Emergency Powers & Pandemics: Federalism and the Management of Public Health Emergencies in Australia. *University of Tasmania Law Review*, 31 (1), 37–57.

Benson, S. and Chambers, G., 2020, PM's Bid to Boost Disaster Powers. *The Australian*, 29 January, p. 1.

Bishop, J. and *Day*, I., 2020. How Many Jobs Did JobKeeper Keep? *Reserve Bank of Australia*, 2020–07.

Brew, N. and Burton, K., 2004. *Australia's Capacity to Respond to an Infectious Disease Outbreak*. Canberra: Parliament of Australia.

CHQI, COVID-19 Hotel Quarantine Inquiry, 2020. *Final Report and Recommendations*. Melbourne: Government of Victoria.

COAG, 2008a. *Communiqué*. Canberra: Council of Australian Governments.

COAG, 2008b. *Model Arrangements for Leadership during Emergencies of National Consequence*. Canberra: Council of Australian Governments.

COAG, 2020. *Communiqué*. Canberra: Council of Australian Governments.

Crowe, D., 2020. Morrison's 3-Step Roadmap to Recovery Is Merely a Menu for the States. *Sydney Morning Herald*, 8 May.

Cumpston, JHL, 1978. *The Health of the People: A Study in Federalism*. Canberra: Roebuck Society.

Dardanelli, P., Kincaid, J., Fenna, A, Kaiser, A., Lecours, A. and Singh, A.K., 2019. Dynamic De/Centralization in Federations: Comparative Conclusions. *Publius*, 49 (1), 194–219.

DCSH, Department of Community Services and Health, 1988. Human Quarantine: The Australian Approach to a World Problem. *In:* ABoS ABS, ed. *Year Book Australia*. Canberra: Commonwealth of Australia. https://www.abs.gov.au/ausstats/abs@.nsf/featurearticlesbytitle/F74D29E8BE724723CA2569DE0024ED5C?OpenDocument

DHA, Department of Health and Ageing, 2011. *Review of Australia's Health Sector Response to Pandemic (H1N1) 2009: Lessons Identified*. Canberra: Commonwealth of Australia.

Fenna, A., 2008. Commonwealth Fiscal Power and Australian Federalism. *University of New South Wales Law Journal*, 31 (2), 509–529.

Fenna, A., 2010. The Return of Keynesianism in Australia: The Rudd Government and the Lessons of Recessions Past. *Australian Journal of Political Science*, 45 (3), 353–369.

Fenna, A., 2017. The Fiscal Predicament of Australian Federalism. *In:* Bruerton, M., Arklay, T., Hollander, R. and Levy, R, eds. *A People's Federation*. Leichhardt: Federation Press, 134–146.

Fenna, A., 2019. The Centralization of Australian Federalism 1901–2010: Measurement and Interpretation. *Publius*, 49 (1), 30–56.

Fenna, A., 2019b. National Competition Policy: Effective Stewardship of Markets. *In* Luetjens, J., 't Hart, P., and Mintrom, M., eds, *Successful Public Policy:Lessons from Australia and New Zealand*. Canberra: ANU Press, 191–206.

Fenna, A. and Anderson, G., 2012. The Rudd Reforms and the Future of Australian Federalism. *In*: Appleby, G., Aroney, N. and John, T., eds. *The Future of Australian Federalism: Comparative and Interdisciplinary Perspectives*. Cambridge: Cambridge University Press, 393–413.

Fenna, A., Phillimore, J. and Ramamurthy, V., 2021. Australian Health-Care Federalism: Beyond the Logic of Autonomy. *In*: Fenwick, T.B. and Banfield A.C., eds. *Beyond Autonomy: Practical and Theoretical Challenges to 21st Century Federalism*. Leiden: Brill, 135–57.

Frydenberg, Hon J. and Cormann, Hon M., 2020. *Final Budget Outcome 2019–20*. Canberra: Commonwealth of Australia, 25 September.

Frydenberg, Hon J. and Morrison, Hon S., 2020. *$130 Billion JobKeeper Payment to Keep Australians in a Job*. Canberra: Commonwealth of Australia, 30 March. https://www.pm.gov.au/media/130-billion-jobkeeper-payment-keep-australians-job

Health, Department of, 2018. *Emergency Response Plan for Communicable Disease Incidents of National Significance: National Arrangements*. Canberra: Commonwealth of Australia.

Home Affairs, Department of, 2019. *Australian Emergency Management Arrangements*. Canberra: Commonwealth of Australia.

Howse, G., 2004. Managing Emerging Infectious Diseases: Is a Federal System an Impediment to Effective Laws? *Australia and New Zealand Health Policy*, 1 (7), 1–4.

Hyslop, A., 1998. Insidious Immigrant: Spanish Influenza and Border quarantine in Australia 1919. *In*: Parry, S., ed. *From Migration to Mining: Medicine and Health in Australian History*. Casuarina: Northern Territory University Press, 201–215.

Karp, P., 2020. Coalition Offers Independent Schools Early Funding if They Return to Face-to-Face Teaching. *The Guardian*, 29 April.

Lee, H.P., Adams, M.W.R., Campbell, C. and Emerton, P., 2018. *Emergency Powers in Australia*. 2nd ed. Cambridge: Cambridge University Press.

LSIC, Legal and Social Issues Committee, 2020. *Inquiry into the Victorian Government's COVID-19 Contact Tracing System and Testing Regime*. Melbourne: Legislative Council, Parliament of Victoria.

Mackellar, D., 1911. My Country. *In* Mackellar, D., *The Closed Door and Other Verses*. Melbourne: Australasian Authors' Agency, 9–11.

McLean, H. and Huf, B., 2020. *Emergency Powers, Public Health and COVID-19*. Melbourne: Parliament of Victoria.

Murphy, K., 2020. Dan Tehan Tried to Pressure Victoria to Reopen Schools, but He Went from Raging Bull to Mewling Kitten. *The Guardian: Australian Edition*, 3 May.

OECD, 2020a. *COVID-19 and Fiscal Relations across Levels of Government*. Paris: Organisation for Economic Co-operation and Development.

OECD, 2020b. *The Territorial Impact of COVID-19: Managing the Crisis across Levels of Government*. Paris: Organisation for Economic Co-operation and Development.

Painter, M., 1998. *Collaborative Federalism: Economic Reform in Australia in the 1990s*. Melbourne: Cambridge University Press.

Paynter, J., 2020. What Victorian Contact Tracing Team Will Learn *from* NSW Visit. *The Australian*, 11 September.

PBO, Parliamentary Budget Office, 2020. *Victorian Budget 20/21: Independent Snapshot*. Melbourne: Parliament of Victoria.

Phillimore, J., and Fenna, A., 2017. Intergovernmental Councils and Centralization in Australian Federalism. *Regional and Federal Studies*, 27 (5), 597–621.

PM, Prime Minister, 2020a. *Address, National Press Club*. Canberra: Commonwealth of Australia, 29 January. Available *from*: https://www.pm.gov.au/media/address-national-press-club [Accessed 8 March 2021].

PM, Prime Minister, 2020b. *Media Release*. Canberra: Commonwealth of Australia, 29 May. Available *from*: https://www.pm.gov.au/media/update-following-national-cabinet-meeting [Accessed 8 March 2021].

PM, Prime Minister, 2020c. *Media Statement.* Canberra: Commonwealth of Australia.

PM, Prime Minister, 2020d. *Press Conference with Premiers and Chief Ministers, Parramatta, NSW: Transcript.* Canberra: Commonwealth of Australia.

PMC, Department of the Prime Minister and Cabinet, 2015. *Reform of the Federation: Green Paper.* Canberra: Commonwealth of Australia.

Poirier, J. and Saunders, C., 2015. Conclusion: Comparative Experiences of Intergovernmental Relations in Federal Systems. *In:* Poirier, J., Saunders, C. and Kincaid, J., eds. *Intergovernmental Relations in Federal Systems: Comparative Structures and Dynamics.* Don Mills: Oxford University Press, 440–498.

PRC, Pew Research Center, 2020. Americans Give the U.S. Low Marks for Its Handling of COVID-19, and So Do People in Other Countries. *Pew Research Center*, 12 September. Available *from*: https://www.pewresearch.org/fact-tank/2020/09/21/americans-give-the-u-s-low-marks-for-its-handling-of-covid-19-and-so-do-people-in-other-countries/ [Accessed 8 March 2021].

RCACQS, Royal Commission into Aged Care Quality and Safety, 2020. *Aged Care and COVID-19: A Special Report.* Canberra: Commonwealth of Australia.

RCNNDA, Royal Commission into National Natural Disaster Arrangements, 2020. *Report.* Canberra: Commonwealth of Australia.

RFWP, Reform of the Federation *White* Paper, 2014. *A Federation for Our Future.* Canberra: Department of the Prime Minister and Cabinet.

Saunders, C., 2020. *A New Federalism? The Role and Future of the National Cabinet.* Carlton: Melbourne School of Government.

Schnabel, J., 2020. *Managing Interdependencies in Federal Systems: Intergovernmental Councils and the Making of Public Policy.* Cham: Palgrave Macmillan.

SCIRP, Special Commission of Inquiry into the Ruby Princess, 2020. *Report.* Sydney: Government of New South Wales.

Treasury, Department of the 2009. Budget Paper No. 1: Budget Strategy and Outlook 2009–10. *Budget Papers 2009–10.* Canberra: Commonwealth of Australia.

Treasury, Department of the, 2020a. *Budget Paper No. 1: Budget Strategy and Outlook.* Canberra: Commonwealth of Australia.

Treasury, Department of the, 2020b. *Budget Paper No. 3: Federal Financial Relations.* Canberra: Commonwealth of Australia.

Van Onselen, P., 2020. The Buck on Quarantine Stops with the Commonwealth. *The Australian*, 25 July.

Victoria, 2020. *Victorian Government Submission to the Senate Select Committee on COVID-19.* Melbourne: Government of Victoria.

Wilkie, M., 2020, *Victims of Failure: How the COVID-19 Policy Response Let Down Australians.* Sydney: Centre for Independent Studies.

Williams, G., 2020. Co-operation Key to the United States of Australia. *The Australian*, 11 May.

4 The impact of COVID-19 on the Austrian federal system

Peter Bußjäger and Mathias Eller

4.1 Introduction

Like other countries, Austria has been hit hard by COVID-19. However, the mortality rate has remained rather low in comparison to other nations. The pandemic strikingly shows not only the vulnerability of society to an invisible exigent adversary which threatens people's physical health but also the difficulties an emergency of this scope poses for legislative and executive bodies. Concerning federalism, at first glance, the impact of the pandemic has been limited so far. For example, until September 2020, there have been no modifications to the Federal Constitution concerning the distribution of competences in legislation or execution. Nevertheless, it is important to investigate the extent to which the federal system in Austria was affected by the virus and how the different levels of government coped with this state of emergency.

Therefore, this chapter is structured as follows: First, the current situation of COVID-19 in Austria is examined, including an assessment of the health and economic costs incurred (2). Second, the distribution of competences on health matters between the Federation and the *Länder* (States) is outlined. The subsequent analysis focuses on the legislative and administrative activities on the federal and *Land* level as well as intergovernmental relations in this context (3). The final section concentrates on the transformations in the practice of federalism in Austria due to the crisis (4).

Numerous governance phenomena occurred in Austria during the crisis. They can be summarized as follows:

1 It is a well-known fact that, in times of crisis, there is a tendency to call for comprehensive and uniform solutions. This has also been the case in Austria;
2 States of emergency trigger the elevation of executive over legislative bodies;
3 *Länder* regulations deviated from Federal Government measures enacted for the whole of Austria due to the differentiated effects of the pandemic in different areas;
4 The Austrian type of cooperative federalism seems to be an effective way to cope with the pandemic;
5 The distribution of competences on health matters between the Federation and the *Länder* has so far not been an obstacle to the sufficient supply of health services.

All in all, it seems that Austria overcame the "first wave" of the pandemic well (Table 4.1). This has surprised various experts who feared the negative effects of the

DOI: 10.4324/9781003251217-4

Table 4.1 Key Statistics on COVID-19 in Austria as of 10 January 2021

Cumulative Cases	Cumulative Cases per 100,000 Population	Cumulative Deaths	Cumulative Deaths per 100,000 Population	Case Fatality Percentage
378,110	4,198.2	6,614	73.4	1.7

Source: World Health Organization Weekly epidemiological update – 12 January 2021. Geneva: WHO, 2021. Available from https://www.who.int/publications/m/item/weekly-epidemiological-update

opaque and complicated distribution of competences, especially in the hospital sector. In an analysis published on the Cambridge Core blog on 12 April 2020, author Thomas Czypionka wrote:

> Despite its fragmented healthcare system, strong federalism, and relatively poor public health capacity, Austria has so far fared surprisingly well in the current crisis. After the swift and decisive introduction of rather drastic measures, infections have shown a considerable decline. As one of the first European countries to impose them, restrictions will be gradually lifted in the coming weeks.

The Austrian form of cooperative federalism has been nevertheless challenged by this new threat and has, so far, passed the test. However, it appears that mistakes have been made in addressing the outbreak, and in the most recent developments, considerable communication problems have arisen between the Federal Government and the Länder. In order to keep the spread of the virus and its impact on the health and economic system in Austria under control, smart Federal Government coordination with responsive and creative *Land* and local governments attuned to their situations will be required in the coming months. The prevalence of the executive bodies on the other hand – especially the Federal Government – fosters to some degree the development of features that normally occur in decentralized unitary states.

4.2 COVID-19 in Austria

The COVID-19 pandemic hit Austria at the end of February 2020, as the new Federal Government formed in January 2020 was only a few weeks into its term. It emerged as a completely unexpected challenge for the coalition of the conservative Peoples' Party and the Greens who had never been in a coalition at federal level before.

As noted above, Austria managed the initial phase of the pandemic comparatively well. After the first wave began at the end of February with the first confirmed infections detected in Innsbruck, it peaked at the end of March with more than a 1,000 infections per day. The lowest level of infections was reached in the middle of June, as the daily infection rate ranged between 20 and 50 new confirmed infections per day.

At the beginning of September 2020, Austria had approximately 28,000 persons in total infected with the virus, with approximately 24,000 recovered, 3,300 active cases, and 726 deaths from COVID-19. At this point in time, the death rate per 100,000 inhabitants in Austria was 8.30 (compared with 0.64 in South Korea; 11.24 in Germany; 5.59 in France; 6.35 in Sweden; 6.76 in the USA; and 62.49 in the UK (Neuwirth 2020)).

As the restrictions imposed on the general public to control the spread of the virus were lifted (such as the restrictions on free movement at the end of May and the re-opening of national borders in June), the infection rate began to increase again. At the beginning of September 2020, Austria faced between 300 and 400 new infections per day. The Federal Government took action to ensure that Austria does not reach the point of exponential growth in cases. Statistics also show that the situation in the hospitals remains stable and does not mirror the growth of infections.

Despite the fairly good performance in controlling infection rates during the first wave of the pandemic, the Austrian economy was hit heavily by the virus control measures. Gross national product sank by about 8 percent. Unemployment increased by leaps and bounds, as did "short-time working,"[1] which is an attempt to encourage companies to retain their employees rather than lay them off. The budgets of the Federation as well as those of the *Länder* and municipalities are out of balance. On the one hand, tax revenues are falling considerably, while on the other hand, expenditures are increasing to mitigate the economic impact of the crisis.

On 4 September 2020, the Federal Government initiated its four-phase "traffic light system" of COVID-19 control measures. The system operates a color-coded scale of the severity of the situation in a given area. "Green" denotes that minimal precautions are required, while "red" indicates that the most stringent controls should be implemented. "Orange" and "yellow" are gradations between the two ends of the spectrum. The system initially assigned "yellow" status to the capital Vienna and the next largest cities in Austria (Graz and Linz) as well as to a district in Tyrol. The rest of Austria was given a "green" status.

A commission provides advice and recommendations to the Federal Minister for Health. Based on its recommendations, the Minister can give instructions to the *Land* Governors who are required to either implement the directives by decrees for the *Land* concerned or instruct the district authorities to implement such measures in their respective territory. The commission is composed of representatives of the Federal Ministry for Health, experts from the Agency for Health and Food Security, medical experts from universities, and representatives of the *Länder* carries out the risk assessment and determines the traffic light of the respective districts. This composition is an example of the functioning of cooperative federalism in Austria.

The "traffic light system" is a challenge for the Austrian federal system as the *Land* Governors have to execute directives of the Federal Minister for Health as well as the recommendations of the commission. It is imperative to note that the *Land* and the federal level may have different interests. In addition, the *Land* Governors are faced with the problem that the legal basis of binding decrees on various matters is weak. The Constitutional Court (14 July 2020, V 363/2020) ruled parts of the decree of the Federal Minister for Health (which regulated the "Lockdown" in March and imposed extensive restrictions of free movement in Austria) to be an infringement of law. As a result of this judgement, the Federal Parliament as the competent legislator modified the existing law in order to make restrictions as they are foreseen in cases of "red" or "orange" compatible with the constitution. At the initiation of the traffic light system in September 2020, this law had not even been discussed in parliament, and it will not enter into force before October 2020.

4.3 COVID-19 and federalism in Austria

4.3.1 Distribution of competences in health matters

According to the Austrian Federal Constitution (B-VG), competences on health matters are distributed between the Federation and the *Länder* (States). However, the Federation has the competence to pass and execute laws concerning public health, except for those concerning the organization of hospitals and municipal sanitation (Art. 10 para 1 n. 12 B-VG). This includes the competence to manage the prevention of epidemics and pandemics. Art. 12 para 1 n. 1, B-VG stipulates that the organization of hospitals is the business of the Federation in regards to the basic legislation, while legislation on implementation and enforcement is the business of the *Länder*. Public hospitals are managed in most cases by *Länder* or municipalities and financed by a very complicated system of social insurance and financial equalization.

According to Art. 10 para 1 n. 12 B-VG, federal administration of public health has to be executed by the *Land* Governors and the subordinated district authorities of the *Länder* (so-called indirect federal administration). According to Art. 103 para 1. B-VG, Governors are bound to the instructions of the Federal Government and individual Federal Ministers (Art. 20). In the case of the pandemic, they are bound to those of the Federal Minister for Health from the Green Party. In order to effect the implementation of such instructions, they are also obliged to employ the powers available to them in their capacity as a functionary of the province's autonomous sphere of competence.

This system of indirect federal administration is characteristic of Austrian federalism and its cooperative element: on the one hand, the Federal Government is legally in a position to enforce its will vis-à-vis the *Land* governors; but on the other hand, the action taken also depends on the capacities of the *Länder* and their commitment to confronting the crisis.

4.3.2 Measures implemented by the authorities on the federal and land level to prevent further spread of the pandemic

Based on the aforementioned provisions, the competent authorities execute the federal Epidemics Act 1950 ("Epidemiegesetz"), which has roots stretching back to 1913. As this law was ill-suited to deal with the current epidemic, various new regulations were passed by the Austrian parliament in the early stages of the pandemic. The most notable of these is the "COVID-19-Maßnahmengesetz" ("COVID-19 Action Law"), which came into force on 16 March 2020. At this stage, the second chamber, the Austrian "Bundesrat," agreed unanimously to all legislative measures proposed by the first chamber. In some fields, such as public procurement law, COVID-19 legislation even led to a temporary loss of state competences.

As a result, the competent authorities on the federal and *Land* level are now entitled to issue decrees prohibiting entry to business premises (for customers, § 1) as well as other specified locations (§ 2). Decrees can be issued by the Minister of Health (no. 1), the Governor of the *Land* (no. 2), and the district administrative authority (no. 3) in their respective jurisdictions (the entire country, the *Land*, the district territory which is an administrative subunit of the respective Land or parts of the district territory).

Based on the COVID-19-Maßnahmengesetz, the enforcement bodies have issued various ordinances that executed the "lockdown" in Austria by prohibiting the "entering of public places." Exceptions have been made for activities required to meet basic daily needs (such as food shopping). The Minister of Health also issued an ordinance on provisional measures to prevent the proliferation of COVID-19, prohibiting access to the customer areas of retail and service premises and of leisure and sports facilities.

On the regional level, Tyrol – the *Land* that had initially been affected by the crisis more than any other – enacted stricter lockdown regulations than those implemented by the Federal Government across the entire Austrian territory. Although the ability of the *Länder* to take independent action ultimately is always dependent on the goodwill of the Federal Government, the Tyrolean approach illustrated a certain degree of flexibility in the management of the crisis. This approach provides the *Länder* with the ability to implement a differentiated COVID-19 response according to local and regional conditions. However, the ordinance that had provided for an even stricter lockdown in the *Land* Tyrol was also recently found to be unlawful by the Constitutional Court (10 December 2020, V 512/2020). In the light of the ruling issued in the summer, this decision was not surprising at all.

The fact that all the legal instruments used to take action during the crisis have already been amended several times reflects the pressure under which the legislative and regulatory bodies have been working as well as the need to continually adapt the legal framework to the dynamic developments.

4.3.3 Intergovernmental relations and cooperative federalism

Intergovernmental relations and the Austrian form of cooperative federalism are closely connected and interdependent. The better the communication and coordination between the different levels of government, the more effective cooperative federalism is. Overall, it can be said that cooperation between the Federation, the *Länder*, and the municipalities proceeded relatively smoothly during the zenith of the "first wave." Not surprisingly, all levels of government emphasized the good cooperation that has been maintained so far during the outbreak. Since the beginning of the crisis, tensions and differences in approach have only emerged in isolated cases. In Vienna, for example, the city opened its parks to the public, while those owned by the Federal Government remained closed.

Perhaps, more prominently, critics have expressed in numerous domestic and foreign media outlets that the authorities of the province of Tyrol reacted inadequately and too slowly to the spread of the virus in the Tyrolean ski resort of Ischgl. The time has not yet come to assign fault for mistakes that might have been made in the response to the outbreak. Since the executing authorities are acting under the responsibility of the Federal Government, their performance should also be examined in due course. To this point, the good cooperation between the Federal Government and *Land* authorities in tackling the crisis does not seem to have been adversely affected by these criticisms.

As the number of Coronavirus infections increased in early September, tensions between the competent authorities became heightened. The *Länder* demanded clearer guidelines in handling the crisis and pointed out that the regional administrative authorities are understaffed. In reaction, additional military personnel were requested by *Land* governments such as Tyrol in order to support the local health authorities and to ensure that the current COVID-19 regulations at the state borders can be executed properly. This example demonstrates the importance of coordination and cooperation between all levels of government as well as a recognition that the competent authorities work under tremendous pressure in emergency situations such as the COVID-19 crisis.

Although the new "traffic light system," introduced at the beginning of September can be seen as a typical example of Austrian cooperative federalism (composed of representatives of federal ministries, *Länder* and experts), its implementation caused various problems. This was due to the lack of transparency in the decision-making process and the unclear legal basis upon which *Land* Governors and district authorities were required to base their regulations. It must be regarded as a failure of the Federal Government that it was not able to elaborate the necessary laws required for the system and present them to parliament in a timely manner.

4.3.4 The role of land governments

Despite the far-reaching powers of the Federal Government, it remains the task of the *Länder* to provide sufficient capacity in hospitals and in relation to testing, for example. To date, this division of responsibility has worked well, especially if you compare Austria to other countries dealing with the crisis. However, as outlined before, as the "second wave" of the pandemic has begun to emerge in Austria, capacity constraints, especially in terms of auxiliary personnel, appear to be becoming increasingly problematic and are engendering tensions between the federal and *Land* authorities.

The pandemic clearly shows the limits of indirect federal administration. The Federation and *Länder* depend on each other: while the Federation has the exclusive competences for legislation, it depends on the *Land* authorities and their willingness and commitment to implement federal regulations.

However, the key role in indirect federal administration is played by the *Land* Governor and not the whole of the *Land* government. The Governor receives the instructions of the Federal Government and passes them to the administrative authorities in their respective jurisdiction. Thus, the role of the *Land* Governments in handling the crisis is limited, despite the fact that it is clear that the respective members of these governments, competent for matters of health or security, play an important role in a crisis such as the COVID-19 pandemic.

4.3.5 The role of local governments

The lowest territorial level in Austria was severely affected by the COVID-19 crisis, particularly with regards to finances. Experts estimate that municipalities will lose up to 2 billion euros as a result of decreased incomes and increased expenditures. The aid packages provided by the Federal Government are currently far from sufficient to overcome the deficits incurred to date.

Although municipalities do not participate directly in the distribution of competences in Austria, Art. 118 para 1 B-VG states that "a municipality has its own sphere of competence and one assigned to it either by the federation or the province." The "own sphere of competence" comprises all matters exclusively or preponderantly the concern of the local community as embodied by the municipality, and suited to performance by the community within its local boundaries. Legislation shall expressly specify matters of that kind as being such which fall within the municipality's own sphere of competence (para 2).

Furthermore, a municipality is guaranteed official responsibility in its own sphere of competence for performance of specific enumerated matters such as local public security administration, the regulation of local public events or local sanitary administration (*örtliche Gesundheitspolizei*), particularly in the field of emergency and first aid services as well as matters pertaining to deaths and interment.

In fact, there was no area of municipal responsibility that remained unaffected by the crisis. The closure of schools, kindergartens, and after-school care centers required a very rapid response and support had to be provided for parents in system-critical professions. In the same vein, important municipal services and facilities had to be closed as well. This not only applied to the cultural and sports sectors but also to waste material collection centers and many municipal offices. Shopping services were organized for the elderly to ensure that vulnerable population groups were protected as best as possible. In addition, the statutory cities[2] were particularly hard hit by the crisis because, unlike ordinary local municipalities, they also had to cope with the tasks of indirect federal administration.

To date, municipalities have been a key player in managing the crisis, and they will remain a crucial partner in keeping the pandemic under control in Austria in the future. It is for precisely this reason that they should be provided with sufficient financial resources to perform the functions necessary in the COVID-19 context.

4.3.6 Measures within the framework of private-sector administration

Both the Federal and *Land* governments are currently attempting to mitigate the economic consequences of the crisis through various financial support measures. If they do so within the framework of private-sector administration, they are not bound by the otherwise applicable division of competences (Art. 10 to 15 B-VG) in line with Art. 17 B-VG. The measures range from aid for "short-time working" to hardship funds and fixed cost subsidies for affected companies.

There is no doubt that the measures taken will have serious budgetary consequences for the federal, *Land*, and local governments. It will therefore be interesting to see how the accumulated debts are distributed among the authorities. According to the latest reports, the next fiscal equalization negotiations, which have the potential to be explosive, will be postponed due to the exceptional situation. Although the extent of the economic consequences of the COVID-19 crisis cannot yet be assessed, there is no question that they are far-reaching.

4.4 Case study of innovation/transformations in COVID-19 and federalism in Austria

Due to its competences regarding legislation and execution of governance functions according to Art. 10 para 1 n. 12 (health care), the Federation was able to impose severe restrictions on daily life in Austria during the first wave of the pandemic.

The authorities of the *Länder* had to execute these provisions under the directive of the Federal Minister for Health. This transferred additional *de facto* power to the Federal Government, even though all proceedings were constitutionally valid. Therefore, during this period, Austria somewhat transitioned from a federal into a decentralized unitary state. The role of the Federation in agenda setting was strengthened. Vertical coordination appears to have to be much more relevant than horizontal cooperation.

On the other hand, new forms of cooperative federalism were introduced or intensified. Video conferences between the staff of the Federal Ministries and the *Land* administrations were held on a daily basis, often with the participation of political representatives.

While the COVID-19 crisis strengthened centralized legislation and emphasized the vertical aspects of Austrian federalism, it also made visible the important role of the *Land* authorities in executing the virus control regulations. Specifically, the district authorities ("Bezirkshauptmannschaften"), which were established as institutions of monarchical administration in 1868 and transferred to the *Länder* in 1920, are functioning as health authorities.

The COVID-19 crisis also seems to have advanced the process of the digitization of Austrian administrative governance. Not only have video conferences become commonplace, but digitization of administrative and judicial procedures has also taken place. It can be anticipated that this will have an enormous impact on the way in which governments will communicate with their citizens in the future.

The impacts of this development of Austrian federalism are not yet clear. In administrative theory, federalism is often seen as an obstacle to efficient E-Government. The COVID-19 crisis might encourage the establishment of new E-Government platforms including services provided by the Federation as well as by the *Länder* and municipalities. This example indicates the growing importance of cooperative federalism in Austria.

Finally, it can be said that the COVID-19 crisis marginalized the role of the federal parliament as well as *Land* parliaments. The National Council and the second chamber of the Austrian parliament, the Federal Council, as well as the *Landtage* (Austria's *Land* parliaments) could only deliver legal empowerment of the Governments. Based on this legal provisions, the governments decreed various incisive restrictions of public life.

Notes

1 Short-time working or short time is a governmental unemployment insurance system in which private-sector employees agree to or are forced to accept a reduction in working time and pay, with the state making up for all or part of the lost wages.
2 A statutory city is vested, in addition to its purview as a municipality, with the powers and duties of a district administrative authority.

Bibliography

Austrian Federal Constitution, 1945. Austria. Available from: https://www.ris.bka.gv.at/GeltendeFassung.wxe?Abfrage=Bundesnormen&Gesetzesnummer=10000138 [Accessed 23 March 2021].Constitutional Court, 2020. *V 363/2020*. Austria, July 14. Available from: https://www.vfgh.gv.at/downloads/VfGH-Entscheidung_V_363_2020_vom_14._Juli_2020.pdf [Accessed 23 March 2021].

Constitutional Court, 2020. *V 512/2020*. Austria, December 10. Available from: https://www.vfgh.gv.at/downloads/VfGH_10.12.2020_V_512_2020_Tirol_Verlassen_des_Wohnsitzes.pdf [Accessed 23 March 2021].

Czypionka, T., 2020. Austria's Response to the Coronavirus Pandemic – A Second Perspective. *Cambridge Core blog*, 12 April. Available from: https://www.cambridge.org/core/blog/2020/04/12/austrias-response-to-the-coronavirus-pandemic-a-second-perspective/ [Accessed 23 March 2021]. Government of Austria, 2020a. *Corona Ampel (COVID-19 Traffic-Light-System)*. *Vienna*, 4 September. Available from: https://corona-ampel.gv.at/ [Accessed 23 March 2021].

Government of Austria, 2020b. *COVID-19-Maßnahmengesetz – COVID-19-MG (StF: BGBl. I Nr. 12/2020 (NR: GP XXVII IA 396/A AB 102 S. 16. BR: AB 10287 S. 903.)*. *Vienna*, 16 March. Available from: https://www.ris.bka.gv.at/GeltendeFassung.wxe?Abfrage=Bundesnormen&Gesetzesnummer=20011073 [Accessed 23 March 2021].

Neuwirth, E., 2020. Erich Neuwirths COVID-19-Analysen. Available from: https://just-the-covid-facts.neuwirth.priv.at/ [Accessed 23 March 2021].

5 Belgium's response to COVID-19

How to manage a pandemic in a competitive federal system?

Peter Bursens, Patricia Popelier and Petra Meier

5.1 Introduction

Belgian federalism is characterized by a 'falling apart' evolution. The centrifugal nature of Belgian federalism is exemplified by six constitutional reforms since 1970, each one resulting in more autonomy and more competences for the federated levels. The state reforms did not follow a masterplan but rather responded to ad hoc demands from the dominant political parties to solve political and policy discord (Deschouwer 2012). The competitive logic of Belgian federalism puts all government levels on equal footing while granting them exclusive powers in allocated competences. The *bricolage* character of the state reforms gave the country a complex division of competences that crosscuts policy domains. Moreover, Belgium ended up with two separate party systems and four electoral colleges resulting in different government coalitions defending diverging interests across the levels of government (Swenden and Jans 2006). The Belgian response to the first two waves of the COVID-19 crisis has been a textbook illustration of how these features (mal) function in practice.

In the remainder of this chapter, we first discuss core data regarding the crisis, such as the number of infections and the economic impact. We present split data for the Belgian government levels and put them within the broader EU context. Next, we briefly present the core institutional set-up of Belgian federalism. The core of this chapter gives an account of how the federal set-up dealt with the response to the COVID-19 threat, during the first wave from March to July 2020 and the second wave from August to December 2020, hence covering both the sanitary, civil protection and economic measures in both waves as well as the exit strategy from the first wave. We end our analysis in the final weeks of 2020 when, after a second peak in the fall, infections stabilized again, be it at a rather high level. The last week of 2020 also marked the symbolical start of the vaccination campaign which started for real in January 2021. Our main conclusion is that Belgium, as many other countries – both unitary and federal – struggled to adequately respond to the pandemic. Yet, some features of its federal set-up impeded an effective Belgian response, especially during the first wave. The dual and, in many ways, competitive character of the system, but also the complex interdependent division of competences, caused burdensome coordination across government levels, leading to calls for another round of state reform, yet, at the same time, also triggered cooperation among the various levels of government (Table 5.1).

DOI: 10.4324/9781003251217-5

Table 5.1 Key Statistics on COVID-19 in Belgium as of 10 January 2021

Cumulative Cases	Cumulative Cases per 100,000 Population	Cumulative Deaths	Cumulative Deaths per 100,000 Population	Case Fatality Percentage
664,261	5,731.5	20,069	173.2	3.0

Source: World Health Organization Weekly epidemiological update – 12 January 2021. Geneva: WHO, 2021. Available from https://www.who.int/publications/m/item/weekly-epidemiological-update

Table 5.2 Percentage of Population, Cases, Hospitalizations, and Fatalities in Belgium in 2020

	Flanders		Wallonia		Brussels	
Population (%)	57		32		11	
	Wave 1	Wave 1+2	Wave 1	Wave 1+2	Wave 1	Wave 1+2
Cases (%)	57	43	30	43	10	13
Hospitalizations (%)	50	48	35	36	15	16
Fatalities (%)	55	50	30	37	15	13

Note: Wave 1 refers to the period until 31 July 2020 and Wave 1+2 refers to the period until 31 December 2020.

5.2 Some data on COVID-19 in Belgium

During the first wave, Belgium was hit quite hard by the virus, compared to other countries in Western Europe. COVID-19 struck Belgium less hard than Spain and Italy, but, in many respects, a lot harder than its neighbors France, Germany, and the Netherlands. The federal scientific health institute Sciensano (2021) reported more than 70,000 cases and nearly 10,000 fatalities on a population of 11.5 million for the five months of the first wave (until 31 July 2020). Over 80 percent of the deaths were 75 years old or older. Half of the fatalities happened in retirement homes. Sciensano argues (2020) that the relative high number is partly due to the method of counting as Belgian statistics also include not confirmed but suspected cases as well as fatalities in retirement homes. After the second wave, the number of detected infections increased to nearly 650,000, mainly caused by a very high second wave peak of cases in the fall and by a much higher number of tests since the summer of 2020. The number of fatalities doubled to almost 20,000 by the end of 2020. Hospitals and intensive care units were put under severe stress during both waves but did not come close to a point of saturation.

The three Belgian regions suffered in an almost equal way during the first wave of the pandemic, measured by the relative number of inhabitants. Nearly 6 out of 10 live in Flanders, 3 out of 10 in Wallonia, and 1 out of 10 in the Brussels Capital Region. The relative number of cases, hospitalizations, and fatalities did not deviate very much from this relative number of inhabitants (see Table 5.2; Sciensano 2021). The share of cases almost perfectly equals the share of the regional population. Yet, Flanders had a slightly lower share of hospitalizations and deaths. The only significant difference was the higher share of hospitalizations and fatalities in the Brussels Capital Region. The second wave hit Wallonia – and to a lesser extent also Brussels – harder than it hit Flanders. By the end of 2020, Wallonia and Flanders had an almost equal share of infections, while Flanders is much more populated. At the same time,

Table 5.3 Economic Forecast for Growth, Budget Deficit, and Public Debt in Belgium, the EU, and the Euro Area for 2020/2021

	Belgium	*EU*	*Euro Area*
GDP Growth forecast (2020/2021) (%)	−8.4/+4.1	−7.4/+4.1	−7.8/+4.2
Budget deficit (2020/2021) (% GDP)	−11.2/−7.1	−8.4/−6.1	−8.8/−6.4

the Flemish share in hospitalizations and deaths decreased less sharply than the Flemish share in cases. Overall, the regional pandemic data do not deviate dramatically from the regional population share.

Economic consequences were correspondingly severe. In its Autumn 2020 Economic Forecast, the European Commission predicted for Belgium an 8.4 percent drop in GDP for 2020, slightly below the EU and Eurozone average. The 2021 growth forecast for Belgium was predicted to be similar to the EU and Eurozone average (European Commission 2020), somewhat more pessimistic than the November 2020 forecast for Belgium of the Belgian Federal Planning Bureau (−7.4 for 2020; 6.5 for 2021). Again, according to the Belgian data, percentages for the Regions differ somewhat, but not spectacularly. In addition, regions that are expected to suffer most in 2020 are also expected to recover more in 2021 (FPB 2020). Belgium has been suffering from a high budget deficit and high public debt for years. Ever since the financial and sovereign debt crisis that hit the Euro area in 2008, consecutive Belgian governments have been struggling to remedy this. Despite continuous problems to install stable federal governments, the figures were evolving slowly toward Euro area requirements (Table 5.3).

The response to COVID-19, however, returned Belgium to base one. In July 2020, Eurostat estimated the 2021 Belgian budget deficit at 7.1 percent of its GDP and its public debt at 117.8 percent of its GDP, significantly above the EU and Euro area averages (European Commission 2020). It will take years to get back on track, despite the NextGenerationEU Recovery Plan (European Commission 2021).

The high numbers of cases and fatalities are remarkable in light of the highly performant health care system, as noticed inside and outside the country (Moens 2020). Next to referring to the counting method, Belgian politicians and medical experts have tried to account for the numbers by pointing to a set of specific features such as the very high population density, the extremely open economy situated on the crossroad of European trade routes, and the effects of returning holiday tourists. This contribution, however, will focus on how the federal institutional set-up has affected the Belgian response to the COVID-19 health crisis.

5.3 Competitive federalism meets pandemic management

Belgium has been transformed from a unitary state to a federal state following six state reforms since 1970. It is an atypical federation featuring a double layer of constituent units. The Belgian territory is divided into three Regions: the Flemish Region, Walloon Region, and Brussels Capital Region. In addition, three Communities – the Flemish Community, the French Community (which calls itself the Federation Wallonia-Brussels), and the German-speaking Community – cover the three language groups. The Flemish Region and Community merged their institutions under the label

Flemish Community. On the French-speaking side, Region and Community have not merged, but increasing efforts strengthen the linkages between French-speaking inhabitants of the Brussels Capital Region and Wallonia, showing not the least in the rebranding. Similarly, the German-speaking Community has steadily extended its competencies in regional matters. Overall, competences that matter differently for different Communities (education, culture) and Regions (economy, environment, agriculture) have been devolved to the constituent units. The federal level is still in charge of large parts of the budget, law and order, infrastructure, and social security, which also greatly affect the Communities and Regions (Meier and Bursens 2020). The underlying logic of the federalization of Belgium has never been to stimulate co-operation between the Regions and Communities nor between the constituent units and the federal level. Competencies were downloaded to pacify conflicting interests (Caluwaerts and Reuchamps 2014), leading to constituting entities that to a large extent function independently from one another. Belgium is characterized by largely exclusive but not coherent packages of policy competences. The result of the pacification of antagonism and tension between ethno-linguistic groups is a competitive state architecture, with a centrifugal dynamic continuously dismantling the center (Popelier 2015). The latter is also exemplified by the juxtaposition of the levels: federal and constituent units' acts stand on equal footing: the exclusive character of allocated competences prevents levels from overruling one another. Compared to the extensive regional political and policy autonomy, fiscal autonomy of the Communities is rather limited (Popelier 2019). Intergovernmental relations are organized along inter-executive and inter-party lines, as political parties as well as the rest of civil society are divided along linguistic lines, except for employer organizations and trade unions. All this has resulted in not only a centrifugal competitive but *de facto* also bipolar federal context (Reuchamps 2013).

The Belgian allocation of competences regarding pandemics is a true patchwork not only because it involves a series of policy domains but also because competences are scattered across different government levels (Van Nieuwenhove and Popelier 2020). With respect to health care policies, the Communities are – among other issues – responsible for specific preventative health care measures (including quarantine measures, track and trace procedures, and the related data-collection) and retirement homes. The federal level and the Communities are each competent for parts of the regulation of hospitals and health care professions. The intricate division is amplified by the institutional complexity of Brussels, resulting in no less than nine responsible ministers, all member of Inter-ministerial Conference for Public Health (Fallon et al. 2020). In addition, the federal level has the competence in matters of civil protection, such as lockdown measures, but problems arise where they touch upon competencies of Communities (schools) and Regions (public transport).

The complex division of competences necessitates effective coordination among government levels. An administrative protocol (Protocol of 5 November 2018) between the federal government and the Communities has created a federal focal point (also as a liaison with the EU and the WHO), a Risk Management Group (RMG, composed of representatives from the various government levels), and a Risk Assessment Group (RAG, composed of medical scientists and other experts). This protocol recognizes the federal level as the coordinating level in case of a pandemic. In addition, stemming from the federal competence for civil protection, the federal level hosts a Coordination and Crisis Centre (CCC). The federal Minister for Internal Affairs can trigger a 'federal phase' of crisis management that activates the RMG and RAG. The latter reports to the evaluation body CELEVAL, which reports to the National Security Council (NSC, composed of core members of the federal government). In other words, the coordination of the complexity is also quite complex.

How did all this play during the first wave of the COVID-19 pandemic? The so-called federal phase of crisis management, also in use after the 2016 terrorist bombings in Brussels, was announced in response to the COVID-19 outbreak on 13 March 2020. This federal phase implied that all decisions to fight the virus were taken by a crisis management committee composed of the federal prime minister, the federal ministers responsible for the relevant policy domains, and the prime ministers of the Regions and Communities. This federal crisis management committee sought advice from several risk assessment groups, including the NSC, CELEVAL, RMG, and RAG. Because COVID-19 affects competences that are scattered among government levels, the prime ministers of the Regions and Communities were also exceptionally added to the NSC.

The federal crisis management committee implemented extensive virus control measures on March 13. These included closing down primary and secondary schools, bars, restaurants, and shops (apart from food shops, pharmacies, and those providing other essential services), cancelling recreational activities, and limiting public transport. These measures were extended on March 18 putting the Belgian territory in a *de facto* lockdown. All non-essential movement, including travel abroad, was forbidden, and companies and administrations were ordered to switch to remote working. The decision to implement these measures was taken only after long and fierce negotiations, pitting Flemish against French-speaking politicians. The former preferred the Dutch approach of remaining relatively open to support economic activities, while the latter leaned toward the French approach of prioritizing public health by installing a far-reaching lock-down (Faniel and Sägesser 2020). The federal crisis management committee decided to prolong the measures (first until April 19 and later until May 3). Alongside the crisis-management measures, both the federal level and the Regions took several measures to support businesses and professions suffering from the lockdown.

At the time of determining the initial series of COVID-19 control measures, the federal government had been for a significant period only administering current affairs, as negotiations to set up a new federal government had been going on for almost a year. Ever since the elections of May 2019, Flemish nationalists and French-speaking social-democrats – the largest parties in Flanders and Wallonia respectively – had been unable to find a compromise. As it was becoming clear that the response to COVID-19 would require decisions affecting civil liberties and engendering major budgetary consequences, the crisis proved to be the catalyst for the installation of a temporary federal government with full powers. The solution was found in upgrading the resigning caretaking government of Prime Minister Wilmès to an emergency government with full powers. While the parties in this government lacked a majority in parliament, it received wide parliamentary support from opposition parties (only the two Flemish nationalist parties and the radical left party refused to support this course of action). In addition to installing a full-blown federal government, the wide parliamentary coalition granted the new government special powers, implying that it would not be required to ask for parliamentary approval for six months in taking urgent measures to fight COVID-19 and mitigate social-economic and administrative consequences. However, in the end, the special powers law was not used for preventative measures. Instead, during the first and the second wave, these measures were based on a simple Ministerial Decree, without parliamentary approval.

Assured by a decreasing number of cases, hospitalizations, and fatalities, the NSC announced on March 24, a phased exit strategy, to start early May, gradually allowing more social and economic activities, including the gradual reopening of schools (a Community competence). During the exit phase, the NSC leaned on advice from a multidisciplinary (i.e., not exclusively medical) expert group (GEES). The advisory body switched again to CELEVAL when the epidemiological situation deteriorated in July.

The control measures taken by the NSC had an impact across all levels of government in Belgium, as they affect law and order and social security (federal competences), territory-related domains (Region competences), and person-related domains (Community competences). This explains why the membership of the NSC was expanded to include the prime ministers from the Regions and the Communities. The ensuing response highlighted the often-complicated division of competences. In some domains, decisions were taken by separate levels of government. For instance, following a federal Ministerial Decree, supported by all levels of government, all three Communities closed down primary and secondary schools within their respective jurisdictions, while the federal level itself closed the borders to non-essential travel. In other policy areas, however, major coordination efforts were necessary to align federal, community, and regional competences. Several examples highlight this complexity. The Regions guaranteed minimal public transport services for local service (buses and trams), while the federal level did the same for national rail network (trains). The Regions put in place a series of financial compensations for businesses that were closed or limited in operation while the federal government extended its temporary unemployment support scheme for employees of those same businesses. The crucial domain of public health presented a major conundrum of policy competences. While the federal level remained responsible for overall crisis management in times of a pandemic, at the operational level, the Community has responsibility. For instance, the three Communities prohibited visits in retirement homes and activated the emergency plans for hospitals. Policies regarding the regulation of pharmaceuticals and health insurance are federal competences, while all levels of government (and some municipalities on top of these) simultaneously engaged in the procurement of medical supplies such as facemasks and protective gowns (see Popelier and Bursens 2021). Major issues regarding quality requirements for materials and usage of testing kits surfaced in mid-April. The responsible federal minister himself complained about 'absurd' situations regarding competences and coordination in this respect (Andries 2020).

One final peculiarity of Belgian federalism relates to its EU membership, which extends the multilevel character of COVID-19 response from two to three levels of government. Some of the EU-level measures must be approved by the Council of Ministers. The Belgian position in the Council must be adopted through a coordination procedure that involves all levels of government. The equality among levels within Belgium necessitates the approval of all governments for all positions and votes taken in the Council. If one or more governments do not agree, the Belgian representative in the Council needs to abstain. This has happened at least once during the first wave of the crisis: Belgium abstained when EU legislation was approved to immediately release €37 billion of EU cohesion funds to strengthen health care systems and support businesses. The abstention was caused by the position of the – by nationalists dominated – Flemish government, which considered the distribution of the funds unbalanced as Wallonia, being a less wealthy region, would receive more than Flanders. In a similar move, the Flemish government, critical toward ambitious EU climate policies in general, blocked Belgian support for a Danish initiative that called for the application of post-COVID-19 investment in a way that would support the European Green Deal.

While the number of infections, hospitalizations, and fatalities stabilized at a low level in May and June, they started to increase again from mid-July, first in the northern province of Antwerp, but soon also in the rest of the country. This evolution prompted the provincial governor of Antwerp to reinstall restrictive measures such as a curfew and mandatory work from home in many professions. Such specific local measures were made possible by a decision of the federal government. When by late summer also other parts of the country were hit by a rise in infections, the federal government reinstalled some of the measures it had taken in the spring, be it in a less severe way. Examples include an extension of mandatory mask wearing in public places and commercial locations (to be identified by local authorities) and a cap on the number of people that were allowed to gather at events and festivities. Similar to the first wave, the renewal of restrictions was taken at the federal level and agreed upon with the regional executives in intergovernmental bodies and based on the scientific reports and recommendations of multidisciplinary advisory bodies. Despite the rapidly deteriorating epidemiological situation, the outcome of the intergovernmental decision-making marked a status quo and, in some areas, even a relaxation of preventative measures.

The start of the second wave in August and September coincided with the final months of the federal care-taker government. Sixteen months after the elections, the leaders of seven political parties were finally able to install a new federal government. Francophone and Flemish social-democrats, liberals, and greens supplemented by Flemish Christian-democrats eventually succeeded in agreeing on a common platform for the remaining years of the legislature. The composition of the federal government reflected notable congruence with the composition of the regional governments in Brussels and the Francophone part of the country and also marked the absence of the Flemish nationalists, the dominant party in the Flemish government.

The incoming federal government changed course in dealing with the pandemic in several ways. Confronted with a rising second wave of infections and hospitalizations, it opted for a gradual tightening of preventative measures, such as the closing of bars and restaurants, restrictions on the number of people present at events, a curfew, and mandatory working at home. Many of these measures were to be implemented by regional and local authorities, resulting in divergent rules in different parts of the country. For instance, the provinces installed different curfew hours. In addition, the new federal government installed new advisory bodies, clearly prioritizing medical expertise above other disciplines. Clearly, the new government wanted to break with the more relaxed approach of its predecessor. While the Flemish nationalists, banned from the federal government, at first opted for fierce opposition to the new approach, they quickly adapted their discourse and behavior. Noticing that a substantial part of the population, also in Flanders, was rather in favor of the restrictions (and of the accompanying economic support measures), they chose for a more cooperative style in the federal led intergovernmental bodies.

Also, in terms of decision-making, the federal government took a new approach. It made clear that the federal structure of Belgium called for continuous cooperation in fighting the pandemic. The government appointed a 'corona commissioner' to streamline cooperation procedures among all levels of government, including local authorities. It also shifted the main decision-making locus to the Concertation Committee, the highest body of intergovernmental relations, composed of the federal prime minister and the prime ministers of all the regional governments, supplemented by the relevant functional ministers. The parties of the new government made explicitly clear that they intended to introduce a more cooperative style of federalism, also beyond the fight against the COVID-19 crisis.

5.4 COVID-19: a wake-up call for more cooperative features in a competitive federal context?

If anything, the COVID-19 outbreak has made clear that coordination and cooperation among government levels are major challenges for the Belgian federal system during public health crises. Representatives of doctors, hospitals, and retirement home networks called for a thorough audit of the division of competences in the public health domain. They additionally berated the absence of unity of command which slows down decision-making and swift response to quickly changing epidemiological evolutions. The practitioners were joined by almost all political parties who advocated either a further devolution of competences to the regional level (the nationalists) or a return to more federal powers. However, not so much the division of competences, but the coordination among levels and the cooperation between actors seems to be crucial. Pandemics affect a plethora of policy domains making coordination necessary in each type of polity, be they unitary or federal. Yet, in federal systems, the underlying principles of constitutional hierarchy between levels and the nature of intergovernmental relations shape the potency of actors to take decisive measures and guarantee their effective implementation. The COVID-19 pandemic will most probably not change the dual and competitive principles of Belgian federalism nor reset its split party system. However, this may not prevent parties and governments to implement more cooperative practices in day-to-day decision-making. Reforms will probably take place within the existing confines, for instance, by means of more formal cooperation such as cooperation agreements regulating coordination horizontally between federated entities and vertically between the federated entities and the federal level. Nevertheless, for the Belgian specific double layer of constituent entities, the Communities and Regions, with their highly interdependent competencies, will keep on turning any effort to achieve efficient coordination into a major challenge.

5.5 Conclusion

Most European countries and EU Member States, in particular, struggled to implement an effective response to the COVID-19 pandemic. Yet, the Belgian approach to COVID-19 crisis management seems to be crucially shaped by its federal structure and related political landscape. In particular, the coordination between government levels, which is indispensable given the heterogeneous allocation of competences across levels, turned out to be spokes in the wheel of an adequate response. Moreover, the dual and competitive nature of its federalism and the resulting party politics posed severe challenges to an effective response to a major public health crisis. These became clear issues at the peak of the first wave, for instance, those related to the understaffing and undersupply of equipment to retirement homes, and the insufficient quality of facemasks delivered by Chinese providers. The second wave coincided with a new federal government that made effective coordination a major goal of its approach. The changes in decision-making bodies and procedures seemed to have increased cooperation among the various levels of government, undoubtedly helped by the temporary political truce from the side of the Flemish nationalists. As soon as the health crisis is over, however, a thorough evaluation will be made of the functioning of the federal system in responding to COVID-19. Our analysis of the response during the first and second wave indeed supports changes in the federal set-up, definitely with respect to reforms that ameliorate coordination and allow for transverse decision-making. At the same time, it would be illusionary to expect that such reform would be overly effective against the background of a complex double layer of Communities and Regions with interdependent competencies and an unchanged party system.

Bibliography

Andries, S., 2020. Interview: Philippe De Backer, 'I've Seen too Many Absurdities. Our System Is Not Working.' *De Standaard*, 30 May. Available from: https://www.standaard.be/cnt/dmf20200529_04976164 [Accessed 8 March 2021].

Caluwaerts, D. and Reuchamps, M., 2014. Combining Federalism with Consociationalism: Is Belgian Consociational Federalism Digging its Own Grave? *Ethnopolitics*, 14 (3), 277–295.

Deschouwer, K., 2012. *The Politics of Belgium*. Basingstoke: Palgrave Macmillan.

European Commission, 2020. European Economic Forecast. *Economic and Financial Affairs*. Available from: https://ec.europa.eu/info/sites/info/files/economy-finance/ip136_en_2.pdf [Accessed 8 March 2021].

European Commission, 2021. *Recovery Plan for Europe*. Available from: https://ec.europa.eu/info/strategy/recovery-plan-europe_en [Accessed 8 March 2021].

Fallon, C., Thiry, A. and Brunet, S., 2020. Planification d'urgence et gestion de crise sanitaire. La Belgique face à la pandémie de COVID-19. *Courrier hebdomadaire de CRISP*, 2453–2454.

Faniel, J. and Sägesser, C., 2020. Le fédéralisme belge à l'épreuve de la pandémie de Covid-19. *Politique, revue belge d'analyse et de débat*, 112, 12–17.

FPB, Federal Planning Bureau, 2020. Regional Economic Outlook 2020–2025 – Statistical Annex. Available from: https://www.plan.be/databases/data-27-en-regional_economic_outlook_2020_2025_statistical_annex [Accessed 8 March 2021].

FPB, Federal Planning Bureau, 2021. Indicators. Available from: https://www.plan.be/indicators/indicators_list.php?lang=en [accessed 8 March 2021].

Meier P. and Bursens, P., 2020. Belgium. The Democratic State of the Federation. *In*: Benz, A. and Sonnicksen, J., eds. *Federalism and Democracy*. Toronto: University of Toronto Press, 180–196.

Moens, B., 2020. Why is Belgium's Death Toll So High? [online]. *Politico*, 19 April. Available from: https://www.politico.eu/article/why-is-belgiums-death-toll-so-high/ [accessed 8 March 2021].

Popelier, P., 2015. Secessionist and Autonomy Movements in Flanders: The Disintegration of Belgium as the Chronicle of a Death Foretold? *In*: Belser, E.M., Fang-Bär, A., Massüger, N. and Oleschak Pillai, R., eds. *Secessionist and Autonomy Movements in Europe*. Bern: Stämpfli Verlag, 215–246.

Popelier, P., 2019. Asymmetry and Complexity as a Device for Multinational Conflict Management. A Country Study of Constitutional Asymmetry in Belgium. *In*: Popelier, P. and Sahadzic, M., eds. *Constitutional Asymmetry in Multinational Federalism. Managing Multinationalism in Multi-tiered Systems.* New York: Palgrave Macmillan, 17–46.

Popelier, P. and Bursens, P., 2021 [Forthcoming]. Managing the Covid-19 Crisis in a Divided Belgian Federation: Cooperation against All Odds. *In*: Steytler, N., ed. *Combating the COVID-19 Pandemic: Federalism a Boon or Bane?*, 88–105.

Reuchamps, M., 2013. Structures institutionnelles du fédéralisme belge. *In*: Dandoy, R., Matagne, G. and Van Wynsberghe, C., eds. *Le fédéralisme belge. Enjeux institutionnels, acteurs socio-politiques et opinions publiques.* Louvain-La-Neuve: Academia-L'Harmattan, 29–61.

Sciensano, 2020. *COVID-19 Surveillance Frequently Asked Questions.* Available from: https://covid-19.sciensano.be/sites/default/files/Covid19/COVID-19_FAQ_ENG_final.pdf [Accessed 8 March 2021].

Sciensano, 2021. Infectious Diseases Data Explorations & Visualizations: COVID-19 [dataset]. Available from: https://epistat.wiv-isp.be/covid/ [Accessed 8 March 2021].

Swenden, W. and Jans, M.T., 2006. Will It Stay or Will It Go? Federalism and the Sustainability of Belgium. *West European Politics*, 29 (5), 877–894.

Van Nieuwenhove, J. and Popelier, P., 2020. De bevoegdheidsverdeling en de co.rdinatie tussen de bevoegde overheden in de strijd tegen de COVID-19-pandemie. *Tijdschrift voor Wetgeving*, 4, 303–313.

6 Federal institutional design and the COVID-19 crisis management in Bosnia and Herzegovina

Nina Sajic

6.1 Introduction

Bosnia and Herzegovina is a federal country consisting of two entities: the Federation of Bosnia and Herzegovina and the Republika Srpska. Sandwiched between the two is a special region: the Brčko District, a multi-ethnic district with its own Government and Parliament. While often characterized by some as a frozen conflict, or a fragile and dysfunctional country that is unstable and in danger of collapse, Bosnia and Herzegovina has evolved since the war ended in 1995 (see Kartsonaki 2016).

However, a lack of mutual trust exists among key political figures at the central level and at the level of constituent units. There are divergent views on the future of the country, and political parties are divided along ethnic/linguistic lines. There is domestic rivalry between those advocating more autonomy and those with centralist aspirations. This rivalry seems to be the primary generator of internal conflict and tensions in Bosnia and Herzegovina.

The Republic Srpska (RS) demands more autonomy because the current constitutional arrangements are not efficient. Bosniak political elites use the same argument to ask for tighter centralization. The complexity of institutional structures of Bosnia and Herzegovina was not, according to Stroschein (2003), produced by accident. Yet, the asymmetric and complex governing institutions were introduced for one simple goal: to ensure that groups, which disagree on the nature of governance, could coexist.[1]

How did the federal architecture of Bosnia and Herzegovina with its asymmetric nature cope with the COVID-19 crisis? The answers found in this chapter show how various orders of government managed the crisis, the contents of their strategy, the nature of their relations, and the roles of constituent units and the central level during the pandemic. There is a brief overview of the pandemic, its impact on the economy, and the people.

The federal institutional design, with its competencies and powers related to the COVID-19 pandemic, guided the measures and actions each order of government took and how those measures were coordinated. One might expect that the fragility of the federal architectural design of Bosnia and Herzegovina would come to the forefront in a time of crisis such as COVID-19. Instead, the chapter concludes that the institutions of Bosnia and Herzegovina responded relatively well regardless of their flaws. All the internal issues did not disappear during the crises; on the contrary, political conflict arose several times between the government's different orders. Some have seen the pandemic as a window of opportunity to strengthen the central level, whereas others saw the pandemic as the chance to strengthen the autonomy of their constituent units. Although at

DOI: 10.4324/9781003251217-6

Table 6.1 Key Statistics on COVID-19 in Bosnia and Herzegovina as of 10 January 2021.

Cumulative Cases	Cumulative Cases per 100,000 Population	Cumulative Deaths	Cumulative Deaths per 100,000 Population	Case Fatality Percentage
115,379	3,516.8	4,305	131.2	3.7

Source: World Health Organization Weekly epidemiological update – 12 January 2021. Geneva: WHO, 2021. Available from https://www.who.int/publications/m/item/weekly-epidemiological-update

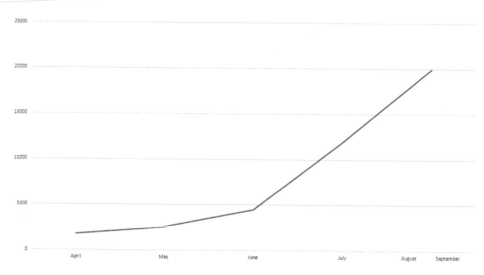

Figure 6.1 Total Number of COVID-19 Cases in Bosnia and Herzegovina from April to September 2020.

Source: The Ministry of Civil Affairs of B&H. Available from: http://mcp.gov.ba/publication/read/epidemioloska-slika-covid-19?pageId=3 [Accessed 4 September 2020].

first, every order of government in Bosnia and Herzegovina sought to act on its own, in the end, the country did respond to the challenge of COVID-19 (Table 6.1).

6.2 COVID-19 in Bosnia and Herzegovina

The first COVID-19 infected patient in the country was registered in Banja Luka, an administrative center of the Republika Srpska, on 5 March 2020. Four days later, the first patient was registered in the Federation of Bosnia and Herzegovina. By the end of March, there were 420 people infected, and the death toll was 13. Figure 6.1 shows the total number of cases in Bosnia and Herzegovina from April to September 2020. As the graph demonstrates, the outbreak was successfully controlled during the spring of 2020 due to the authorities' restrictive measures and the approach taken at all levels. To ease pressure on the relatively under-resourced health care system and avoid the scenarios played out in Italy and Spain, the entities in Bosnia and Herzegovina introduced preventive and restrictive measures at the early stages of the epidemic. The restrictive public health measures were gradually lifted, beginning in May.

Although the health sector is highly decentralized in Bosnia and Herzegovina, the epidemiological situation is managed, monitored, and reported by several orders of

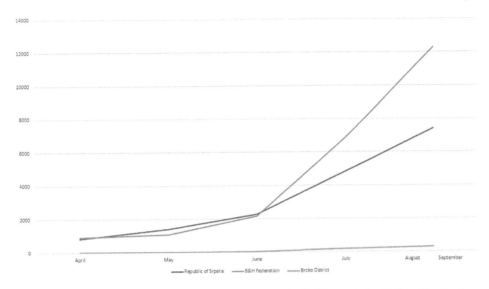

Figure 6.2 Distribution of COVID-19 Cases in FB&H, RS, and the Brčko District in 2020.

Source: The Ministry of Civil Affairs of Bosnia and Herzegovina. Available from: http://mcp.gov.ba/publication/read/epidemioloska-slika-covid-19?pageId=3 [Accessed 2 September 2020].

government: the entities, the cantons, and the Brčko District. Figure 6.2 shows the distribution of COVID-19 cases in the entities and the Brčko District.

As both graphs show, early July 2020 marked the resurgence of COVID-19 cases within the entire territory of Bosnia and Herzegovina. There were 20,804 people infected and a death toll of 636 at the beginning of September 2020. The new surges in cases were a result of non-compliance with protective measures. Not wearing masks and not practicing physical distancing drove the surge, according to the officials and medical practitioners.

While the aggressive strategy was aimed to reduce human and health costs, it has nevertheless contributed to a negative impact on the economy. The country was headed into a recession, together with other Western Balkan countries. Despite its troubled past, Bosnia and Herzegovina is an upper middle-income country, according to the World Bank's classification (World Bank 2020), although it now has a significant unemployment rate of 15.7 percent (Agency for Statistics of Bosnia and Herzegovina). Bosnia and Herzegovina had a slow recovery from the economic crisis of 2008. In 2014, the country was affected by unprecedented floods with damages and losses that cost around 15 percent of its annual GDP (World Bank Group 2020).

As in many other European countries, not all the sectors and economic activities were affected in the same way. Some sectors, such as medical suppliers and pharmacies, which were considered essential, remained fully active and even had increased economic activities. Those considered non-essential, such as tourism, leisure, hotels, restaurants, beauty salons, and educational facilities, were completely shut down and have suffered the most. Between these two categories were sectors not closed by the any government, but their activities were reduced due to other confinement measures.

These sectors included legal and accounting activities, various manufacturing activities, plus imports, and exports.

While there are still no reliable data accounting for the impact of COVID-19 on the overall economic costs of the virus, officials estimate that the overall GDP in Bosnia and Herzegovina will fall between 3.5 percent and 5 percent. The unemployment rate since the beginning of the pandemic until the end of June went up by 4.6 percent (Labour and Employment Agency of Bosnia and Herzegovina 2020). The income from exports was down by 15.1 percent and import income declined by 18 percent in the first half of the year (Banjaluka.net 2020). Industrial production in April and May was about 16 percent below the output levels of 2019 (European Commission 2020). The economic tolls of COVID-19 can also be seen through value-added tax (VAT) collection. From January to August 2020, VAT collection was 10.6 percent lower than in the same period of 2019, resulting in a lower distribution of VAT revenues (Indirect Taxation Authority of Bosnia and Herzegovina 2020)[2] than in 2019. For the Federation of Bosnia and Herzegovina, it was 12.1 percent lower. For Republika Srpska, it was 7.4 percent lower, and for the Brčko District, it was 12.4 percent lower (Indirect Taxation Authority of Bosnia and Herzegovina, 5 September 2020).

6.3 COVID-19 and federalism in Bosnia and Herzegovina

Although the Constitution of Bosnia and Herzegovina does not define the country as a federal state *per se*, its institutional architectural features and characteristics are common to all federal countries (General Framework Agreement for Peace in Bosnia and Herzegovina 1995).[3]

The federal institutional design was introduced, or rather, imposed, by the international community in Dayton, Ohio, USA, in 1995 in order to resolve a four-year civil conflict in Bosnia and Herzegovina. The constitution recognizes Bosniaks, Croats, and Serbs (along with Others) as constituent peoples. The two entities of the country – the Federation of Bosnia and Herzegovina (mostly inhabited by Bosniaks and Croats) and the Republic of Srpska (with a Serb majority) – each have their own presidents, governments, parliaments, and constitutions. The Republic of Srpska is centralized, while the Federation of Bosnia and Herzegovina is further divided into ten cantons, each having its own government, parliament, and judicial powers.

The decentralization of the Federation of Bosnia and Herzegovina is based on the so-called Washington Agreement (The General Framework on the Federation 1994) between Bosniaks and Croats signed in 1994. As a result of that agreement, there are five cantons with a Bosniak majority, three with a Croat majority and two are "ethnically mixed." There is also the Brčko District, a self-governing administrative unit under the sovereignty of Bosnia and Herzegovina, whose territory is shared by both entities. One of the particularities of this asymmetrical federal institutional design of Bosnia and Herzegovina is a rotating Presidency. There are three members of the Presidency, each representing one of the constituent peoples – Bosniaks, Croats, and Serbs. These three presidents are *primus inter pares* (first among equals) and are directly elected for a four-year mandate.

The powers of the state institutions are clearly specified, and residual powers remain with the governments of the entities. All the powers not expressly granted to the central government are vested in two entities: the Republic of Srpska and the Federation of Bosnia and Herzegovina. In the Federation of Bosnia and Herzegovina, these powers are distributed between the entity and the cantons in such a way that all the powers that are not expressly given to this entity by its constitution are vested in the cantons. The federal institutions have limited competencies in the health sector, including the definition of international strategies, the coordination and harmonization of the plans of the two entities, and the establishment and supervision of a unified market for medical devices. The entities and the Brčko District, on the other hand, have extensive powers in the health sector. The Republic of Srpska has a centralized healthcare system, while in the Federation of Bosnia and Herzegovina, healthcare is a shared competence between the entity government and the ten cantons.

Most of the other powers related to COVID-19 crisis management do not belong to the central level, but fall under the jurisdiction of the entities:

- Internal restrictions on movement of people and goods
- Education
- Financial stimulus packages
- Work permits and working hours
- Public transportation
- Social welfare
- Curfews
- Economic recovery and development measures

In the Federation of Bosnia and Herzegovina, these powers are also shared competencies with cantons. The powers that belong to Bosnia's central government include international loan arrangements, border control, repatriation of citizens, use of the armed forces, coordination of entities' civil protection units, and harmonization of their plans in the event of natural or other disasters in Bosnia and Herzegovina.

The COVID-19 crisis has been managed mostly by the entities, cantons, and the Brčko District, with a somewhat limited role of the central government institutions. In the Republic of Srpska, the pandemic risk manager has been the Emergency Situation HQ. This is an *ad hoc* committee, chaired by the Republic of Srpska prime minister, which comes together to manage emergencies during times of crisis. In the Federation of Bosnia and Herzegovina, the Federal Department of Civilian Protection has managed the response to the COVID-19 outbreak. Each canton has its own crisis units or disease control centers within their respective ministries of health. In the Brčko District, the Protection and Rescue HQ chaired by the district's mayor has managed the crisis. Crisis Units within local communities are responsible for taking on measures such as business hours and closing or opening of economic activities. Orders and decisions taken by these Crisis Units may override decisions taken by higher orders of government it they are more restrictive and until a state of emergency has been declared.

From the onset of the pandemic, there was a lack of coordination and cooperation between the entities. However, both have taken a cautious approach and early control strategy to fight the pandemic. The Republic of Srpska was first to introduce preventive and restrictive measures. It imposed a ban on all public gatherings, closed the universities, schools and kindergartens, and limited business hours in certain cities. The Federation of Bosnia and Herzegovina followed the Republic of Srpska's example after a few days of delay. This delay, in turn, caused strong reactions from that entity's officials, who felt that this would undermine their own measures' effectiveness. On 16 March 2020, the Republic of Srpska declared an emergency and the Federation of Bosnia and Herzegovina declared a status of disaster. The first institution of Bosnia's central government to react to the pandemic was the tripartite Presidency of the country, which adopted 18 measures regarding the COVID-19 crisis. These included, among other things, orders to the Bosnia and Herzegovina Armed Forces to put all of their resources at the disposal of the government to tackle the crisis, a request to the central Council of Ministers to declare a situation of natural or other disaster in the whole territory of the country, and support for introducing a quarantine at border crossings (Presidency 2020). The Bosnia and Herzegovina Council of Ministers declared a state of natural or other disaster in the country. The council first restricted the entry of people from countries affected by the pandemic, before deciding to temporarily shut down borders for all foreigners with few exceptions, and organized the repatriation of citizens of Bosnia and Herzegovina who were abroad. To help domestic companies, the central government's Council of Ministers adopted a decision to give preference to domestic companies bidding on public tenders. This decision will be effective for one year (Council of Ministers 2020).

In Bosnia's central government, the preventive measures adopted were not always coordinated and respected by other levels of government. A case in point is the Bosnia and Herzegovina Presidency's initiative to introduce quarantine stations near border crossings for people entering the country. At first, this initiative was only implemented by the Republic of Srpska. The Federation of Bosnia and Herzegovina took action on this measure following two weeks of delay, and only after the federal Presidency decided to shut border crossings that did not have quarantine stations.

COVID-19 mitigation measures were taken by both entities – measures such as the introduction of curfews, the closing down of shops, provision of financial and other assistance to the economy, and the organization of online courses for pupils and students. Exemptions were made for pharmacies and grocery stores. The measures were quite similar between the two entities[4] and were taken simultaneously. This was not so much a result of the coordination between the entities, but more due to the competitive nature of their relations. There have also been cases of conflict-laden and tense inter-governmental relations between the Federation of Bosnia and Herzegovina and its cantons, especially those with a Croat majority. At the beginning of the pandemic, Canton 10 (which has a Croat majority) banned the entry and transit of Bosnia and Herzegovina citizens through its territory. While for this cantonal government, the measure was introduced to protect its population, for the Prime Minister of the Federation of Bosnia and Herzegovina (a Bosniak), this measure was an "attack on constitutional order," (Fena News Agency 2020). The cantonal order was revoked almost immediately, however, because it was seen as an attempt of the Croat majority canton to strengthen its autonomy.

Declaring a state of emergency at the beginning of April 2020 allowed the Republic of Srbska to enact decrees and regulations related to the pandemic with faster legal force, including to the provision of business subventions and assistance. The Federation of Bosnia and Herzegovina passed the so-called "Corona Law" a month later to help the economic recovery of affected businesses. The Brčko District also adopted the "Corona Law" at the beginning of May 2020.

There has been no coordination between the entities on their plans to ease the lockdown measures. The Federation of Bosnia and Herzegovina revoked its curfew and quarantine stations a few weeks before the Republic of Srpska did, which once again sparked intense opposition in the Republic.

Constituent units have mostly managed the economy during the crisis because Bosnia's central government has practically no jurisdiction over the economy. There are still no exact figures on the financial resources that will be spent by all governments in Bosnia and Herzegovina. However, all governments have implemented measures to fight the pandemic – the entities, the cantons, the Brčko District, and local communities. According to the available data, the entities have spent around 25 million euros each to purchase medical equipment and supplies (International Monetary Fund 2020). For the Federation of Bosnia and Herzegovina, this spending was around 1 percent of its annual budget and for the Republic of Srpska around 1.5 percent. As a first wave response to fight COVID-19, the Republic of Srpska allocated around 5 percent of its annual budget (RTRS 2020), which included the purchase of the medical equipment and measures to mitigate the economic impact of the pandemic. In the Federation of Bosnia and Herzegovina, these figures are even less precise as both their government, and the governments of its cantons have financed various measures during the pandemic. Local communities also have taken their share of the financial burden. For example, Banja Luka, the second-largest city in the country, allocated around 3.5 percent of its annual budget as a response to the pandemic (BL Portal 2020).

The entities introduced similar fiscal measures, although once again without any coordination and consultation. For example, the Republic of Srpska covered personal income tax and social security contributions for about 40,000 workers in the sectors that were closed by government decision from March to May 2020. The Republic of Srpska also paid minimum salaries for all employees in these sectors in April, totalling about 1.6 percent of its annual budget (Policy Tracker 2020). The Federation of Bosnia and Herzegovina subsidized contributions and taxes and paid minimum wages for employees of the companies impacted by COVID-19 but only if their headquarters was registered in that entity (Policy Tracker 2020). This measure led to discrimination by the Republic of Srpska against the companies that also operate in the Federation of Bosnia and Herzegovina since these companies were excluded from the subsidies. However, companies from the Federation of Bosnia and Herzegovina that operate in the Republic of Srpska had equal treatment there. Both entities set up special funds to mitigate the pandemic's economic impacts and facilitate access to funds for companies once again without any prior coordination or consultation.

The conflictual and even obstructive nature of intergovernmental relations in Bosnia and Herzegovina resurfaced over the acquisition of medical equipment and supplies and in relation to international aid. Bosnia's central government first tried to obstruct one of the constituent units.[5] Then, internal disputes between Bosniak and Croats also led to blocking an emergency loan from the International Monetary Fund. The IMF emergency loan was aimed to help Bosnia and Herzegovina address the COVID-19 crisis. However, the Bosniak ministers at the Council of Ministers objected to it, primarily because of their disagreement over the distribution of money between the Federation of Bosnia and Herzegovina and its ten cantons.

6.4 Conclusion

In cooperative decision-making among different governments, trust is the "oil" which makes the process go smoothly. "Without it, gridlock and polarization are more likely to surface and to remain a feature of politics, notwithstanding the arrival of a (fragile) agreement" (Swendon 2013). The competitive nature of federalism in Bosnia and Herzegovina, coupled with the lack of trust and the presence of animosity among Bosniaks, Croats, and Serbs, creates a space for disputes over powers and responsibilities as well as conflicts of interest. As Marciacq (2015) rightly observes, the three constituent peoples of Bosnia and Herzegovina have divergent views on their country's future and how the state should evolve. Their mutual level of trust remains relatively low, especially at the grassroots levels (Marciacq 2015).

For any federal state's functioning, intergovernmental cooperation is required, but in multinational federations such as Bosnia and Herzegovina, achieving harmonious collaboration among the central authorities and the constituent units often represents a challenge. This is especially the case in matters that directly concern or fall under the jurisdiction of constituent units, as do many aspects of COVID-19 crisis management.

The COVID-19 crisis did not bring about any new transformation in the practice of federalism in Bosnia and Herzegovina; if anything, it has only deepened the existing divisions and polarizations. However, Bosnia and Herzegovina managed to do relatively well during the first wave of the pandemic despite all the flaws and complexity of its federal institutional design. This was partly due to the competitive intergovernmental relations and partly because the constituent units in Bosnia and Herzegovina, during the COVID-19 crisis, were left on their own as was the case with many European countries. At the onset of the crisis, there was a complete absence of solidarity and cooperation in Europe, even within the EU, where some of its member states introduced export bans on certain medical supplies.[6] The constituent units took the "every man for himself" strategy as their immediate response to the crisis. For those advocating more autonomy, such as the Republic of Srpska and the cantons with a Croat majority, this was a window of opportunity to pursue that goal. The others have tried to strengthen the central government with the obstruction of various measures. The COVID-19 crisis was not the first crisis that tested the country's federal institutional design. During the unprecedented floods that affected Bosnia and Herzegovina in 2014, the constituent units managed the crisis with the central government being inefficient and obstructive. We are yet to see to what extent the COVID-19 pandemic may lead to any reassignment of new responsibilities or the creation of more effective mechanisms of intergovernmental cooperation.

Notes

1 The Federation of Bosnia and Herzegovina refers to one of the constituent units (entities) of Bosnia and Herzegovina. Contrary to what its name suggests, it does not refer to the whole country of Bosnia and Herzegovina, but just to one part. The Federation of Bosnia and Herzegovina is further divided into ten cantons.

2 The VAT system was introduced in Bosnia and Herzegovina in 2006. Distribution of VAT revenues between the central government, the entities, and the Brčko District is regulated by the Law on Payments into the Single Account and Distribution of Revenues as well as decisions on a partition coefficient that is being determined every year. For more, see Indirect Taxation Authority of Bosnia and Herzegovina http://www.new.uino.gov.ba/en/General-information-on-VAT-system-in-Bosnia-and-Herzegovina.

3 "...two orders of government, distribution of legislative and executive authority defined by a constitution, allocation of revenues between two orders of government, representation of constituent units in central decision-making institutions, a supreme constitution that cannot be amended without a consent of significant proportion of its constituent

units, an arbitrary or umpire to decide on potential disputes between different orders of government, arrangements (institutions or processes) for intergovernmental cooperation." Ronald L. Watts, *Comparing Federal Systems* (London, Montreal and Kingston: McGill-Queen's University Press, 1999), 7.

4 In the Federation of Bosnia and Herzegovina, some of these measures were introduced by Cantons as they fall directly into their jurisdiction.

5 As an illustration, one could highlight the international aid provided to the Republic of Srpska by Hungary and the Russian Federation upon the request of the Serb member of the Bosnia and Herzegovina Presidency. The B&H Minister of Foreign Affairs (Bosniak) officially complained to the ministers of Foreign Affairs of these countries, as well to the EU, for not also sending medical aid to the other entity as well, although the Federation of Bosnia and Herzegovina never formally requested any assistance from Russia or Hungary.

6 For example, France requisitioned both the stocks and production of protective masks in the country.

Bibliography

Agency for Statistics of Bosnia and Herzegovina [dataset]. Annual indicators 2019, Available from: https://bhas.gov.ba/Home/ [Accessed 15 August 2020].

Banjaluka.net, 21 July 2020. Analiza: Korona vise usporila uvoz nego izvoz [online]. Available from: https://banjaluka.net/analiza-korona-vise-usporila-uvoz-nego-izvoz-iz-bih/ [Accessed 16 March 2021].

BL Portal, 10 September 2020. Korona odnijala milione iz lokalnih budzeta u RS [online]. Available from: https://www.bl-portal.com/drustvo/korona-odnijela-milione-iz-lokalnih-budzeta-u-rs/ [Accessed 16 March 2021].

Council of Ministers of Bosnia and Herzegovina, 29 May 2020. *Council of Ministers Holds Its Extraordinary Phone Session.*

European Commission: Directorate-General for Economic and Financial Affairs, July 2020. *EU Candidate Countries' & Potential Candidates' Economic Quarterly (CCEQ), 2nd Quarter 2020, Technical Paper 042.* Available from: https://ec.europa.eu/info/sites/info/files/economy-finance/tp042_en.pdf [Accessed 16 March 2021].

Fena News Agency, 22 March 2020. Novalic: The Order Issued by Canton 10 an Attack on the Constitutional Order [online]. Available from: https://www.fena.news/bih/novalic-the-order-issued-by-canton-10-an-attack-on-the-constitutional-order/ [Accessed 16 March 2021].

General Framework Agreement for Peace in Bosnia and Herzegovina 1995 available from the U.S. Department of State https://2009-2017.state.gov/p/eur/rls/or/dayton/52577.htm

General Framework on the Federation 1994, available from the UN Peacemaker https://peacemaker.un.org/sites/peacemaker.un.org/files/BA_940301_FrameworkAgreement OnTheFederation.pdf

Indirect Taxation Authority of Bosnia and Herzegovina, 2021. General Information on VAT System in Bosnia and Herzegovina. Available from: http://www.new.uino.gov.ba/en/General-information-on-VAT-system-in-Bosnia-and-Herzegovina [Accessed 16 March 2021].

Indirect Taxation Authority of Bosnia and Herzegovina. Information Received by Email Correspondence, 5 September 2020.

International Monetary Fund, 2020. Policy Tracker: Bosnia and Herzegovina, Key Policy Responses as of August 13, 2020. Available from: https://www.imf.org/en/Topics/imf-and-covid19/Policy-Responses-to-COVID-19#B [Accessed 20 August 2020].

Kartsonaki, A., 2016. Twenty Years after Dayton: Bosnia-Herzegovina (Still) Stable and Explosive. *Civil Wars*, 18 (4), 488–516.

Labour and Employment Agency of Bosnia and Herzegovina, 5 August 2020. *Labour Market Overview, Situation as of 30 June 2020.*

Marciacq, F., 2015. Sub-state Diplomacy in Malfunctioning States: The Case of the Republika Srpska, Bosnia and Herzegovina. *Regional and Federal Studies*, 25 (4), 340.

Ministry of Civil Affairs of Bosnia and Herzegovina, 2020. *Epidemiološka slika (Covid 19)*. Available from: http://mcp.gov.ba/publication/read/epidemioloska-slika-covid-19?pageId=3 [Accessed 4 September 2020].

Policy Tracker: Bosnia and Herzegovina. "Key Policy Responses as of August 13, 2020."

Presidency of Bosnia and Herzegovina, 16 March 2020. BiH Presidency Holds Its 56th Extraordinary Session. Available from: http://predsjednistvobih.ba/zaklj/sjed/default.aspx?id=87858&langTag=en-US [Available 16 March 2020].

RTRS 3 June 2020. Available from: https://lat.rtrs.tv/vijesti/vijest.php?id=386742 [Accessed 16 March 2020].

RTRS, 3 June 2020. Vidovic: Sredstva of MMF-a bice ulozena u zdravstvo i privredu.

Stroschein, S., 2003.What Belgium Can Teach Bosnia: The Use of Autonomy in 'Divided House' States. *Journal of Ethnopolitics and Minority Issues in Europe*, 3, 22.

Swenden, W., 2013. Conclusion: The Future of Belgian Federalism-between Reform and Swansong? *Regional and Federal Studies*, 23 (3), 370.

The World Bank, 2020. The World Bank in Bosnia and Herzegovina [online]. Available from: https://www.worldbank.org/en/country/bosniaandherzegovina [Accessed 1 August 2020].

"Washington Agreement," 1995. Peace Agreements Digital Collection. *United States Institute of Peace*. Available from: http://www.usip.org/sites/default/files/file/resources/collections/peace_agreements/washagree_03011994.pdf [Accessed 16 March 2021].

Watts, R.L., 1999. *Comparing Federal Systems*. London, Montreal and Kingston: McGill-Queen's University Press, 7.

World Bank Group, 2020. Stories of Impact: Building Back Better in Bosnia and Herzegovina. Available from: http://documents1.worldbank.org/curated/en/689131494237342559/pdf/114809-BRI-PUBLIC-soi-bosnia-and-herzegovina.pdf [Accessed 1 August 2020].

World Health Organization Weekly epidemiological update – 12 January 2021. Geneva: WHO, 2021. Available from https://www.who.int/publications/m/item/weekly-epidemiological-update

7 Brazilian federalism

Facing the COVID-19 pandemic[1]

*Eduardo Henrique Corrêa da S.P. Néris and
Rodrigo Ribeiro Bedritichuk*

7.1 Introduction

Contrary to several predictions of a prosperous year, 2020 was instead marked by a global fight against a new virus which has killed many across the globe.

In Brazil, the COVID-19 crisis has led to several conflicts among many of the 26 states and the federal capital as well as between the federal central government, the states, and the municipalities. Faced with uncertainty, political actors adopted blame-avoiding strategies, duplicating the most restrictive actions taken elsewhere as a way of seeking legitimacy among the people. As federated units adopted different criteria to intensify or soften restrictive measures, judicial activism was a mark of the period. A wave of lawsuits flooded state and federal courts, and the range of policies was frequently decided by judges.

Nevertheless, the COVID-19 pandemic in Brazil had ambiguous outcomes. Despite the uncoordinated control measures and a huge number of deaths, by the end of January 2021, Brazil seemed to have achieved the goal of flattening the virus transmission curve. Crucially, there was no collapse of the healthcare system (Table 7.1).

7.2 COVID-19 in Brazil

The first confirmed COVID-19 case on Brazilian soil was a Brazilian businessman who returned to the country from Italy on 21 February 2020 (Ministry of Health 2021). His infection was verified as COVID-19 on February 26 at a hospital in São Paulo. At the time, it was assumed that the virus would not spread rapidly in a tropical climate and, therefore, that the situation was under control.

However, the monitoring of several suspected cases was already underway, and the Ministry of Health announced new methods of consolidating information on possible cases across Brazil. At the time, there was still no evidence of the circulation of the

Table 7.1 Key Statistics on COVID-19 in Brazil as of 10 January 2021

Cumulative Cases	Cumulative Cases per 100,000 Population	Cumulative Deaths	Cumulative Deaths per 100,000 Population	Case Fatality Percentage
8,013,708	3,770.1	201,460	94.8	2.5

Source: World Health Organization Weekly epidemiological update – 12 January 2021. Geneva: WHO, 2021. Available from https://www.who.int/publications/m/item/weekly-epidemiological-update

DOI: 10.4324/9781003251217-7

virus in the national territory, since all those infected came from countries in which the virus was spreading widely.

On 5 March 2020, the first case of community transmission was recorded. To reduce the spread of the virus, in early March, the government concluded the first major contract for the purchase of N95 protective masks and surgical masks to be used by public health professionals.

On 21 March 2020, the President of the Republic Jair Bolsonaro issued an order designating essential services for the functioning of the country that could not be interrupted even in the midst of the pandemic. These included public security, health assistance, fuel, electricity, and water supply, and telecommunications and internet, among others. In the same month, Bolsonaro also created a "Crisis Committee at the national level" to manage Brazil's response to the pandemic.

As the pandemic spread to almost all Brazilian municipalities, the states also focused their attention on controlling the virus and, in turn, created their own Crisis Committees. These bodies were created by decrees standardized by the heads of the Brazilian states and the President of the Republic to streamline decision-making between different government sectors.

Furthermore, it was observed that the spread of COVID-19 from large cities to smaller municipalities evolved over time. The climate greatly impacted the rate of the spread of the virus. As winter approached, there was a decrease in the number of patients suffering from respiratory conditions in the tropical North and Northeast regions and an increase in cases in the temperate Midwest and South of the country.

As of 8 September 2020, the virus R number was 0.94 (less than one) (Our World in Data 2021). In terms of deaths per hundred thousand inhabitants, Brazil then ranked tenth, recording lower death rates than European countries such as the United Kingdom and Spain as well as some South American countries such as Peru and Chile (Coronavirus Resource Center 2021).

Between September and the end of 2020, however, Brazil experienced a challenging period as COVID-19 continued to spread throughout the country despite the control measures implemented by governments. Like many other countries that experienced infection spikes in the final third of the year, cases and deaths rose over this period (Table 7.2).

As a means of organizing information essential for the management of the crisis in the medical field, the federal Ministry of Health launched an interactive platform on Public Health in Brazil, called "Localiza SUS." This platform contains data on new COVID-19 cases, the number of deaths, the availability of hospital beds for the treatment of COVID-19 patients as well as information about health professionals, respirators, medicines, Personal Protective Equipment, etc.

Table 7.2 Cases of COVID-19 in Brazil as of 31 December 2020

Brazil	
Total cases	7,675,973
Cases per 100,000 inhabitants	3,611
Total deaths	194,949
Deaths per 100,000 inhabitants	91.76

Source: https://ourworldindata.org/coronavirus/country/brazil?country=~BRA

The pandemic had a major impact on the Brazilian economy in 2020. The unemployment rate reached 13.3 percent (8.9 million people lost their jobs) in September 2020. GNP decreased by 9.7 percent in the second quarter, and the federal debt is estimated at more than BRL 700 billion (compared to BRL 95 billion in 2019).

Federalism in Brazil worked as expected in the economic crisis: the federal government enacted social programs to relieve unemployment and helped subnational units with extra financial transfers. Due to the state of public emergency declared by the Congress, the government was not obliged to meet the primary fiscal balance target in 2020 and was thus able to finance a series of economic measures to maintain the fiscal balance of the federation. Some of the measures included the interruption of debt payments between the states and the federal government and debt renegotiation between federal constituent units and the banks. For four months, the federal government also provided financial support to the health system via transfers to the State Participation Fund (FPE) and the Municipality Participation Fund (FPM) in order to ensure that their revenues were equivalent to 2019 levels. Specifically, by federal law number 14,041 of August 18 (2020), BRL 12.124 billion (US\$ 2,824 billion) was allocated as financial support to FPE and FPM due to the loss of their tax collection revenue.

The federal government also instituted the Federative Program to Confront Coronavirus in May 2020. Through special federal law number 173, debt payments were temporarily suspended between the States and the Federal Government (BRL 12.6 billion or US\$ 2.5 billion), and BRL 60 billion (US\$ 12 billion) was transferred to subnational entities. The criteria for the distribution of resources among the federal constituent units were based on population size and the incidence of COVID-19 cases. Program expenses were also linked to health actions to combat the pandemic.

The most distinctive action on the economic front was *Auxílio Emergencial*, a federal program that provided assistance to informal sector workers and unemployed members of low-income families. *Auxílio emergencial* transferred BRL 600 (US\$ 120) per month to each family from April to August and BRL 300 (US\$ 60) from September to December. The aid was provided to more than 67 million people.

The federal government created a Crisis Committee to address strategic issues related to the pandemic. The Committee gave its attention to diverse issues, including the repatriation of Brazilians from abroad; the testing and provision of equipment for public security forces; and the special care provided to indigenous communities. In addition to the Crisis Committee, the COVID-19 Crisis Combat Operations Center (CCOP) was established, whose role was to implement the decisions of the Crisis Committee. Seeking greater articulation with subnational entities, the Special Secretariat for Federative Affairs (SEAF) instituted bi-weekly meetings with the Crisis Committees of the states. SEAF also met with municipal associations to better understand the particularities and needs of municipalities in the context of the crisis.

7.3 Brazilian federal system

Brazil's federal system has three constitutionally recognized levels of government: the federal (central) government; 26 state governments and the federal district; and 5,570 municipalities.

Some studies link federal arrangements to lower social spending, a lack of coordination, and inefficient policies attributed to political fragmentation and subnational government veto powers. Brazil does not fit this analysis. Despite the three-level federal system with more than 5,000 constituent units, Brazil has a strong federal government, significant social spending and, in some areas, successful intergovernment coordination (Machado 2014). How can this apparent paradox be explained?

It is important to note that federalism was adopted in Brazil to divide power in what was once a unitary state. In cases like this, a tendency toward centralization is not uncommon, even when power is shared among federated units. This is the case in Brazil, where power and legislative authority are shared with subnational units, not delegated to them.

The 1988 Constitution endows the federal government with an extensive array of exclusive powers and legislative authority. The Constitution also assigns the federal government, states, and municipalities concurrent powers and legislative authority over certain policy areas. However, the Constitution does not prescribe a specific decision-making process on federal matters. Constitutional amendments require only a three-fifths majority and two roll-call votes in the national parliament. They do not require national referenda or an approval of a qualified majority of state-level legislatures as is the case in other federal countries. The institutional model of Brazilian federalism endows the federal government with extensive power to initiate legislation. Since there are few veto points, Presidents are likely to be successful in passing legislation, even if it would change federal matters (Arretche 2013).

Conflicts between federal constituent units are resolved by the Brazilian Supreme Court (STF). Historically, STF has struck down state and municipal legislation when it is in conflict with the federal Constitution or national legislation. It is rare, if not impossible, to find an STF decision that invalidates federal legislation for infringing on powers reserved for states or municipalities.

Finally, political circumstances reinforce tendencies toward centralization. By the 1990s, almost all Brazilian states had large public debts and were on the verge of declaring bankruptcy. The federal government assumed states' debts but required them to adopt a series of measures in return, such as limiting personnel costs, restricting state borrowing, and privatizing state banks. Constitutional amendments and national legislation were passed to limit the expenditures of subnational units. With lower fiscal capacity, in practice, these units do not have the political autonomy as formally granted to them by the 1988 Constitution (Rosenn 2005).

These political circumstances explain why the federal government in Brazil is so strong, despite Brazil being a three-level federation and the decentralization tendency introduced by the 1988 Constitution. But can the federal government coordinate policy action among federal constituent units and deliver nationwide services? The answer to this question is complex and varies according to policy area.

Brazil adopted a universal healthcare system in 1988 – a great challenge considering the continental size of the country and a population of more than 200 million inhabitants. Healthcare and other social policies are part of cooperative federalism, meaning that the federal government, states, and municipalities all share power to enact programs in these areas. Mechanisms of coordination among federal constituent units evolved in the 1990s. These mechanisms succeeded in facilitating decentralization of health spending and coordination of efforts among different municipalities, states, and the federal government.

The federal government ensures coordination of efforts in healthcare through the use of conditional transfers to subnational units, requiring recipients to fulfill general guidelines enacted by the Ministry of Health. States and municipalities participate in the decision-making process on health policy through councils and joint committees. Today, almost all ambulatory (outpatient) expenditures are carried out by municipalities, while the federal government sets the general direction of health care policy by conditional transfer of funding.

7.4 Federalism and COVID-19

Conflicts between federal constituent units, as well as between the executive and the judicial branches of the government, were common during the pandemic. Policy review in the courts was a mark of the pandemic's first wave.

While countries in Europe and Asia were already suffering the damage caused by COVID-19, Brazil remained in apprehensive anticipation, waiting for the first case of the virus to arrive. Federal Law n° 13.979, enacted on 6 February 2020, was one of the first concrete measures adopted by the government. The law stipulated actions that could be taken by authorities to control the spread of the virus such as social isolation, quarantine, and mandatory tests or vaccines. Meanwhile, the federal Ministry of Health held meetings with state Secretaries of Health to align actions and coordinate efforts. The main recommendation was to flatten the virus transmission curve, although there was no consensus on how to achieve this goal.

As the pandemic approached Brazil, authorities at different levels of government began to take action independently and impose disproportionately restrictive measures, thus creating a panic scenario and stimulating conflict between federal constituent units. Trying to avoid blame in such situations could motivate authorities to emulate the most restrictive actions taken elsewhere (Elkins and Simmons 2005). Electoral strategies also may have a role in the conflicts between constituent federal units, which can be seen as conflicts between political actors. Local elections held in November 2020, and the anticipation of political coalitions in the 2022 general election led to public disagreements and accusations between the President, governors, and mayors regarding pandemic control measures and the related economic costs.

In March 2020, when the pandemic was in the early stages in Brazil, some states closed airports, ports, and highways, consequently isolating themselves from the rest of the country. These actions could have stopped the delivery of food, drugs, and other essential goods throughout the nation. On March 20, the President enacted an executive decree (MP 926) to centralize actions in this area, requiring technical advice of a federal agency before any restriction on transportation could be enacted. The President also stated that it was up to him to declare the essential activities that should continue even under isolation measures. To resolve this evident conflict between federal constituent units, the Supreme Court was called upon to resolve this deadlock in federalism.[2]

The STF decided that the actions taken by authorities to control COVID-19 are a common power of all three levels of government. Thereby, the Court endorsed the executive decree enacted by the President and also recognized that states and municipalities could adopt their own measures and policies according to regional or local needs. This decision gave judicial support to measures adopted by governors and mayors, reinforcing the spirit of cooperative federalism. On one hand, the STF's decision granted political autonomy to federal constituent units in tackling the pandemic, but on the other hand, it intensified uncoordinated actions.

Nevertheless, the Supreme Court went further in the analysis, stating that, to achieve coordination, a federal constituent unit could not act against a restrictive guideline enacted by a superior federal constituent unit. Effectively, what this means is that a municipality can adopt more stringent control measures than those adopted by the state, but not less stringent ones. Even if a municipality proves that its health-care situation allows for a relaxation of control measures, such as reopening schools, the mayor of such a municipality cannot enact this if it contravenes the state guideline. In this case, autonomy seems to be a one-way street, given that the units in the federation must comply with the STF's decision.

As would be expected, a wave of lawsuits flooded state and federal courts because each federal constituent unit adopted different criteria for the intensification or relaxation of virus control measures. As conflicts were referred to the justice system, the courts defined a range of policies related to the pandemic. By the end of August 2020, the Supreme Court had issued rulings in over 4,890 lawsuits regarding governmental actions to tackle COVID-19 (STF 2021).

Nevertheless, a number of joint actions were observed and encouraged by the federal government in a system of articulation and cooperation with states and municipalities. States initiated their own plans prepared by multidisciplinary teams of experts designed to mitigate the impacts of the new coronavirus. In an example of horizontal cooperation, the state of Amazonas offered support to the state of Roraima when its hospitals were reaching capacity treating COVID-19 patients. The state of Amazonas had already gone through its worst moment of the crisis and had, at that time, spare capacity in its hospitals to receive patients from Roraima.

7.5 Conclusions and transformation in Brazil

The COVID-19 pandemic resulted in thousands of deaths in Brazil and a huge economic damage. Despite this, the Brazilian health system did not collapse, and the case-fatality rate was low compared to that of a number of other countries around the world (Coronavirus Resource Center 2021). This outcome may suggest that Brazil achieved the goal of flattening the transmission curve. Uncoordinated actions do not necessarily lead to wrong actions.

Monetary and fiscal reforms go hand in hand with the redefinition of powers among federal constituent units. These issues are permanently debated in Brazil. However, the pandemic has brought a sense of urgency to the discussion, and it may affect the speed of approval of reforms by the legislatures. Conflicts between federal constituent units and judicial activism created a climate of uncertainty. This was a scenario in which every mayor, judge, or prosecutor thought that they had the right answer on how to deal with the pandemic. In this context, the model of federalism in Brazil may change in the short term, either by institutionalizing coordination among federal constituent units or providing subnational entities with more defined administrative and financial powers.

It is not clear whether jurisprudence shifted the Brazil's federal model toward decentralization or if the Supreme Court decisions reinforced decentralization only in certain policy areas. Regardless, it is important to strengthen mechanisms of negotiation on federal affairs in Brazilian federation.

Another important point of transformation due to the COVID-19 crisis is the shift toward result-orientation by public institutions. Brazil has a strong bureaucratic structure, resulting in significant resources being dedicated to verifying and monitoring processes that contribute little to the organization's purpose. The pandemic has shown that institutional processes with flexible, well-planned, and results-oriented structures are better able to serve the public interest, ensuring good public sector governance.

Notes

1 The authors would like to thank Deborah Aroxa, Hanna Cruz, Julio Queiroz, and Luciana Lopes for helpful comments.
2 Direct Unconstitutionality Action (ADI) 6134 and Claim of Non-compliance with Fundamental Precept (ADPF) 672.

Bibliography

Arretche, M., 2013. Demos-Constraining or Demos-Enabling Federalism? Political Institutions and Policy Change in Brazil. *Journal of Politics in Latin America*, 2, 133–150.

Coronavirus Resource Center, 2021. Mortality Analyses. *Johns Hopkins University and Medicine*. Available from: https://coronavirus.jhu.edu/data/mortality [Accessed 16 March 2021].

Elkins, Z. and Simmons, B., 2005. On Waves, Clusters, and Diffusion: A Conceptual Framework. *The ANNALS of the American Academy of Political and Social Science*, 598 (1), 33–51.

Johns Hopkins Coronavirus Resource Center Data, 2021. Brazil. Baltimore. *Johns Hopkins University of Medicine*. Available from: https://coronavirus.jhu.edu/map.html [Accessed 13 February 2021].

Machado, J.A., 2014. Federalismo, poder de veto e coordenação de políticas sociais no Brasil pós-1988. *O&S*, 21 (69), 335–350.

Ministry of Health, 2021. Covid-19 in Brazil [dataset]. Available from: https://www.gov.br/saude/pt-br [Accessed 16 March 2021].

Our World in Data, 2021. Brazil: Coronavirus Pandemic Country Profile [dataset]. Available from: https://ourworldindata.org/coronavirus/country/brazil?country=~BRA [Accessed 16 March 2021].

Ribeiro, J. and Moreira, M.R., 2016. The Crisis of Cooperative Federalism in the Health Policies in Brazil. *Saúde Debate*, 40, 14–24.

Rosenn, K.S., 2005. Federalism in Brazil. *Duquesne Law Review*, 43. STF, Sipremo Tribunal Federal, 2021. Painel De Ações COVID-19. Available from: https://transparencia.stf.jus.br/extensions/app_processo_covid19/index.html [Accessed 16 March 2021].

World Coronavirus Statistics Data, 2021. *COVID-19 Alert: Coronavirus Disease*. Available from: https://www.google.com/search?client=firefox-b-d&q=world+coronavirus+statistics+data [Accessed 14 February 2021].

Worldometers.info, 2021. *Countries in the World by Population, 2021* [online]. Dover, Delaware USA. Available from: https://www.worldometers.info/world-population/population-by-country/ [Accessed 14 February 2021].

8 Reduced acrimony, quiet management

Intergovernmental relations during the COVID-19 pandemic in Canada

André Lecours, Daniel Béland and Jennifer Wallner

8.1 Introduction

Federalism is a defining feature of Canada both as a political system and a community of peoples (Smiley 1987). Accordingly, the country's experience of the COVID-19 pandemic was very much mediated by the rules and practices of the federal system. The virus hit the westernmost province of British Columbia first but eventually affected the two largest provinces of Québec and Ontario most. Federalism allowed provincial and territorial governments to tailor the response to the pandemic to particular situations. At the same time, the federal government enacted country-wide measures to contain the spread of the virus, like closing the international border with the United States and introducing key income replacement measures to mitigate the socio-economic consequences of the pandemic. There was a unity and diversity quality to Canada's response to the pandemic.

Interestingly, Canada's often acrimonious intergovernmental relations calmed down during the first wave of the pandemic, as some Premiers historically at odds with Prime Minister Justin Trudeau found political incentives to collaborate. Indeed, approval ratings of virtually every Premier rose in the Spring of 2020 (Dart & Maru/Blue 2020). A good degree of intergovernmental collaboration facilitated Canada's response to COVID-19.

This chapter first paints the picture of the health and socio-economic impact of COVID-19 on the Canadian federation. It then details the role played by the two orders of government in the response to the virus and analyzes how a combination of structural and circumstantial factors helped keep intergovernmental conflict low. Finally, the chapter explains how the pandemic has increased, probably temporarily, the frequency of intergovernmental contacts, which have occurred along the lines of pre-existing structures and practices unlikely to be fundamentally transformed by the fight against the virus (Table 8.1).

Table 8.1 Key Statistics on COVID-19 in Canada as of 10 January 2021

Cumulative Cases	Cumulative Cases per 100,000 Population	Cumulative Deaths	Cumulative Deaths per 100,000 Population	Case Fatality Percentage
644,348	1,707.2	16,707	44.3	2.6

Source: World Health Organization Weekly epidemiological update – 12 January 2021. Geneva: WHO, 2021. Available from https://www.who.int/publications/m/item/weekly-epidemiological-update

DOI: 10.4324/9781003251217-8

8.2 The health and economic impact of COVID-19

COVID-19 had a significant impact on Canada's public health and economic situation. As of 19 January 2021, Canada had registered nearly 720,000 detected COVID-19 cases.[1] The number of cases varied greatly from one province to the next. For instance, Quebec, the country's second largest province (8.6 million inhabitants), had the highest number of detected cases (245,734). Ontario, the largest province by far (14.7 million inhabitants), registered the second largest number of cases (242,277). Among the four most populous provinces (Alberta, British Columbia, Ontario, and Quebec), British Columbia performed the best in controlling the number of cases. In part because of pro-active public health measures enacted early on, it only registered 61,912 cases, which is good considering its population of about 5 million. Among the less populous provinces, the four Atlantic Provinces (Newfoundland and Labrador, New Brunswick, Nova Scotia, and Prince Edward Island) did much better than Manitoba and Saskatchewan, becoming the most successful region of the country in the fight against the pandemic, with the exception of the three territories, which were unevenly affected by it (relatively few cases in the Northwest Territory and Yukon but a more challenging situation in Nunavut, at least during the second wave of the pandemic). Overall, some regions of the country were more affected by the virus than others, something that is attributed to a mixture of factors, including exposure to international travel, population density as well as the nature and timing of policy decisions about issues such as quarantine, self-insolation, and the staffing of long-term care facilities, where more than two-third of infected people died and close to a quarter of all Canadians who have tested positive for COVID-19 lived. This situation has triggered a national debate about long-term care policies in Canada (Béland and Marier 2020).

Like in many other countries, the pandemic and the public health measures enacted in response to COVID-19 have created a sudden economic downturn in Canada. For example, during the second quarter of 2020, "the economy is estimated to have plunged 39.8 percent," a dramatic and unprecedented development (Deloitte 2020, p. 5). For the year 2020, a downturn of nearly 6 percent was expected. Some sectors of the economy were hit especially hard, including accommodation and food services, construction, manufacturing, retail, arts, entertainment, and recreation (Deloitte 2020). Because of a sharp decline of economic activity in these key areas, unemployment increased rapidly. From February to March 2020, the national unemployment rate jumped from 5.6 to 7.8 percent before reaching 13 percent in April and 13.7 percent in May. In part, because of a gradual and partial reopening of key sectors of the economy, the unemployment rate declined slightly in June to reach 12.3 percent, which was still more than twice as high as the figure for February. Simultaneously, while the economic shock affected the entire country, as was the case for the pandemic itself, some demographics such as women, were more affected by the economic downturn and the job losses (Wright 2020). Regional variation also proved significant. For example, in Alberta, a province already facing economic difficulties before the COVID-19 crisis due in part to lower oil prices, unemployment increased rapidly from 7.2 percent in February to 15.5 percent in May, and it did not decline in June, as it did nationally and in most other provinces. Although the economy recovered partly during the summer and fall of 2020, the national unemployment rate sat at 8.5 percent in November, which is much higher than before the pandemic.

Such a swift economic downturn led to the rapid enactment of temporary yet massive federal emergency measures to help families, workers, and employers despite the presence of a minority government in Ottawa. These expensive, large-scale measures, coupled with massive revenue loses, led to a sudden and unprecedented increase in the size of the federal deficit, which is anticipated to reach 381 billion dollars CDN in 2020–2021 compared to only 14 billion dollars CDN in 2018–2019 and 34.4 billion CDN in 2019–2020. A possible second wave of COVID-19 could slow down a revenue-generating economic recovery while pressuring the federal government to spend even more on emergency economic and social policy measures, a situation that would further increase the federal deficit. As far as fiscal challenges are concerned, the provinces, territories, and municipalities are especially vulnerable, a situation leading to calls to reform fiscal federalism in order to help these governments struggling to pay growing bills with lower revenues and a fiscal capacity much more limited than the federal government's (Béland et al. 2020). There is significant variation in the fiscal situation of provincial governments. For instance, while a poorer province facing a resource bust like Newfoundland and Labrador is in a dire situation, a wealthier one like British Columbia is in a much better position to weather the crisis. Still, calls to reform fiscal federalism and, in effect, to increase federal transfers to the provinces in key areas such as health care and long-term care are getting louder (Béland et al. 2020).

8.3 The intergovernmental management of the pandemic

Canada is a decentralized federation both from a public policy and a fiscal point of view (Lecours 2019). The ten provinces have exclusive or primary legislative and administrative power in the fields of education, health care, employment relations, civil law, law enforcement, and natural resources. The federal government has exclusive or primary legislative and administrative power in the fields of currency, defense, agriculture, citizenship and immigration, foreign affairs, criminal law, and employment insurance. From a fiscal perspective, approximately 80 percent of provincial revenues are own-source, and the major fiscal transfers from the federal government are either unconditional (equalization) or very weakly conditional (the Canada Health Transfer [CHT] and the Canada Social Transfer [CST]). The three territories have powers similar to those of provinces but no constitutional existence, as they owe their autonomy to the Parliament of Canada rather than to a constitutional division of powers. Municipalities also lack constitutional standing; they are under the authority of provincial governments.

Health care and emergency management were foremost fields of jurisdiction during the pandemic. Health care, in all its forms, is a provincial responsibility. Provincial health care systems have to conform to broad principles contained in the 1984 federal *Canada Health Act* and the federal government funds about 20 percent of provincial health care costs through the CHT. There are no specific emergency management powers listed in the Canadian Constitution aside from the federal authority over quarantine (*British North America Act*, section 91-11), which was not invoked by the federal government during the pandemic. Similarly, the federal *Emergencies Act* was not invoked, after provincial governments clearly signaled they considered such a move unnecessary. There is a federal Disaster Financial Assistance Arrangements program, but it explicitly excludes pandemics.

Both orders of government played important roles during the pandemic.[2] On public health, provinces were on the front lines, managing the health care system and long-term care homes; deciding on confinement and de-confinement as well as on the use of masks in indoor public spaces; controlling movement within their territory as well as to and from other provinces; and choosing when to close and open schools as well as how to structure learning in the exceptional circumstances. Provinces also decided on the opening and closure of businesses, and some of them formed regional 'bubbles' for the purpose of inter-provincial movement. The federal government managed international travel and the border with the United States. It also oversaw vaccine development efforts and procurement. Moreover, at the request of the Québec and Ontario governments, it deployed members of the Canadian Armed Forces in the two provinces' long-term care homes. Most of the federal government's action focused on mitigating the economic impact of the pandemic through temporary programs that included the Canada Emergency Response Benefits (CERB) to support the unemployed; the Canada Emergency Student Benefit (CESB), to support post-secondary students; and the Canada Emergency Wage Subsidy (CEWS), to help employers rehire laid off workers. Provinces were generally receptive to these temporary programs, even if they were sometimes not given much forewarning before their announcement and implementation. Some provincial governments formulated smaller and complementary, assistance programs (for example, Québec developed an incentive program for retaining workers deemed essential during the pandemic such as grocery stores employees). Overall, the management of both the public health and the economic dimensions of the pandemic occurred in respect of the constitutional division of powers. Typical of Canadian federalism, when the federal government sought to impose conditions for a special one-time transfer of almost 20 billion dollars CAN, the provinces pushed back to reduce or outright eliminate these conditions (Marquis 2020).

Although the federal government possesses a fiscal might far superior to that of the provinces, the large federal deficit generated by the creation of numerous, and sometimes far-reaching, temporary programs will place the federal government in Ottawa in a difficult fiscal position for years to come. In the context of such large budgetary deficits, any effort to centralize the economy in anyway is highly unlikely. Instead, provinces have already shown their intention to double-down on their traditional demand for an increase in federal transfers for health care; the catastrophic situation in long-term care homes in Ontario and, especially, Québec seems to have provided new ammunitions to provincial governments in their pursuit of increased health care funding (Béland and Marier 2020).

Intergovernmental relations during the pandemic were generally harmonious and collaborative. This is somewhat surprising considering that federal–provincial relations were quite tense just before the pandemic. Several of the country's Conservative Premiers (Doug Ford of Ontario, Jason Kenney of Alberta, and Scott Moe of Saskatchewan) had openly attacked Liberal Prime Minister Justin Trudeau for his carbon-taxing policy and his perceived reluctance to develop pipeline capacity to transport oil from producing provinces (primarily Alberta) to the Canadian West and East coasts, where it could then be taken to Asian and European markets, respectively (Béland and Lecours, forthcoming). Québec's conservative nationalist Premier François Legault (*Coalition Avenir Québec*) had publicly rowed with Trudeau over his province's secularism legislation, which the Prime Minister criticized. Yet, during the first wave of the pandemic, most of these Premiers refrained from any serious criticism of the federal government, with some even praising the federal government and collaborating in intergovernmental relations (Grenier 2020).[3]

At least three factors explain how Canada was able to have low intergovernmental conflict during the pandemic. First, Canadian political parties are overall weakly integrated through the levels of government, with the federal and provincial Conservative parties not being integrated at all (Thorlakson 2009). Consequently, Conservative Premiers were not structurally driven to oppose the federal Liberal government for the purpose of helping the federal Conservative party to score political points. As the pandemic offered a chance for some Conservative Premiers to improve their approval rating in their province, they were free to adopt a collaborative approach with the federal government if they judged it could help them politically.[4]

Second, Canada's parliamentary system allowed the Prime Minister to use the tools of Cabinet government (Lijphart 2012, p. 10) to conduct relations with Premiers with whom he had previous or ongoing tensions. For example, Trudeau tasked a powerful minister in his cabinet from Ontario, Chrystia Freeland (Minister of Intergovernmental Affairs and also Deputy Prime Minister, before becoming Minister of Finance), to assume primary responsibility for relations with that provincial government.[5] Moreover, the federal Liberal government's parliamentary minority (a relatively uncommon situation in Canada) provided incentives to forge harmonious intergovernmental relations, with the expectation of either prolonging the life of the minority government (notoriously short in Canada) or placing the Liberals in a good position to gain a majority at the next elections. For the federal government, reducing conflict with the provinces typically involves refraining from unilateral action, national standards, and conditional transfers. Prime Minister Trudeau often stated that the federal government was there to help provinces in whichever way it could, presenting a supportive yet not overbearing position.

Third, the existence of a dense network of federal–provincial relations (especially at the bureaucratic level) facilitated the transition toward more intense intergovernmental contact. At the political level, intergovernmental relations have long been dominated almost exclusively by executives; as such, so-called executive federalism is an important element of continuity in the Canadian federation (Wallner 2017). The practice of First Ministers Meetings (typically, but not always, held annually), which is at the apex of executive federalism, served as a template for the weekly conversation between Canada's Prime Minister and provincial Premiers. These conversations, though largely dedicated to information-sharing, produced some coordination in the response to COVID-19, which allowed Canada to have an overall effective management of the pandemic. They facilitated greater inter-provincial communication than is typically the case in Canadian federalism, as provincial governments could explore opportunities for common positions on different aspects of the management of the pandemic, including the closing/opening of the border with the United States, procurement of medical and testing equipment, and the possibility of the federal government invoking the *Emergencies Act*. In addition to consensus-seeking negotiations and information-sharing, inter-provincial relations also included instances of material collaboration (e.g., Alberta donating medical equipment to other provinces).

Provincial governments played a prominent role during the pandemic. Their constitutional powers over health care, education, municipal institutions, and private property allowed them to be the main decision-makers on many questions that directly impacted the everyday life of Canadians. The room for autonomous action by municipalities depended upon the specific governance approach of the province since municipalities are constitutionally required to operate within the provincial legislative framework. For example, on masks in indoor public spaces, the Québec government issued an order for compulsory use effective 11 July 2020 while the Ontario government left that decision up to municipal and local authorities.

Federalism performed well in Canada during the first wave of the pandemic, as autonomous federal and provincial action structured by the constitutional division of powers was complemented by increased intergovernmental communication and information-sharing. Canada was created as a federation, and just like it is unimaginable to think of this multinational state (Burgess and Pinder 2011) as anything but federal in normal times, it is equally unthinkable that it would have performed better, or as well, without federalism during the COVID-19 crisis. The virus affected regions of the country quite differently, and federalism allowed for responses tailored to specific situations to be implemented.

8.4 Innovations, transformations, and missed opportunities in IGR

There can be no denying the fact that the effort to contend with the COVID-19 pandemic has transformed the frequency of intergovernmental meetings in Canada. As soon as the lockdown was announced on 13 March 2020, the Prime Minister and the Premiers met weekly via telephone conference calls. In December 2020, the Prime Minister also convened a formal First Ministers' Meeting on fighting COVID-19 and strengthening health care. For the most part, during the first wave of the pandemic, many Premiers voiced largely positive responses in reaction to the efforts of the Prime Minister and members of his government. As noted above, Deputy Prime Minister Chrystia Freeland received considerable positive feedback from various Premiers.

Disagreements have nevertheless arisen in some unexpected ways. For example, the effort to mobilize technology and create a voluntary contact tracing application in Canada has been complicated by intergovernmental conflict. Specifically, the federal government has been working to create a centralized, 'national' application while individual provinces and territories launched similar initiatives. On 19 June 2020, CBC News reported that New Brunswick Premier Blaine Higgs was told to stop working on a provincial app in favor of a single federally backed application using Bluetooth technology provided jointly by Apple and Google (MacKinnon 2020). And, on 13 July 2020, Alberta Premier Jason Kenney accused the federal government of preventing tech companies from working with provinces to improve contact tracing apps (Major 2020). This example exposes the classic blame avoidance or buck-passing dynamic long associated with intergovernmental relations in federations.

This pandemic also marks the first time we see the rise of personal communications among politicians in addition to the concerted use of social media to communicate intergovernmental responses to a major emergency. To start, a growing number of politicians are eschewing the traditional formal lines of communication, set through staff, in favor of rapid texting and Blackberry phone calls. Premier Doug Ford, for example, has been calling and checking in with Minister Chrystia Freeland virtually every other day since the early days of the pandemic in March 2020 (Hains 2020). The Premiers who are most sympathetic to the federal government re-tweeted and posted information from the Government of Canada rather than drawing upon their own provincial resources. For example, the Premier of

Newfoundland and Labrador regularly posted content drawn from federal ministers and the Chief Public Health Officer, unlike the Premier of Saskatchewan who did not post or re-tweet anything with content from the Government of Canada. However, as also noted above, even the most combative Premiers toned down their rhetoric throughout the pandemic and scaled back the frequency of their critiques against the federal government.

One of the most striking responses to the pandemic was the intermittent closures of internal borders enacted by provincial and territorial governments under the auspices of public health. This is a marked and a dramatic departure from the long-standing guarantee of internal mobility rights throughout the federation. Interestingly, throughout the first wave of the pandemic, Ontario was the lone province that did not impose generalized border restrictions for interprovincial travel or requirements to self-isolate if visiting from another region in the country. What is more, in the lead-up to the First Ministers Meeting held in December 2020, Premier Doug Ford started publicly asking whether or not the federal government would move from the mandatory 14-day quarantine to rapid testing of new arrivals to expedite the reopening of borders (McGrath 2020). Others, however, have installed varied arrangements, tailored to local needs, establishing regionalized practices that carved out specific areas of the country. Atlantic Canada created a 'regional bubble,' while Manitoba postponed some of its plans to ease restrictions in response to public feedback to its proposals. Specifically, as reported by Cameron MacLean (2020), the plan included relaxing the 14-day self-isolation requirement for travelers from eastern and southern Ontario, Quebec, and Atlantic Canada. However, overwhelming responses from Manitobans indicated that the public wanted to see the restrictions remain in place, and so the Manitoba government opted to maintain the status quo. What is remarkable here is that all of these provisions and restrictions on internal mobility have been enacted largely without any controversy or conflict. It is a clear indicator of the seriousness with which Canadians took the need to stop the spread of the COVID-19 virus.

As Canada is deep into the 'second wave' of the pandemic and now facing the challenges of vaccinating the population, while managing existing infections and trying to hold off the increasingly contagious iterations of COVID-19 emerging around the world, a series of missed opportunities are apparent. Throughout the first wave of the pandemic and into the period of uncertain stability of a 'new normal,' little has been heard from the sectoral level tables or the Council of the Federation (COF), a body composed of 13 provincial and territorial Premiers created to strengthen horizontal cooperation. Traditionally the workhorses of intergovernmental relations in Canada, according to the Canadian Intergovernmental Conference Secretariat, while teleconferences and videoconferences for various tables have occurred throughout the first wave, only a few public statements have been released. In the meantime, despite issuing a few intermittent statements, the provincial and territorial Premiers decided to forgo the annual meeting of the COF, indirectly (and likely unintentionally) confirming to outside observers that the COF is essentially a body to coordinate lobbying efforts as opposed to mobilizing meaningful horizontal collaboration. Moving forward, researchers will need to determine if decision-makers and public officials throughout the country used this period to bolster the capacity of these bodies, share valuable information, develop coherent strategies, and begin to anticipate future problems as Canada and the world adapts to a new reality.

Canadians are also learning that some provincial decisions about how to mobilize federal funds and vaccinate residents vary considerably. Since the start of the pandemic, the Premiers were clear in their opposition to any notion of the federal government enacting the Emergencies Act: "That's not their jurisdiction," said Premier Ford in response to a question posed by a journalist. "We don't need the nanny state telling us what to do" (quoted in McGrath 2020, n.p.). Consequently, money transferred by the federal government to the provinces for COVID-19 health spending, support for employers or individuals, and a general contingency fund, arrived without any strings. While some provinces may have used the money allocated to them, according to the *Globe and Mail*, Ontario was still holding onto $12 billion in contingency funds when the second wave hit in the Fall of 2020 (Gray 2020). During the First Ministers Meeting in December, the federal government committed to covering 100 percent of the cost of procuring the vaccine and the supplies needed for vaccination. That month, as vaccines arrived in the country, provinces began to administer them. However, decisions on whom, when, and how to administer vaccines showed signs of inconsistency and a general lack of clear details in terms of the overall roll-out and execution strategies (The Canadian Press 2020). Assuring the efficient and effective vaccination of Canadians is a critical step in combatting this pandemic. The use of the contingency funds afforded by the federal government to provinces in order to insure, for example, the safety of children in schools and essential workers who cannot work from home, could have been more clearly detailed by provincial and territorial governments to their populations.

8.5 Conclusion

Overall, certain elements of federalism appear to have worked well, especially during the first wave of the COVID-19 pandemic. Using its superior fiscal clout, the federal government moved quickly to enact new economic measures to support individual Canadians and certain economic sectors through the shutdown. Furthermore, additional grants were issued to provinces and territories to support re-opening. Provinces and territories, in the meantime, found ways to curb the spread of the virus within their respective populations. Missteps certainly occurred, particularly on long-term care homes, and some provinces did a much better job than others in the terms of public health measures. Yet, federalism and intergovernmental relations worked relatively well during the pandemic, which helped mitigate its impact on Canadians. The discourse among political leaders was also generally positive through the first wave of the pandemic, though it remains unclear if such agreeable relations will remain in place subsequently. What is certain is that Canada's federal system needs to continue to find ways to foster intergovernmental collaboration in order to facilitate the implementation of policies necessary to navigate future public health and economic challenges.

Notes

1 Unless indicated, all the statistics in this section were retrieved from federal government (including Statistics Canada) websites in January 2020.
2 Municipalities' school boards and local public health officials implemented and adapted provincial directives.

3 That was the case for Ontario's Doug Ford and Alberta's Jason Kenney. Québec Premier François Legault thanked Prime Minister Trudeau for accepting to deploy the Canadian Armed Forces in the province's long-term retirement homes.
4 This was the case for Doug Ford who was unpopular in Ontario until the pandemic.
5 Premier Ford then spoke glowingly of Minister Freeland and the job she was doing.

Bibliography

Béland, D. and Lecours, A., [Forthcoming]. L'Alberta, l'aliénation de l'Ouest et le programme fédéral de péréquation: identités territoriales, cadrage idéologique et inscription à l'agenda politique. *Politique et Sociétés*.

Béland, D., Lecours, A., Paquet, M. and Tombe, T., 2020. A Critical Juncture in Fiscal Federalism? Canada's Response to COVID-19. *Canadian Journal of Political Science* [online]. Available from: https://www.cambridge.org/core/journals/canadian-journal-of-political-science-revue-canadienne-de-science-politique/article/critical-juncture-in-fiscal-federalism-canadas-response-to-covid19/E4F8184DACB186C41C1E8839A7A89BB6 [Accessed 8 March 2021].

Béland, D. and Patrik, M., 2020. COVID-19 and Long-Term Care Policy for Older People in Canada. *Journal of Aging & Social Policy*, 32 (4–5), 358–364.

Burgess, M. and Pinder, J., eds, 2011. *Multinational Federations*. London: Routledge.

Dart & Maru/Blue Voice Canada Poll, 2020. *Canadian Premiers' Quarterly Approval Rating Tracking*, Q2 June. Available from: https://dartincom.ca/wp-content/uploads/2020/06/Premiers-Release-Chart-Q2-F-2020-.pdf [Accessed 8 March 2021].

Deloitte, 2020. *Unprecedented in Every Way; Economic Outlook: June 2020*. Toronto: Deloitte Canada. Available from: https://www2.deloitte.com/content/dam/Deloitte/ca/Documents/finance/ca-economic-outlook-report-june-2020-aoda-en.pdf?icid=juneReport_en [Accessed 8 March 2021].

Gray, J., 2020. Ontario Had $12-Bilion in Unspent Contingency Funds as COVID-19's Second Wave Hit, Report Says [online]. *Globe and Mail*, 8 December. Available from: https://www.theglobeandmail.com/canada/article-ontario-had-12-billion-in-contingency-funds-as-covid-19s-second-wave/ [Accessed 8 March 2021].

Grenier, É., 2020. The Pandemic Is Breaking Down Political Barriers between Provincial and Federal Governments [online]. *CBC News*, 5 April. Available from: https://www.cbc.ca/news/politics/grenier-provincial-federal-cooperation-1.5521531 [Accessed 8 March 2021].

Hains, D., 2020. How Doug Ford and Chrystia Freeland Became Canada's Political Odd Couple [online]. *iPolitics*, 28 December. Available from: https://ipolitics.ca/2020/12/28/how-doug-ford-and-chrystia-freeland-became-canadas-political-odd-couple/ [Accessed 8 March 2021].

Lecours, A., 2019. Dynamic De/centralization in Canada, 1867–2010. *Publius: The Journal of Federalism*, 49 (1), 57–83.

Lijphart, A., 2012. *Patterns of Democracy: Government Forms and Performance in Thirty-Six Countries*. 2nd ed. New Haven: Yale University Press.

MacKinnon, B., 2020. Province's Plans for COVID-19 Contact-tracing App Denied by Ottawa [online]. *CBC News*, 19 June. Available from: https://www.cbc.ca/news/canada/new-brunswick/covid-19-contact-tracing-app-new-brunswick-national-1.5618973 [Accessed 8 March 2021].

MacLean, C., 2020. Travel Restrictions for Visitors from Eastern Provinces Stay in Place after Pushback from Manitobans [online]. *CBC News*, 23 July. Available from: https://www.cbc.ca/news/canada/manitoba/manitoba-covid-19-update-thursday-july-23-1.5660359 [Accessed 8 March 2021].

Major, D., 2020. Alberta Premier Jason Kenney Accuses Feds of Getting in the Way of Fixing Contact Tracing App [online]. *CBC News*, 13 July. Available from: https://www.cbc.ca/news/politics/kenney-covid-pandemic-contact-tracing-1.5648056 [Accessed 8 March 2021].

Marquis, M., 2020. Réouverture de l'économie: Trudeau s'entend avec les provinces et les territoires. *La Presse*, 16 July. Available from: https://www.lapresse.ca/affaires/economie/2020-07-16/reouverture-de-l-economie-trudeau-s-entend-avec-les-provinces-et-territoires.php [Accessed 8 March 2021].

McGrath, J.M., 2020. This Is a Global Crisis: Why Is Doug Ford Talking about Who Has Jurisdiction? *TVO*, 13 November. Available from: https://www.tvo.org/article/this-is-a-global-crisis-why-is-doug-ford-talking-about-who-has-jurisdiction [Accessed 8 March 2021].

Smiley, D., 1987. *The Federal Condition in Canada*. Toronto: McGraw-Hill Ryerson.

The Canadian Press, 2020. A Look at What Provinces and Territories Have Said about COVID-19 Vaccine Plans [online]. *CityNews*, 18 December. Available from: https://toronto.citynews.ca/2020/12/18/a-look-at-what-provinces-and-territories-have-said-about-covid-19-vaccine-plans-16/ [Accessed 8 March 2021].

Thorlakson, L., 2009. Patterns of Party Integration, Influence and Autonomy in Seven Federations. *Party Politics*, 15, 157–177.

Wallner, J., 2017. Ideas and Intergovernmental Relations in Canada. *PS: Political Science & Politics*, 50 (3), 717–722.

Wright, T., 2020. Feds Probing Ways to Address COVID-19 Impact on Women. *CTV News*, 23 May. Available from: https://www.ctvnews.ca/politics/feds-probing-ways-to-address-covid-19-impact-on-women-1.4951560 [Accessed 8 March 2021].

9 Federalism and the COVID-19 crisis

The perspective from Ethiopia

Zemelak Ayitenew Ayele

9.1 Introduction

The COVID-19 pandemic emerged when Ethiopia was at a political crossroads. The Ethiopian Peoples' Revolutionary Democratic Front (EPRDF), the party that ruled the country in a centralized manner for almost three decades, was forced to undergo a fundamental makeover as a result of the 2015–2018 public protests. The protests saw the rise to power of Abiy Ahmed, the current Prime Minister, who pledged to transform the country to a democratic state. The party underwent not only a change in leadership but also in name (now, it is called Ethiopian Prosperity Party (EPP)), structure (it is no longer a coalition of ethnic-based regional parties), and ideology (it has abandoned revolutionary democracy). The Tigray Peoples Liberation Front (TPLF) – the founder and the nucleus of the EPRDF – has been pushed from the center of political power and is reduced to being a single-region party. The sixth general elections, which were viewed as a litmus test on whether the country was indeed transforming into a democratic state, was scheduled for August 2020. It is in such a national political context that COVID-19 emerged.

This chapter argues that the rise of COVID-19 not only has stalled political reforms in Ethiopia but also exposed certain flaws in the design and operation of the Ethiopian federal system. Severe ongoing disagreements between the EPP and the TPLF erupted into full-scale armed clashes on 4 November 2020, and the conflict is still ongoing at the time of writing. The chapter begins by describing when and how COVID-19 began spreading in Ethiopia and the rate at which it is spreading. It then discusses the Ethiopian federal system, and the role each level of government is expected to play in containing the spread of the virus and whether and how it is discharging its responsibilities in this respect. It concludes with a discussion of how the emergence of COVID-19 is impacting on the Ethiopian federal system (Table 9.1).

Table 9.1 Key Statistics on COVID-19 in Ethiopia as of 10 January 2021

Cumulative Cases	Cumulative Cases per 100,000 Population	Cumulative Deaths	Cumulative Deaths per 100,000 Population	Case Fatality Percentage
127,792	111.2	1,985	1.7	1.6

Source: World Health Organization Weekly epidemiological update – 12 January 2021. Geneva: WHO, 2021. Available from https://www.who.int/publications/m/item/weekly-epidemiological-update

DOI: 10.4324/9781003251217-9

9.2 COVID-19 and the extent of infection

The first case of COVID-19 in Ethiopia was reported on 13 March 2020, a mere two days after the virus was declared a global pandemic by the World Health Organization (WHO). Since then, the number of those infected has been growing. Although the virus has been spreading at a decreasing rate, it has reached every state of the federation. Addis Ababa, the country's capital and largest city, has seen the highest COVID-19 positivity rates, accounting for two-thirds of the country's total case count.

As of January 2021, there were close to 136,000 confirmed cases of COVID-19 in Ethiopia, and a little over 2,000 people have died due to the virus (Ministry of Health 2021). In a country with a population of 115 million, the number of confirmed cases is indeed relatively low. However, the actual number of infected persons might be much higher, and the low rate of infection and death seems merely a reflection of the limited testing taking place in the country. At the beginning of the pandemic, the country did not even have the technology to conduct tests, and samples were sent to South Africa for assessment. Subsequently, Ethiopia was able to ramp up testing capacity to around 20,000 tests per day and at the time of writing about 1.7 million people had been tested (Ministry of Health 2021). It is thus evident that the testing capacity is far from where it should be despite the federal and state governments' efforts to increase their testing daily capacity since the first confirmed case was reported.

9.3 Ethiopia's federal system

9.3.1 A dual federal system

In Ethiopia, the federal and state governments both enjoy explicit constitutional recognition (Fiseha 2007). The federation has a bi-cameral Parliament, House of Peoples Representatives, and House of Federation (HoF), even though the latter does not exercise legislative powers (see Ethiopian Constitution 1995). It has also a parliamentary form of government. The federation is composed of ten states[1] each of which has a state council and parliamentary form of government. The states are organized principally along ethnic lines even though none of the states is ethnically homogenous. Local government, which is composed of rural *woredas* and cities, enjoys no explicit constitutional recognition (Ayele and Fessha 2012).

9.3.2 Controlling pandemics in the constitutional division of powers

The federal government's authority to control pandemic diseases emanates from two constitutional sources. As per Article 51(3) of the 1995 Constitution, the federal government "establishes and implements national standards and basic policy," among others, on public health (see Fiseha and Ayele 2017). This provision therefore gives the federal government policy and legislative responsibility for public health issues, including pandemics. Moreover, a pandemic is a health risk which is often associated with people traveling across national and international borders. As the level of government charged with controlling the country's ports of entry and exit, the federal government is responsible for containing pandemics by determining whether one should be granted entry into the country based on health considerations (Art. 51(18), Ethiopian Constitution 1995).

Almost all federal agencies seem to have some role to play in containing the virus even though some agencies play a more direct role. The Ministry of Health (MoH) exercises an overall authority on public health related matters (Art. 27, Proclamation 1097). The Ethiopian Food and Drug Control Authority (EFDCA)[2] and Public Health Institute (PHI) which work under the MoH have mandates that are linked to fighting pandemics. For instance, the PHI has the mandate to collect, analyze, and disseminate information on, among others, 'epidemic prone diseases' (FDRE 2013). It is also authorized to investigate and verify the outbreak of pandemics and alert concerned organs and supporting state and local government in dealing with pandemics (FDRE 2013). It also exercises regulatory functions in relation to quarantine and communicable diseases (Art. 72(2), Proclamation 1112). The EFDCA is in charge of controlling ports of entry and exits, among others, with the purpose of preventing pandemics. It is empowered to deny individuals entry or exit or subject them to be quarantined in the case of a pandemic (Art. 4(15), Proclamation 661). The Ministry of Peace (MoP), with National Disaster and Risk Management Commission (NDRMC), a federal agency which is answerable to the former, plays certain roles in controlling the COVID-19 outbreak. A National Emergency Coordination Centre (NECC) has been established within the NDRMC 'to coordinate the multi-sector response' to the humanitarian and logistical issues that are linked with containing COVID-19. The NECC, among others, has established quarantine centers and food banks in border areas. Federal and state police and other security agencies play the role of guarding quarantine centers. Moreover, both the federal and state governments are constitutionally empowered to declare a state of emergency (SoE) (Art. 93, Ethiopian Constitution 1995) as a method of containing pandemic diseases, and federal and state police are expected to enforce the SoE.

The states have the power to adopt state-wide policies on social matters and, thus, on matters relating to public health (Art. 52(2)(c), Proclamation 661). The Constitution authorizes them to declare an SoE if doing so is necessary for controlling the spread of endemic diseases (Art. 93(1)(b), Ethiopian Constitution 1995). In practice, a state bureau of health plays a primary role in terms of controlling pandemics. The competence of the local government in the area of public health is not clearly stated in the Constitution nor is it defined in state constitutions and laws even though the latter authorize *woredas* and cities to prepare and implement their own plan on social and economic matters (Ayele 2014). In any case, in practice, *woredas* and cities are in charge of providing primary healthcare and establishing health centers (Art. 93(1)(b), Ethiopian Constitution 1995). The local government agency which is responsible for health related matters, and therefore COVID-19, is the *woreda*/city office of health.

9.3.3 Federal and state responses to COVID-19

9.3.3.1 Measures to contain the pandemic

After the first case of COVID-19 was confirmed, the federal and state governments began taking restrictive measures, short of declaring a state of emergency, to contain the spread of the virus. Federal agencies, such as MoH and PHI, began administering temperature checks at airports. The federal government closed all federal offices and asked all non-essential federal employees to work from home. Ethiopian Airlines was forced to gradually suspend all international flights, save for cargo flights. On

20 March 2020, the Council of Ministers (CoM) decided to close the borders of the country save for those who agree to submit themselves for 14 days quarantine at their own expense.

Similarly, the states and some local governments put restrictions on public movements. For instance, Bahr Dar, the capital of Amhara state, imposed a two-week lockdown, starting from 31 March 2020. Several cities in Oromia, such as Adama and Assela, also suspended all public transportation.

The Tigray state was the first and the only state to invoke a state power to impose a state of emergency as per Article 93 of the Constitution. It declared an SoE with the objective of containing the virus. The state suspended public movements to and from rural areas within the state and ordered the closure of coffee houses, cafeterias, and other similar establishments for the duration of the SoE (*Addis Standard* 2020). It also required anyone entering the state to be tested. The Tigray SoE was followed five months later by a federal SoE, which was declared on 8 April 2020.[3] The federal SoE imposed several restrictions and obligations.[4] It ordered the closure of the borders of the country except for Ethiopian citizens. It required everyone to wear masks in public spaces, banned gatherings of more than four people and forbade shaking hands. It also required buses, trains, and other vehicles to use only half their capacity to transport people and for passengers to pay double the normal fee. Schools, clubs, bars, theatres, and cinemas were closed. Cafeterias, restaurants, and hotels were allowed to provide limited services. Sports and games involving more than two people were banned.

The SoE expired in August 2020, and many of the restrictions have been eased, at least in practice, despite the fact that the virus is still spreading at a growing rate. Ethiopian Airlines has resumed flights, and there is evident laxation in public movements within Addis Ababa despite the city being the epicenter of the virus.

Initially, there were problems in terms of coordinating the measures that the state and the federal government took to contain the spread of the virus. This was mainly due to the absence of formally established intergovernmental relations (IGR) fora in Ethiopia. Indeed, federal agencies had informal and *ad hoc* communication with their counterparts at state level on common issues. In the absence of formal IGR fora, it is these informal communication channels which are now being used for coordinating the effort to contain the virus. In this regard, the MoH is playing the principal role by liaising with states bureaus of health which, in turn, liaise with local offices of health. Information regarding testing and infection rates is sent by state bureaus of health to the MoH which produces a national report and makes it public every afternoon. As mentioned, the NECC, which is active under the NDRMC coordinates the humanitarian responses that are linked to the COVID-19 outbreak.

9.3.3.2 *Measures taken to ease adverse socio-economic impacts of COVID-19*

Ethiopia has been registering double-digit economic growth beginning from the early 2000s showing great progress in terms of poverty reduction. All that has been achieved in this regard is now threatened due to the emergence of COVID-19 which is not only undoing these achievements but also creating new economic and social challenges.

The Federal Job Creation Commission report shows that 330,000 jobs have been lost thus far due to COVID-19 (see Ethiopian Reporter 2020; Bundervoet, Abebe and Wieser 2020). Likewise, a survey that the World Bank conducted in two rounds on the impact of COVID-19 on 550 business firms in Addis Ababa shows that 41 percent of them completely ceased operation even though this number decreased to 29 percent in the second round of the survey (Dione 2020). Up to 40 percent of the firms reported zero earning mainly due to up to 80 percent drop in demand for goods and services these firms provide (Dione 2020). A UN Ethiopia report indicates that, by causing up to a 4 percent drop in the country's GDP, COVID-19 will increase the number of those who live under the national income poverty line – currently 10 million – by 2.2 million (UN Ethiopia 2020). A survey by the World Bank shows that 45 percent and 55 percent of urban and rural households, respectively, have suffered income loses due to COVID-19 (Dabalen and Paci 2020). The government has reduced its own estimate of the country's economic growth for 2020, from 9 to 5.2 percent. Moreover, the virus emerged close to the main rainy season of the country which is gravely affecting the agriculture sector, the backbone of the country's economy and food security. The situation is worsened by the occurrence of a major locus infestation in six of the nine states (Tigray, Amhara, Somali, Afar, Oromia, and SNNP). Food inflation is thus hovering around 30 percent (WFP 2020).

The federal government is playing the most dominant role in terms of dealing with the adverse economic and social consequences of COVID-19. It has taken various measures aimed at alleviating the adverse economic impacts of COVID-19, including tax exemption on imported materials and equipment that can be used in containing the spread of the virus. It also gave tax exemptions to affected companies as well as cancelations of interest and penalties for unpaid taxes which were due between 2015 and 2018. Moreover, it introduced price controls on basic commodities. The National Bank also injected ETB 15 billion (USD 450 million) liquidity to private banks so that they could provide grace periods or 'debt relief and additional loans to their customers in need' (Samuel 2020). Employers are banned from dismissing their employees except in accordance with a protocol issued by the Ministry of Social Affairs. States and local governments are also introducing tax exemptions to small traders and businesses.

The full economic and social impacts of the virus are yet to be seen. It is evident though that the measures, such as tax exemptions and debt relief, which are being introduced by the federal and state governments, are likely to lead to a reduced public revenue which will directly impact the capacity of the federal, state, and local governments to provide basic services to the public.

9.4 COVID-19 and its impacts on the Ethiopian federal system

The federal system has indeed allowed each level of government to take steps that it deemed appropriate to contain the spread of the virus without waiting for instruction from the central government. A good example in this respect is the decision of the Tigray state to declare an SoE and implement various measures to restrict the spread of the virus. The various responses of the other states and cities also show how the federal system has allowed some degree of flexibility to authorities at different levels in terms of responding to the virus. Yet, the emergence of the virus has also exposed some serious flaws in the design of the Ethiopian federal system.

First, as mentioned, formally established IGR fora are non-existent in the country. In the main, state and federal agencies interact with each other on *ad hoc* basis (Wakjira 2017). The absence of a properly institutionalized IGR system had thus made the responses of the two levels of government to the spread of the virus unsystematic and uncoordinated despite some improvement in this regard. For instance, initially, the report of the MoH on the number of infected people did not include reports from some states, most notably from the Tigray state which declared its report using its own media.

Second, according to many analysts, the emergence of COVID-19 has exposed a flaw in the constitutional adjudication system of the country. In Ethiopia, the HoF, the upper house of Parliament, is charged with resolving constitutional disputes, assisted in this respect by the Council of Constitutional Inquiry which is composed of judges and other legal experts (Art. 62(1) and 82–84, Ethiopian Constitution 1995). The HoF is a political organ which is composed on a partisan basis. In the past, various scholars had criticized this system of constitutional umpiring as unworkable. However, the framers of the constitution maintained that given the fact that the constitution is a political document, as much as it is a legal document, its interpretation could not be entrusted with unelected judges.

The COVID-19 pandemic therefore highlighted two major constitutional issues notably the flaw in the constitutional adjudication system of the country and the need for an independent constitutional umpire. The first issue has to do with the postponement of the sixth national elections. The national elections that were supposed to be held in May 2020 were postponed to August 2020 due to breakdown of law and order in different parts of country. As was mentioned in the introduction, the country came out of three years of public protest after the rise to power of Abiy Ahmed in April 2018, and the breakdown of law and order continued in different parts of the country months after the protests ceased. After the first case of COVID-19 was confirmed in Ethiopia, the National Elections Board of Ethiopia (NEBE) determined that it would be unable to administer the elections in August 2020. This presented a dilemma since the term of the sitting Parliament and state councils were set to expire on 10 October 2020. The Constitution provides barely any guidance on how the country would be governed after the expiry of the term of the current parliament and in the event of such a postponement of elections. Major opposition parties, including the TPLF, the Oromo Federalist Congress (OFC), and the Ethiopian Democratic Party (EDP), maintained that the current government will have no constitutional basis to continue governing the country after 10 October and that there was a need to politically settle the issue of how the country is to be governed until the next elections are held. The government ignored this call and asked the HoF to settle this issue by using its power of constitutional interpretation.

The HoF, based on the advice of the Council of Constitutional Inquiry, determined that the sixth general elections could be postponed until, with the advice of the MoH and the NEBE, the HPR determines that it was safe to hold elections. Put differently, the HoF authorized the government to unilaterally decide if and when to hold the next elections and, in the meantime, to exercise undiminished political powers (Council of Constitutional Inquiry 2020). This decision put the government on a collision course with the opposition and caused much unrest.

The second constitutional issue has to do with the decision of the Tigray state to hold its own elections. The TPLF insisted on the elections being held before the expiry of the term of Parliament and state councils. After the NEBE rejected its request to administer a state-wide election in Tigray, the Tigray state adopted its own election law and established a state election board. Tigray state's resolution in this respect was constitutionally questionable. This is because all matters relating to elections lie within the competences of the federal government and that all elections are administered by the NEBE (Art. 51(15) and 102, Constitution Act 1995). The failure to resolve this deadlock through the normal process of constitutional adjudication created a constitutional crisis. The already strained relations between Tigray state and the federal government deteriorated rapidly precipitating an intensive armed confrontation. Following Tigray's decision to defy the HoF's and the federal government's formal overture and press ahead with state elections, in November 2020, federal forces were dispatched to enforce what the Prime Minister called the 'rule of law.' At the time of writing, federal forces had established control of the state capital.

9.5 Conclusion

The COVID-19 pandemic has already posed immense political, economic, and social challenges in Ethiopia. It has stalled a political process that was hoped to transform the country into a democratic state. It has undone progress made in terms of poverty reduction. It has also shown some major flaws in the design of the Ethiopian federal system. Yet not everything is doom and gloom. There is unprecedented debate on traditional and social media on the design and future of the country's federalism among academics and the people at large. This indicates the growing awareness of, and public interest in, matters relating to the country's federal system.

Notes

1 The original nine states were Tigray, Afar, Amhara, Oromia, Somali, Hareri, Gambella, Benishangul-Gumuz, and Southern Nations and Nationalities and Peoples (SNNP). The tenth state, the Sidama was created in June 2020.
2 In its establishing proclamation, this authority was called 'Ethiopian Food Medicine and Healthcare Administration and Control Authority. Food, Medicine and Health Care Administration and Control Proclamation 661 (2009) and Food and Medicine Administration Proclamations 661(2009) and 1112(2009).
3 State of Emergency Proclamation Enacted to Counter and Control the Spread of the COVID-19 and Mitigate Its Impact Proclamation No 3 (2020).
4 A Regulation issued by the Council of Ministers to implement the State of Emergency Proclamation 3(2020).

Bibliography

Addis Standard, 2020. Tigray Region Declares State of Emergency to Prevent Spread of #COVID19 [online]. *Addis Standard*, 26 March. Available from: https://addisstandard. com/news-alert-tigray-region-declares-state-of-emergency-to-prevent-spread-of-covid19/ [Accessed 12 March 2020].
Ayele, Z., 2014. *Local Government in Ethiopia: Advancing Development and Accommodating Ethnic Minorities*, Baden-Baden-Nomos Verlagsges.
Ayele, Z. and Fessha, Y., 2012. The Place and Status of Local Government in Federal States: The Case of Ethiopia. *African Today*, 58 (4), 89–109.

Bundervoet, T., Abebe, G. and Wieser, C., 2020. Monitoring COVID-19 Impacts on Firms in Ethiopia: Results from a High-Frequency Phone Survey. *World Bank Group*, 6 June. Available from: http://documents1.worldbank.org/curated/en/939631591634604256/pdf/Results-from-a-High-Frequency-Phone-Survey-of-Firms.pdf [Accessed 12 March 2021].

Constitution of the Federal Democratic Republic of Ethiopia, 21 August 1995. Chapter 6, Article 51(15), Article 51(18), Article 62(1), Articles 82–84, Article 93, Article 93(1)(b), Article 102.

Dabalen, A. and Paci, P., 2020. How Severe Will the Poverty Impacts of COVID-19 be in Africa? *World Bank*, 5 August. Available from: https://blogs.worldbank.org/africacan/how-severe-will-poverty-impacts-covid-19-be-africa [Accessed 07 August 2020].

Dione, O., 2020. Tackling the Impacts of COVID-19 Is Imperative to Ethiopia's Journey to Prosperity [online]. *World Bank*, 29 October. Available from: https://blogs.worldbank.org/africacan/tackling-impacts-covid-19-imperative-ethiopias-journey-prosperity [Accessed 14 December 2020].

Ethiopian Reporter, 2020. የሥራ ፈጠራ ኮሚሽን በኮሮና ወረርሽኝ ምክንያት በሚሊዮኖች የሚቆጠሩ ሥራዎች ሊታጡ እንደሚችሉ ሥጋቱን ገለጸ (The Federal Job Creation Commission Fears that Millions of Jobs Could Be Lost Due to COVID-19). Ethiopian Reporter, 26 July. Available from: https://www.ethiopianreporter.com/article/19417 [Accessed 12 March 2021].

FDRE, 2013. Ethiopian Public Health Institute Establishment Regulation 301, Article 6.

FDRE Council of Constitutional Inquiry, May 2020. Recommendations on Constitutional Issues that the House of Peoples Representatives Sent to the CCI in Relation to the Postponement of to the 6th General Elections due to COVID-19 (የኢ.ፌ.ድ.ሪ የሕግ መንግስት አጣሪ ጉባኤ የኢ.ፌ.ድ.ሪ የሕዝብ ተወካች ምክር ቤት በሆገራችን በኮቪድ-19 ወረርሽኝ ምክንያት 6ኛውን ጠቅላላ አገራዊ ምርጫ አስመልክቶ ለሕገ መንግስት አጣሪ ጉባኤ በላከው የሕገ መንግስት ትርጉም ጥያቄ ላይ የቀረበ የውሳኔ ሃሳብ (አዲስ አበባ: ግንቦት 2012)). Available from: https://www.cci.gov.et/?lang=en [Accessed 12 March 2021].

Fiseha, A., 2007. *Federalism and the Accommodation of Diversity in Ethiopia: A Comparative Study.* Nijmegen: Wolf Legal Publishers.

Fiseha, A. and Ayele, Z., 2017. Concurrent Powers in the Ethiopian Federal System. *In*: Steytler, N., eds. *Concurrent Powers in Federal Systems: Meaning Making and Managing.* Leiden: Koninklijke Brill NW, 241–260.

Ministry of Health, 2021. የበሽታው ስርጭት በከተሞች (Spread of the Disease in Cities) [dataset]. *Federal Democratic Republic Ethiopia*. Available from: https://www.covid19.et/covid-19/ [Accessed 14 December 2020].

Proclamation 661, Federal Democratic Republic of Ethiopia 2009, Article 4(15), Article 52(2)(c).

Proclamation 1097, Federal Democratic Republic of Ethiopia 2018, Article 27.

Proclamation 1112, Federal Democratic Republic of Ethiopia 2019, Article 72(2).

Samuel, G., 2020. State Avails Stimulus Package to Rescue Banking Industry: The Gov't Avails 15 Billion ETB to Banks through the National Bank of Ethiopia. *Addis Fortune*, 28 March. Available from: https://addisfortune.news/state-avails-stimulus-package-to-rescue-banking-industry/ [Accessed 7 September 2020].

UN Ethiopia, 2020. *Socio-Economic Impact of COVID-19 in Ethiopia.* Addis Ababa: UN Ethiopia. Available from: https://reliefweb.int/sites/reliefweb.int/files/resources/UN%2520Socio-Economic%2520Impact%2520Assessment%2520-%2520FINAL%2520DRAFT%2520%2520-%252014May20.pdf [Accessed 29 July 2020].

Wakjira, K., 2017. Institutionalization of IGR in the Ethiopian Federation: Towards Cooperative or Coercive Federalism? *Ethiopian Journal of Federal Studies*, 4 (2), 121–160.

WFP, World Food Programme, May 2020. *WFP Ethiopia Market Watch: Food Security Analysis.* Available from: https://reliefweb.int/sites/reliefweb.int/files/resources/WFP%20Ethiopia%20Market%20Watch%20-%20May%202020.pdf [Accessed 8 September 2020].

10 Germany's response to COVID-19

Federal coordination and executive politics

Sabine Kropp and Johanna Schnabel

10.1 Introduction

Germany was praised for its effective management of the first wave of the COVID-19 pandemic, which occurred from March to May 2020 (e.g., Oltermann 2020). Overall, infection and death rates remained relatively low, and hospitals were never overwhelmed. The second wave, however, hit Germany much harder. The country lost the gains made in the first wave in handling the crisis. Infection and death rates escalated in November and December 2020, and governments struggled to bring them down. Some hospitals had to stop admitting patients into emergency care. Despite several shutdowns, Germany's economy did reasonably well, however.

After the first cases occurred at the end of January 2020, the first measures by governments in Germany were introduced in March 2020. They were similar to those in most other countries: bans on gatherings and events; closures of schools, restaurants, (non-essential) shops, and other premises; travel restrictions and closing of international (and some domestic) borders; procurement of protective personal equipment (PPE), ventilators, and tests.

After a relaxation of most measures in summer, another partial lockdown was imposed in November, when the second wave hit, eventually turning into a hard lockdown including night-time curfews in hotspots (i.e., districts with a high incidence rate). In addition to these containment measures, a range of economic stimulus measures were adopted, such as support for businesses, tax cuts, and a furlough scheme.[1]

Although Germany is a rather centralized federation (Kaiser and Vogel 2019), the distribution of powers in the event of a public health crisis puts most responsibility on the *Länder*, Germany's constituent units. The *Länder* decided on the introduction and easing of most measures. However, they coordinated their decisions, under the leadership of the federal government – especially in the beginning of the crisis and again, after a bumpy start, during the second wave. Rather similar measures were introduced, though the specifics and the timing varied. Coordination occurred mostly via the Conference of the Premiers of the *Länder* (*Ministerpräsidentenkonferenz* or MPK), which met frequently with the chancellor. Despite an, overall, coordinated approach to crisis management (Marx 2020), the *Länder* competed in lifting restriction measures in June. Some *Länder* also deviated from agreements with the federal government at the beginning of the second wave in October. Balancing fundamental rights and health protection, administrative courts overturned some measures. This further increased regional variation.

DOI: 10.4324/9781003251217-10

The heavy reliance on *Länder* action to contain the virus does not mean that the federal government was inactive. Besides coordinating *Länder* decisions, the federal government procured PPE and had to bear the bulk of the economic and fiscal burden. Major friction has not occurred, even though disagreements took place about the easing of measures. During the second wave, further tightening of restrictions caused some tensions. The crisis has not led to a shift of authority either. It mainly confirmed the emphasis on coordination and collaboration characteristic of German federalism (Hegele and Behnke 2017; Kropp 2010; Lhotta and von Blumenthal 2015). However, the important role played by the *Länder* was rather unusual. It met a widespread attitude of German citizens expecting to find uniform solutions throughout the country, even if problems vary regionally.

10.2 COVID-19 in Germany: phases and data

The first COVID-19 case was reported on 28 January 2020, in Bavaria, after an infected businessperson returned from a trip to China. Within six weeks, infections spread rapidly across all 16 *Länder* – though Bavaria, Baden-Württemberg, and North Rhine-Westphalia were more severely affected than the other *Länder*. During the first wave, infection rates peaked at the beginning of April, with 6,174 confirmed cases. By 10 January 2021, Germany, the 19th largest country in the world by population (Worldometers 2021), had the 9th highest total number of COVID-19 cases: 1,908,527 (Table 10.1). The highest seven-day-average of new German cases per day was 25,612 on 22 December 2020 and was on a downward slope to 6,723 on 15 February 2021 – 39th in the world for its seven-day average of new cases (Table 10.2).

The number of deaths in Germany from COVID-19 was 65,829, 10th highest in the world (Statista 2021). The case-fatality rate on 14 February 2021 was 2.8 percent, the 6th highest in the world (Table 10.3).

Table 10.1 Key Statistics on COVID-19 in Germany as of 10 January 2021

Cumulative Cases	Cumulative Cases per 100,000 Population	Cumulative Deaths	Cumulative Deaths per 100,000 Population	Case Fatality Percentage
1,908,527	2,277.9	40,343	48.2	2.1

Source: World Health Organization Weekly epidemiological update – 12 January 2021. Geneva: WHO, 2021. Available from https://www.who.int/publications/m/item/weekly-epidemiological-update

Table 10.2 Cases of COVID-19 in Germany as of 15 February 2021

Germany	
Total Cases – February 15, 2021[a]	2,352,756
New Cases – February 15, 2021[a]	5,132
Seven-day avg New Cases – February 15, 2021[b]	6,723

a Total cases and new cases source: https://coronavirus.jhu.edu/map.html
b Seven-day-avg new case source: https://www.google.com/search?client=firefox-b-d&q=world+coronavirus+statistics+data

Table 10.3 Case-Fatality Ratio and Total Deaths in Germany

Germany	
Case-fatality ratio – February 14, 2021[a]	2.8%
Total deaths – February 15, 2021[b]	65,829

a Case-fatality ratio source: https://www.dw.com/en/as-germans-continue-to-circulate-covid-death-rate-rises/a-56240918
b Total deaths source: https://coronavirus.jhu.edu/map.html

Measures were taken early enough to contain the virus effectively, albeit with some delay. It took some time until governments realized the dynamics triggered by an exponential increase of infections. Minor time lags were caused by the need to coordinate the crisis responses. Due to the hard restrictions adopted on 16 March 2020, the curve flattened significantly. The measures were eased in late April. During the second phase, in summer, the number of infections dropped to about 300 new cases, sometimes even fewer, a day. Trust in government and among citizens was reasonably high and even increased during the first months of the pandemic (Kühne et al. 2020). Surveys revealed that a majority of the citizens either supported the measures adopted or even wanted harder restrictions (see infratest dimap 2020).

In September, the number of infections grew rapidly again. Restrictions were tightened. In late October, after the number of infections had reached more than 18,000 cases a day, Germany finally entered another partial lockdown, which included the closure of restaurants and bars (except for take-away), hotels, sport clubs, and gyms as well as restrictions on gatherings and contacts. Schools and shops remained open. Measures were renewed and further tightened in late November. Nevertheless, the second partial lockdown failed to generate the desired effects. The incidence rate remained high, though with considerable regional variations.

At the beginning of December 2020, Germany had seen more than 1 million registered infections and bemoaned more than 17,000 deaths.[2] Hospitals still had some capacity for treatment, but capacities started to max out due to staff shortage. Therefore, a stricter lockdown was decided on 13 December, which included the closure of non-essential shops, hair salons and barber shops, schools (or move to online teaching), and childcare centers as well as stricter social distancing rules. These measures applied, in a first instance, until 10 January 2021 – with some lifting over the Holidays, to be decided by each *Land* and depending on infection rates.

While decisions were made rather smoothly during the first wave, the management of the second wave was more difficult. On the one hand, education ministers were blamed for failing to prepare the schools, during the summer break, for a second wave. On the other hand, the *Länder* governments were more hesitant to tighten restrictions when containment measures became increasingly contested. One measure was particularly criticized. Right before the fall break, statutory orders, adopted months before, had to be implemented unexpectedly. These regulations stipulated that as of an incidence rate of 50 infected persons (out of 100,000 inhabitants) in a given county, travelers from this county could not stay in hotels and apartments outside their *Land*. The effect was a *de facto* ban on travel within the federation, right during holiday time. In addition, Germany witnessed a considerable number of demonstrations against the restriction measures. Even though motivations and attitudes of the protesters differed, a significant share of this movement is linked to the extreme right. As a consequence, some *Länder* governments in Eastern Germany (particularly Thuringia, Saxony, Saxony-Anhalt) were hesitant to impose stricter measures. In these *Länder*, citizens tend to be more skeptical of state intervention and the share of seats won by the right-wing party known as Alternative for Germany (*Alternative für Deutschland* or AfD) in *Länder* parliaments is large. The reluctance of governments in the Eastern *Länder* to tighten restrictions faded in late November 2020, however, after Saxony and Thuringia had become extreme hotspots with counties having an incidence rate of more than 600.

The economic costs caused by the crisis were tremendous. The GDP decreased by approximately 5.0 percent in 2020. After a quick recovery during summer, economic growth came to an end again in November. The federal government adopted several large support packages to assist businesses, individuals, and families and to stimulate the economy. This included various kinds of subsidies as well as a temporary VAT reduction. Two stimulus packages, adopted in March and June, amounted to an impressive €156 billion (March) and €130 billion (June) or 4.9 percent of GDP and 4 percent of GDP, respectively (IMF 2021). During the second lockdown, the federal government generously compensated lost profits of restaurants and hotels, including one-off financial assistance set at 75 percent of revenues in November and December 2019 ("*November und Dezemberhilfe*"). The *Länder* focused on SME and the self-employed providing direct support and loan guarantees.

After years of budget surpluses, public debt will be the highest in Germany's postwar history (see *tagesschau* 2020). As of September 2020, the federal debt increased by 20.3 percent (€241.5 billion) within one year, while the debt of the *Länder* grew by 9.1 percent (€52.4 billion). Public spending of all levels of government exceeded the previous year's level by 26.9 percent (BMF 2020). The "black zero," a metaphor for Germany's constitutional debt brake (Articles 109, 115 of the Basic Law), was suspended for 2020 and 2021. Germany's fiscal rule can be temporarily suspended in the event of "unusual emergency situations beyond governmental control and substantially harmful to the state's financial capacity" (Article 109, paragraph 3, Basic Law), which the *Bundestag* decided on 25 March 2020. It is not an overstatement to assume that the fiscal burden will cause conflicts about how to readjust distributive justice as a basic principle of the German welfare state.

10.3 COVID-19 and federalism in Germany

10.3.1 *General features*

Germany's federal system comprises the federal government and 16 constituent units, called *Länder*. It can be described as a prime example of cooperative and interlocking federalism (Kropp 2010), which is bolstered by a strong unitary culture and pressures for harmonization. Centralizing trends can be observed in the legislative sphere, but not in the administrative sphere (Kaiser and Vogel 2019). But even if responsibilities have shifted to the federal level, this did not cause centralization in the classical meaning, that is, activities are not concentrated under the federal authority. Indeed, the *Länder* participate in federal legislation via the second chamber, the *Bundesrat*, which consists of the *Länder* governments.

The main feature of Germany's interlocking federalism is administrative federalism, due to a functional distribution of power (Behnke and Kropp 2020; Hueglin and Fenna 2015), whereby the *Länder* implement federal legislation as their own responsibility and at their own cost. When federal legislation directly affects them, for instance, because they must implement or (co-)finance policies, the Länder have a power of veto ("consent laws," about 40 percent of all federal legislation) because a majority of votes (which are counted *en bloc* for each *Land*) is needed in the *Bundesrat*. Complex negotiations between the federal government and the *Länder* are common and often involve *Länder* governed by different parties than those in power at the federal level.

As a consequence of interlocking federalism, there is a strong emphasis on coordination and collaboration. Vertical coordination, between the federal government and the *Länder*, is needed given the functional distribution of powers. It is also required because the *Länder* participate in federal decision-making via the *Bundesrat*. The cooperative nature of German federalism is reflected in the ministerial conferences through which the federal government and the *Länder*, or the *Länder* themselves, coordinate a broad range of policies (Hegele and Behnke 2013, 2017; Lhotta and von Blumenthal 2015). The premiers of the *Länder* meet at least four times a year (as the *Ministerpräsidentenkonferenz* or MPK), of which two meetings include the German chancellor. In times of crisis, the frequency of meetings is higher. Alongside MPK, several policy-specific councils cover a range of policy areas such as education, economy, finances, and health (Hegele and Behnke 2013, 2017). Some of these conferences are purely horizontal institutions while others include the federal government.

The constitutional mandate to achieve equivalent living conditions, the absence of linguistic or ethnic pluralism, and a strong commitment to fiscal equalization have created strong pressures for harmonization and a general aversion to policy diversity. This has been a driver of both centralization and coordination.

10.3.2 Distributions of responsibilities during the pandemic

The governance arrangements in the event of a public health emergency confirm the main features of Germany's federal system. However, they give the *Länder* a much stronger role than its overall features would suggest.

The core piece of legislation is the Infection Protection Act (*Infektionsschutzgesetz*, IfSG, adopted in 2001), a federal law. The IfSG authorizes the *Länder* to impose restriction measures such as bans on gatherings or school closures in the event of a public health crisis. Although the *Länder* introduce measures by issuing statutory orders, which corresponds to administrative federalism, the situation somewhat deviates from the usual pattern. Under the IfSG, the federal government is able to coordinate crisis management, but it cannot decide on restriction measures. Indeed, the decision lies entirely with each *Land*. In contrast to other countries, Germany did not have a national stockpile of PPE run by the federal government. Yet, the federal government maintains the responsibility over borders and international travel.

In March 2020, the IfSG was reformed after proving insufficient to fight the pandemic. A first draft of the amended law would have authorized the federal health minister to issue statutory orders without the consent of the *Bundesrat*. It was widely regarded as a blunt attempt of the federal health minister to empower himself. Despite enormous pressure of time, the federal parliament, the *Bundestag*, was able to alter the draft so that parliament, not the government, would declare and end the 'epidemic situation of national scope.' The federal health minister was granted responsibilities, "considering the responsibilities of the *Länder*" (IfSG §5) though, to maintain the health sector. An evaluation clause was also included. Moreover, the provisions were to expire in April 2021. Thus, while the law empowered the federal health minister, it also aimed at setting narrow limits on executive action.

However, even the revised IfSG contained provisions that were not sufficiently specified. The courts again and again overturned restrictions on the grounds that they were not well-founded, appropriate, and effective. According to the "materiality principle" (*Wesentlichkeitstheorie*), which is a basic legal principle developed by the German Federal Constitutional Court, all relevant decisions, particularly those encroaching onto fundamental rights, must be made by parliament. Statutory orders are not sufficient. Consequently, the IfSG was reformed again in November 2020 (see IfSG 2000). § 28a now contains a list of specific measures that the *Länder* are allowed to take such as bans on events and gatherings; travel bans; the requirement to wear face masks; and the closure of shops and other premises. These measures are bound to specific thresholds (incidence of 35 or 50) and are subject to further conditions. *Länder* statutory orders are limited to a duration of four weeks. People must not be socially isolated. A reference to regional circumstances must be given. In that, the law explicitly denies uniform decisions which restrict citizens equally when regions are affected by the pandemic differently.

Counties and cities, which form part of the *Länder*, can also take measures to prevent and fight infections. They are either in charge of executing measures to prevent and fight infections decided by the *Länder* or act on their own responsibility. This includes testing and tracing, the closing of schools, and restrictions on gatherings and movements of individuals. Local health authorities, however, often suffer from staff shortage, which is why the federal armed forces can provide support. Hospitals are a shared jurisdiction, with the *Länder* notably being in charge of hospital planning.

Germany's public health agency, the Robert Koch Institute (RKI), is a federal government body. It operates under the Federal Ministry of Health. Its main tasks are to provide evidence; to advise the federal government; and to develop norms and standards for health protection and the containment of diseases. Although it is mentioned in the IfSG, the RKI has no monopoly on advising governments.

10.3.3 Implementation of measures

In the first phase of the first wave, coordination prevailed. Bans on gatherings and events; quarantine; shops; the closing of restaurants; the return to classroom teaching; and semester times at universities were all decided by the *Länder* – but only after discussion with each other and the federal government. Both the federal government and the Länder procured PPE when hospitals, care homes, and surgeries reported shortages. Temporarily, the *Länder* and local authorities competed in ordering masks and PPE, thereby driving the costs of already rare goods. Procurement by the federal government was coordinated with the *Länder*. While this could be expected, coordination occurred even in areas for which the federal government is responsible and could, in principle, have acted alone – such as borders. Sometimes, the federal government coordinated bilaterally with the relevant *Länder*.

The federal government adopted several economic stimulus measures (summarized above). Some measures included co-funding (e.g., *Kinderbonus*, day care) or were administered by the *Länder* (e.g., temporal help for small and medium-sized enterprises). The federal government also compensated local governments and the *Länder* for losses in revenues and assisted the Länder in supporting public transport. These measures sometimes led to the establishment of a formal intergovernmental agreement (*Verwaltungsabkommen*).

The only decisions that were not coordinated concerned the closing of schools – though a certain imitation effect materialized with Saarland being the first *Land* to do so on 13 March 2020, and the others following quickly thereafter. The federal government's decision to reopen borders to EU/Schengen members and the United Kingdom was not coordinated either. Mecklenburg-West Pomerania and Schleswig-Holstein decided to close their domestic borders without consulting the entirety of the *Länder*. None of these decisions led to serious intergovernmental conflict, however.

In the easing, or second, phase of the first wave, coordination persisted. For instance, the *Länder* reached agreement with the chancellor that larger events would still be banned. Overall, fewer decisions were coordinated, however, and fewer intergovernmental meetings were held. This can be explained by the declining infection and death rates, and it never really undermined crisis management or led to serious intergovernmental conflict. In fact, policy diversity remained relatively small. Some tensions could be observed when (some of) the *Länder*, particularly Thuringia, Saxony, or North Rhine-Westphalia, pushed for an easing of restrictions while the federal government, especially the chancellor, as well as Bavaria and Mecklenburg-West Pomerania, were more hesitant. Eventually, the federal government gave in, but agreement that the *Länder* would lift restrictions on their own was reached mainly because the *Länder* had given the federal government no choice. Rather than intergovernmental or partisan disagreement on crisis management, these tensions mainly related to upcoming elections in six *Länder* and the 2021 federal elections. For example, with the leadership of the CDU up for grabs and chancellor Angela Merkel (CDU) not running in the 2021 federal elections, the crisis provided an opportunity for the premiers of two of the largest *Länder* – Armin Laschet (CDU) in North Rhine-Westphalia and Markus Söder (from CDU's sister party CSU) in Bavaria – to gain visibility and credit.

In October, in light of an increasing number of infections, conflicts within the MPK became evident. The federal government insisted on hard restrictions again. The chancellor was not able to convince all premiers that recommendations were insufficient to flatten the curve, however. Tensions also occurred between the reluctant premiers and those who wanted a stricter lockdown. Although agreement to introduce a partial lockdown was finally reached in late October 2020, the *Länder* decided to deviate from the joint resolution. For example, some *Länder* decided to reopen hotels over Christmas. Others, for example, Bavaria and Berlin, reduced the number of persons that are allowed to meet privately.

Another episode also underlined the new assertiveness of the *Länder*. When a federal government draft resolution proposing further tightening of restrictions was leaked in late November 2020, the premiers bluntly rejected the federal government's plan. As a consequence, decisions were delayed at a crucial point of time. However, the pressure on the premiers to come up with a proposal of their own increased. In the end, the *Länder* had no choice but to suggest stricter measures. When it became clear that the partial lockdown was insufficient to avoid an escalation of infection and death rates, governments also quickly reached agreement to impose a full lockdown. This shows that Germany's intergovernmental relations deliver when swift and effective action is required.

Although coordination – closer at times and looser at others – prevailed throughout the pandemic, the *Länder* maintained their ability to tailor measures to local circumstances, which is one of federalism's main *raisons d'être* after all. Coordination did not produce uniformity but left scope for adaptation. For example, some *Länder* with higher exposure to the virus (e.g., Bavaria, Saxony) adopted stricter measures while others with lower infection rates (e.g., Schleswig-Holstein) were able to impose fewer restrictions. However, since October, the chains of infection could neither be traced by the overstrained local health offices nor could outbreaks be contained locally and regionally. The critical public opinion and the opposition parties, among them the Green Party, the Liberal Party and the Left Party, pushed for uniform measures and a centralization of health policy more emphatically than during the first wave of the pandemic. Federalism itself came under pressure.

10.3.4 Intergovernmental relations

The overall pattern of crisis management was coordination, which occurred both vertically, between the federal government and the *Länder*, and horizontally, among the *Länder*. The depth of coordination varied, however. Sometimes, agreement was reached that restrictions would be imposed or lifted, and sometimes coordination also included more specific aspects, such as specific limits or details on protective measures. But sometimes coordination just meant consultation (e.g., in regard to borders).

To coordinate their crisis management, the federal government and the *Länder* relied on existing forums, and especially the MPK. In the first phase of the first wave, the German chancellor and the premiers held weekly meetings, followed by joint press conferences. Decisions on primary and secondary education, including protective measures, were discussed by the Conference of Ministers of Education (*Kultusministerkonferenz*, KMK), and the Conference of Ministers of the Economy (*Wirtschaftsministerkonferenz*, WMK) coordinated the reopening of restaurants. All these conferences are institutions of the executive branch of government. The MPK was convened more frequently in times when problems grew more acute, while the body was rather inactive in summer when infection rates were low.

The Robert Koch Institute provided information necessary for decision-making on both levels of government (Kuhlmann 2020, p. 296). The *Länder* also established advisory boards. In addition, most governments resorted to the expertise of independent epidemiologists and sought economic, sociological, ethical, or legal expertise. Ultimately, federalism and decentralization functioned as an institutionalized learning tool, forcing the actors at all levels of government into a permanent discourse ('yardstick federalism,' Benz 2012). Conflicting research results were publicly debated, and (mostly preliminary) findings continually evaluated, leading to a revision of doctrines and measures, if necessary. An example is the debate on the effectiveness of face masks in containing the pandemic. Prescribing masks in the public as early as in April 2020, the city government of Jena succeeded in avoiding a further increase of the infection rate. This measure was subsequently considered as best practice. Later, masks were made mandatory throughout the country, with some regional variations though.

The crisis also revealed the inherent ambivalence of federalism as a learning tool. Learning also implies drawing lessons from failures, but failures can have dramatic consequences. For example, the premiers of Saxony, Saxony-Anhalt, and Thuringia refused to take strict measures at the beginning of the second wave. Later, they had to admit having been wrong in their evaluation of the exponentially increasing infection rates. In light of dramatic incidence rates and death numbers, the three *Länder* governments readjusted their initial course and adopted even harder restrictions than the other *Länder*. This example shows that self-rule may allow for serious errors of individual governments. In contrast to potential failures of centralized decision-making, the consequences of these errors are more contained, however. In Germany's unitary culture, there is often a criticism of trial and error, as institutionalized by federalism, as leading to a diversity of messages that would confuse citizens and undermine public support of the restrictions.

Opportunistic strategies that are deemed typical for federations (Bednar 2009) materialized throughout the pandemic, to some extent. For example, some premiers (e.g., Bavaria, Berlin) argued that the federal government should assume more responsibility; some waited until the MPK had taken measures, arguing that they were somehow obliged to follow. The federal government occasionally attempted to encroach onto the *Länder* responsibilities (i.e., on school policy), and *Länder* governments blamed each other for their failures. Federal politicians, such as the CDU/CSU party group leader in the *Bundestag*, demanded more fiscal engagement of the *Länder* in supporting the economy during the crisis, evoking the opposition of the entirety of the *Länder*.

Overall, strongly institutionalized intergovernmental bodies turned out to be a considerable advantage. These bodies can be convened immediately. Moreover, federal negotiations take place as an iterated game. Actors are usually able to take the interests and positions of others into consideration. This tended to decrease the level of conflict and helped contain defective strategies. Yet, during the second wave, it became apparent that even the MPK struggled to make the *Länder* comply with joint resolutions. Some *Länder* governments adopted deviating policies immediately after MPK meetings, concerning *inter alia* the reopening of schools, which is a core responsibility of the Länder and was highly contested.

10.4 Conclusions

Despite these issues, rather than hindering effective crisis management, Germany's cooperative federalism seems to have helped it. The decentralized approach to restriction measures meant that they could be tailored to local circumstances. The most severely affected *Länder* could impose stricter measures than others with fewer cases. Intergovernmental coordination ensured that decentralized decision-making nevertheless would not lead to contradictory measures or harmful policy diversity – which, in Germany, tends to have a negative connotation and is referred to as a "patchwork of measures." Federalism here functioned as a learning tool, forcing responsible actors and experts into permanent debates about what would be appropriate, effective, and legitimate action. Although this is a considerable advantage when knowledge is not consolidated, contradictory debates and diverging policies have partly unsettled the population and decreased trust in political leadership.

Similar to other federations (see chapters by Fenna, Freiburghaus, Mueller, and Vatter in this volume), executive federalism prevailed since parliaments, particularly on the *Länder* level, were side-lined for most of the pandemic. Consequently, some *Länder* parliaments demanded more veto powers. Berlin adopted a so-called "Covid-19 parliamentary participation law" (*Parlamentsbeteiligungsgesetz*) empowering the *Land* parliament to raise an objection against statutory orders or to change existing ones. The *Land* parliament must also agree to extensions of statutory orders affecting basic rights. Yet, it can happen that more parliamentary participation will finally be at the expense of effective crisis management.

The management of the COVID-19 pandemic did not substantially change federal relations. The pandemic revealed the importance of the *Länder* as providers of public policy, however, and the premiers gained importance and visibility. This does not mean that there was no discussion on the distribution of relevant powers, with some commenters and even politicians seeing a need to centralize powers so as to strengthen the role of the federal government. The crisis uncovered existing shortcomings in public service delivery at the *Länder* level, for instance, regarding digitalization in primary and secondary education. The advantages and disadvantages of federalism in times of a public health crisis were critically discussed, with the overall opinion being, during the first wave, that Germany's federal system has been rather conducive to its successful crisis response (Behnke 2020; Kropp 2020). This changed during the second wave. Federalism itself was criticized as being ineffective, rigid, and conducive to egoistic behavior by the *Länder* premiers. Intergovernmental cooperation, which has helped contain any solo efforts by the *Länder* governments, is likely to become more complicated when party competition intensifies.

Notes

1 The furlough scheme that was in used was the *Kurzarbeit* program, which had been in place before the COVID-19 pandemic to help companies prevent layoffs during temporary drops in sales of products or services.
2 At the end of December, the number of infections increased to 1,7 million and more than 33,000 deaths were recorded.

Bibliography

Bednar, J., 2009. *The Robust Federation. Principles of Design*. Cambridge: Cambridge UP.

Behnke, N., 2020. Föderalismus in der (Corona-) Krise? Föderale Funktionen, Kompetenzen und Entscheidungsprozesse. *Aus Politik und Zeitgeschichte*, 70 (35–37), 9–15.

Behnke, N. and Kropp, S., 2020. Administrative Federalism. *In*: Kuhlmann, S., Proeller, I., Schimanke, D. and Ziekow, J., eds. *Public Administration in Germany*. Houndmills Basingstoke: Palgrave Macmillan, 35–51.

Benz, A., 2012. Yardstick Competition and Policy Learning in Multi-level Systems. *Regional and Federal Studies*, 22 (3), 251–267.

BMF, December 2020. Current Economic and Financial Situation: Overview of the Current Situation. Available from: https://www.bundesfinanzministerium.de/Monatsberichte/2020/12/Inhalte/Kapitel-4-Wirtschafts-und-Finanzlage/ueberblick.html [Accessed 28 January 2021].

Hegele, Y. and Behnke, N., 2013. Die Landesministerkonferenzen und der Bund – Kooperativer Föderalismus im Schatten der Politikverflechtung. *Politische Vierteljahresschrift*, 54 (1), 21–49.

Hegele, Y. and Behnke, N., 2017. Horizontal Coordination in Cooperative Federalism: The Purpose of Ministerial Conferences in Germany. *Regional & Federal Studies*, 27 (5), 529–548.

Hueglin, T.O. and Fenna, A., 2015. *Comparative Federalism: A Systematic Inquiry*. 2nd ed. Toronto: University of Toronto Press.

IfSG, Infection Protection Action, 2000. Law for the Prevention and Control of Infectious Diseases in Humans, 20 July. Available from: http://www.gesetze-im-internet.de/ifsg/index.html [Accessed 23 November 2020].

IMF, International Monetary Fund, 2021. Stimulus Packages in 2020. Available from: https://www.imf.org/en/Topics/imf-and-covid19/Policy-Responses-to-COVID-19#G [Accessed 25 January 2021].

infratest dimap, 2020. ARD-DeutschlandTREND Extra "Corona measures": Representative Study on Behalf of ARD from November 5, 2020. Available from: https://www.infratest-dimap.de/umfragen-analysen/bundesweit/ard-deutschlandtrend/2020/november-extra-coronamassnahmen/ [Accessed 1 December 2020].

Kaiser, A. and Vogel, S., 2019. Dynamic De/Centralization in Germany, 1949–2010. *Publius: The Journal of Federalism*, 49 (1), 84–111.

Kropp, S., 2010. *Kooperativer Föderalismus und Politikverflechtung*. Wiesbaden: Springer.

Kropp, S., 2020. Zerreißprobe für den Flickenteppich? VerfBlog, 23 November. Available from: https://verfassungsblog.de/zerreissprobe-fuer-den-flickenteppich/ [Accessed 16 February 2020].

Kuhlmann, S., 2020. Between Unity and Variety: Germany's Responses to the Covid-19 Pandemic. *In*: Joyce, P., Maron, F. and Reddy, P.S., eds. *Governance in a Global Pandemic*. Brussels: IIAS-IISA, 291–304.

Kühne, S., Kroh, M., Liebig, S., Rees, J. and Zick, A., 2020. Zusammenhalt in Corona-Zeiten: Die meisten Menschen sind zufrieden mit dem staatlichen Krisenmanagement und vertrauen einander. DIW Aktuell, 49.

Lhotta, R. and von Blumenthal, J., 2015. Intergovernmental Relations in the Federal Republic of Germany: Complex Co-operation and Party Politics. *In*: Poirier, J., Saunders, C. and Kincaid, J., eds. *Intergovernmental Relations in Federal Systems. Comparative Structures and Dynamics*. Don Mills: Oxford University Press, 206–238.

Marx, I., 2020. Corona-Maßnahmen: Welches Bundesland regelt was wie? Tagesschau.De. Available from: https://www.tagesschau.de/inland/bund-laender-beschluss-uebersicht-101.html [Accessed 16 February 2020].

Oltermann, P., 2020. Germany's Devolved Logic Is Helping it Win the Coronavirus Race [online]. The Guardian, 5 April. Available from: https://www.theguardian.com/world/2020/apr/05/germanys-devolved-logic-is-helping-it-win-the-coronavirus-race [Accessed 20 November 2020].

Statista., 15 February 2021. Number of Coronavirus (COVID-19) Cases, Recoveries, and Deaths among the Most Impacted Countries Worldwide as of February 15, 2021. Available from: https://www.statista.com/statistics/1105235/coronavirus-2019ncov-cases-recoveries-deaths-most-affected-countries-worldwide/ [Accessed 16 February 2021].

tagesschau, 2020. Almost 2.2 Trillion Euros in National Debt [online]. tageschau, 22 December. Available from: https://www.tagesschau.de/wirtschaft/konjunktur/schulden-haushalt-deutschland-corona-101.html [Accessed 18 January 2021].

Worldometers.info, 2021. Countries in the World by Population, 2021 [online]. Dover, Delaware USA. Available from: https://www.worldometers.info/world-population/population-by-country/ [Accessed 16 February 2021].

11 Federalism and the COVID-19 crisis

Center-state apposite relations in India

Rekha Saxena

11.1 Introduction

The COVID-19 pandemic around the world has put both healthcare and federal structures to the test. A key feature of India's response to the COVID-19 outbreak has been the close collaboration and cooperation between the Union (central) and state governments. The pandemic has underlined the necessity for strengthening cooperative federalism since no single jurisdiction or level of government has the capability to deal with the crisis on its own. In India, as in most federations, the constitution lists healthcare a responsibility assigned to state governments. In extraordinary circumstances such as the outbreak of COVID-19, the constitution provides for the Union government to take the lead in coordinating between and supporting the states. The legal framework for these interventions is provided by two laws, the 1897 *Epidemic Diseases Act* and the 2005 *Disaster Management Act* (Table 11.1).

11.2 COVID-19 first wave in India

During the first phase of the pandemic, India began with a very stringent and rigid lockdown in the months of March-April-May 2020 and then in subsequent months, unlocking measures to protect the economy and prevent the livelihood crisis of Indians in itself invites a case study. As of January 2021, India stands as the seventh most affected country in the world if we consider the number of active cases country-wise. However, fatalities and total cases put India third and second respectively. While the recovery rate in India is on a persistent improvement rate (94.74 percent), the fatality rate is at 1.45 percent. The rise in active cases has varied across the states/UTs. From Maharashtra to Kerala to West Bengal and then to Delhi, the rise in caseload has continuously varied. The states/UTs with worst fatality rates have been Punjab (3.15 percent), Maharashtra (2.57 percent), and Gujarat (2.23 percent). As many as

Table 11.1 Key Statistics on COVID-19 in India as of 10 January 2021

Cumulative Cases	Cumulative Cases per 100,000 Population	Cumulative Deaths	Cumulative Deaths per 100,000 Population	Case Fatality Percentage
10,450,284	757.3	150,999	10.9	1.4

Source: *World Health Organization Weekly epidemiological update* – 12 January 2021. Geneva: WHO, 2021. Available from https://www.who.int/publications/m/item/weekly-epidemiological-update

DOI: 10.4324/9781003251217-11

13 states have witnessed their fatality rates higher than the national average. While Maharashtra has been the most affected states, the southern states of Karnataka, Andhra Pradesh, Tamil Nadu, and Kerala have followed with most affected states. Despite that, there is another level of variation when it comes to highest test positivity rate (percentage of tested people turning out to be positive for COVID-19 infection). Though Maharashtra with 16.29 percent still leads the pack, it is followed by the Goa (13.45 percent), Chandigarh (11.77 percent), Nagaland (9.96 percent), and Kerala (9.62 percent). However, highest number of tests per million population has been carried out the most into Delhi, Jammu and Kashmir, Andhra Pradesh, Karnataka, and Kerala (Business Standard 2020).

The Center has allowed the states to devise ways for the safe reopening of the schools and coaching centers post mid-October. However, such a move needed to be given a second thought given the high prevalence of COVID-19 infections among children in the states of Tamil Nadu and Andhra Pradesh. How viable would the unlocking measures be in improving the lives of the people would witness the test of times as continued transmission is still witnessed in the states of Kerala and Tamil Nadu due to careless attitudes among the people. The fifth round of India's unlockdown in October 2020, also called unlock 5.0, further extended the opening of activities in the fields of education, entertainment cinema, and business conferences. This was allowed at the time when the rise of COVID-19 cases was still high in many cities. Although the new cases of infection are still piling up, the country witnessed a decline in the case load compared to the previous months, especially during July, August, and September (Johns Hopkins Coronavirus Resource Center 2021). What is unique and uncommon in the case of India is the two varied line of measures adopted in dealing with the pandemic.

11.3 COVID-19 and federalism in India

The 1897 *Epidemic Diseases Act* constitutionally empowers both the central and state governments to regulate the spread of epidemic diseases. According to the act, the Union is empowered to take preventive steps with respect to epidemic diseases at ports of entry and exit. At the same time, it also empowers the state governments to take preventive and regulatory measures to curb the spread of epidemic diseases within their own jurisdiction. Consequently, the act enables states to impose bans on public gatherings, close educational institutions including schools, colleges, and universities, and instruct companies to devise work-from-home strategies within their territories. The state of Karnataka became the first to invoke the act and put the powers assigned under it into action on 11 March 2020. The states of Haryana, Maharashtra, Delhi, and Goa followed suit shortly thereafter. In due course of time, consequently, the central government also asked all the states to invoke provisions of section 2 of the act, so that health ministry advisories could become enforceable.

Another significant act is the 2005 *Disaster Management Act*. Constitutionally, Disaster Management is part of residuary power of legislation which according to Article 248 of the 1949 *Constitution of Indian* rests with the Parliament of India. While the 2005 *Disaster Management Act* was brought out through entry 23 of the concurrent list namely, "Social security and social insurance, employment and unemployment," it was framed to deal with disasters at both central and state levels. It was on 14 March that the Union government classified COVID-19 as a "notified disaster." The act empowers both the central and state governments to impose a complete lockdown and regulate movement of people.

In India, as in most federations, the constitution lists healthcare a responsibility assigned to state governments. In extraordinary circumstances such as the COVID-19 outbreak, the constitution provides for the Union government to take the lead in coordinating between and supporting the states. In hindsight, the initial response of the center, as evident from the pan-India imposition of the first and second phases of lockdown without making any consultation with State governments, had appeared to be centralizing. The all-pervasive notifications and guidelines issued by Union had only encroached upon areas strictly falling within the domain of the State (State list in 7th Schedule of the Constitution). This included the State government offices (Entry 41), hospitals (Entry 6), shops and markets (Entry 28), industries (Entry 24), agriculture (Entry 14), etc., the encroachment of which ultimately paralyzed State finances.

However, an argument can be made that gradually, through Prime Minister's video meetings with various Chief Ministers, Administrators and Lieutenant Governors, inputs and suggestion were sought from states. This signified the larger reinvigoration of leeway of the state. Moreover, when it comes to easing of restrictions and extending relaxations, lockdown 4.0 was different from the earlier ones. In contrast from the earlier lockdown phases, states were given greater autonomy, for example, with respect to classification of red, orange, and green zones, respectively. Furthermore, states could also seal their borders (e.g., UP, Haryana, and Karnataka) to restrict the entry of people from other states in order to contain the outbreak. With the onset of new phase Unlock 1.0 from 1 June 2020, both center and state started to play a pivotal role in further opening up the economy with alacrity. More autonomy was extended to States in declaring any area as buffer zone within their territories and thereupon impose containment restrictions.

From the standpoint of executive federalism, it was fascinating to see India's attempt to handle this pandemic through an executive order, which has been in line with similar approaches adopted by many federal countries. All previously enacted laws have been used to deal with the situation. The Legislature did not come into the picture unnecessarily.

The more apprehensible understanding of federal framework requires light not only on extant division of powers between center and states but also on available laws for containing the outbreak. In the majority of the federal countries, including India, the constitution lists healthcare as a responsibility of state governments, but during pandemics, when the life of citizens is at stake, the central government takes up an upbeat role as witnessed in the event of lockdown which in turn, however, has exacerbated the economy. Since 'economic and social planning' is in the concurrent list, it is the central government that assumed responsibility for the overall management of the economy amidst this lockdown.

11.4 Responses to the first wave

The slugfest of efforts that various levels of governments have put in containing the pandemic is in themselves noteworthy. The central government has persistently widened the COVID-19 testing and made interventions in the economic sector to alleviate the growing public concerns. The announcement of a financial support package worth USD 22.6 billion to help people during the crisis was one of those interventions. This stimulus included free food grains and cooking gas for the poor for three months (which was later extended for another five months) and cash incentives to women and poor senior citizens for the same period.

The simultaneous efforts of the various states and the innovative ways that they adopted in dealing with the pandemic also call for appraisal. In terms of declaring relief measures, steps taken by the state governments reiterate the significance of a strong federal structure for effective governance. For instance, Kerala was the first state to announce an economic package of INR 200 billion (USD 2.6 billion). Yet another important initiative was taken by the state of Odisha even before COVID-19 cases started surfacing in the state. The state government reached out to people in smaller towns and villages asking everyone who had returned home since the outbreak of COVID-19 to self-quarantine at home – an estimated 84,000 people were put under home quarantine to contain the virus in the state. Furthermore, it created an online portal which all people entering the state were required to register with in order to facilitate contact tracing and health screening. Punjab Government's micro-containment and house-to-house surveillance strategy in tackling the outbreak received plaudits from Prime Minister Narendra Modi, further asking the other states to replicate the same model (The Tribune 2020).

District administrations have also been very proactive in the context of the COVID-19 outbreak and its management. The efforts and initiates of Bhilwara district administration in Rajasthan and Dharavi Model of Maharashtra have stood out. The Bhilwara district administration adopted an aggressive approach to containing the spread of this virus. More than 2.2 million people were screened in Bhilwara. The district's success is attributed to the collective efforts of dedicated local officials and has encouraged the central government to embrace the 'Bhilwara model of containment' across the country, particularly in the most-affected districts in different states of India. In Dharavi, the Brihan Mumbai Municipal Corporation started to screen people on a massive scale by visiting houses and setting up fever camps in localities. Temperatures were taken by infrared thermometers, and blood oxygen levels were read by pulse oximeters. By screening about 0.4 million people helped in taking out suspect cases – some 15,000 – from the system. Among those suspected to be carrying the COVID-19 virus, those with symptoms were quarantined and subsequently tested. The ones who tested positive were sent to hospital isolation wards; those negatives remained at the quarantine centers for 14 days. While 'test-test-test' was the mantra of the experts, on ground in Dharavi, it was 'screen-test-screen-test.' This was at the heart of the Dharavi model. It showed how smart testing could be a way out of shortages of resources and kits (Kaur 2020).

The Agra city administration's proactive tactics in categorizing cases, rigorous testing, conducting door-to door surveys, and stringent quarantine procedures was proven to be effective. The city administration adopted the policy of preparing a list of people returning from foreign tours and classifying their family and other intimate contacts. The neighborhoods in which confirmed cases resided were designated 'hotspots,' with a 3-km radius containment zone established around them and a further 5-km radius area designated as a buffer zone. Signifying the spirit of cooperative federalism, the Union health ministry was highly engaged in supporting the administrations' containment plans. At least 2,000 health workers were found working constantly in fighting the outbreak, and over 3,000 ASHA (Accredited Social Health Activist) were enlisted to help with door-to-door surveillance of over 160,000 households comprising more than 1 million city residents. This did make Agra yet another case study for other states and cities to emulate.

But the crescendo of cooperative federalism was witnessed in COVID-19 case management in Delhi. With the exponential rise in infected cases in the month of June, taking Delhi into the grip of the pandemic, both Central Government and Government of NCT, jointly and unitedly, came together in ameliorating the situations in Delhi (PTI 2020).

During the lockdown, the pandemic also provided much impetus to intergovernmental collaboration. Over the period of three months, multiple video conferences took place between the prime minister and the chief ministers. While affirming their support for an extended lockdown, states also sought for additional financial support from the central government to alleviate their own challenging fiscal situations. Time and again, Prime Minister acknowledged the collective decision-making that had gone into extending the lockdown till the month of May.

11.5 Moments of intergovernmental contentions

However, in between lockdown, the decision by state of Kerala to allow limited reopening of restaurants and local public transit brought it into conflict with the Union Ministry of Home Affairs which considered such measures violative of lockdown guidelines. Furthermore, in developing a more graded understanding of the COVID-19 situation across the country, the Union Ministry of Home Affairs also identified some districts where the spread was "especially serious." These places included seven districts in the state of West Bengal, Delhi, and Indore in Madhya Pradesh, Pune, and Mumbai in Maharashtra. Inter-Ministerial Central Teams were sent to these places to assess and suggest additional mitigation measures. However, the state government of West Bengal raised objections to Centre's interventions, having lack of clarity on deploying these teams under the 2005 *Disaster Management Act*. Without clarifying the criteria for the basis of selection of those districts in West Bengal, the state government opined those measures violative of the spirit of federalism.

During unlock 3.0, the center took a grim view of relentless restrictions issued by most of the states on interstate and intrastate movement of people and goods. Such curbs, according to the Center, only created roadblocks in economic activity as well as employment. Thereupon, Ministry of home Affairs expressed concerns to all the states and UTs over local level restrictions imposed by latter that curtailed the movements of people across various districts. The Chief Secretaries of the states were warned not to go against paragraph 5 of the unlock 3.0 guidelines of the central government and were told not to restrict interstate and intrastate movements (Express News Service 2020).

Come unlock 4.0, local lockdown could not be imposed by the states/UTs beyond the containment areas without the prior approval of MHA. Furthermore, no restrictions on the interstate and intrastate movement of the people and goods was to be strictly adhered to. This provision was also extended to the cross-border trade between states and neighboring countries. Most importantly the provision of e-permit or e-pass for the movement across the state and states was to be done away with (The Hindu 2020).

The coordination, determination, and maintenance of standards of higher education is bestowed upon University Grants Commission (UGC) in India. In pursual of its duties and functions, in the month of July, the UGC released its guidelines for the conduct of final year examinations in the country. These guidelines were prepared by an expert committee whose perspicacity recommended the conduct of terminal semester/final year examinations, by universities/institutions by the end of September 2020 in offline (pen and paper)/online/blended (online and offline) mode. Such a decision by the UGC brought objections from multiple quarters. Not only students but many state governments condemned the guidelines and took the matter to the Indian Judiciary (NDTV 2020).

The State Governments of Maharashtra and Delhi attempted to cancel the examinations by invoking the 1897 *Epidemic Diseases Act* and the 2005 *Disaster Management Act*. However, UGC was of the view that these acts could not be invoked to make the statutory provisions of the *University Grants Commissioner Act* inconsequential. The decisions by respective states could have affected the standards of higher education. This was considered by the UGC as an encroachment on the legislative field of coordinating and determining the standards of higher education-exclusively reserved for Parliament under Schedule VII of the Constitution. The Supreme Court in its ruling on 28 August 2020 held that state governments would not be allowed to promote students without holding final year university examinations amid the COVID-19 pandemic. However, the Court gave states the discretion to approach the UGC for an extension of the deadline by which final year exams should be completed (Mahajan 2020).

Furthermore, the tussle between center and states continued over the conduct of medical entrance exam NEET and engineering entrance JEE. The center extended full autonomy to National Testing Agency (NTA) which is a premier, specialist, autonomous and self-sustained testing organization of central government to conduct entrance examinations for admission/fellowship in higher educational institutions (NTA 2021). NTA went on to conduct the exams after months of postponement inviting a call for further postponement from many states.

West Bengal Chief Minister Mamata Banerjee urged all Chief Ministers to collectively move the Supreme Court to postpone the NEET and JEE citing the safety of students. Thereupon, seven chief ministers of non-BJP ruled states decided to jointly move the Supreme Court on the issue. Among the chief ministers who attended the meeting were West Bengal's Mamata Banerjee (TMC), Maharashtra's Uddhav Thackeray, who is heading the Shiv Sena-NCP-Congress government, Punjab's Amarinder Singh (Congress), Jharkhand's Hemant Soren (JMM), Rajasthan's Ashok Gehlot (Congress), Chhattisgarh's Bhupesh Baghel (Congress), and Puducherry's V Narayanasamy (Congress). However, NTA wrote to the state governments to extend support in local movement of the candidates so that they could be able to reach their examination centers on time. Despite states' apprehension about the spread of infection, with judgment of Indian judiciary in its favor, NTA conducted the exams successfully. The state inadvertently supported the conduct of exams. Health secretaries were asked to help NEET officers. District Magistrates and cops were asked to ensure ease of movement and manage crowds as well as maintain law and order. The whole episode of conflict between center and state turned into a story of coordination and cooperation for protecting the future of the students (Gosh 2020).

11.6 Mapping the road ahead

India is receiving appreciation worldwide for its handling of the outbreak considering its vast population density but there were criticisms regarding the hasty imposition of a nationwide curfew-like Lockdown. From federal perspicacity, the outbreak could have been dealt in a better way by consulting the states from the very beginning. Instead of an abrupt lockdown, a few days' time would have allowed industries and manufacturers to make alternative arrangements. Most importantly, migrant workers and citizens should have been given deadline to go back to their homes a time bound manner.

Moreover, it would have been more appropriate to transfer funds from PM-CARES and PM RELIEF FUND to state governments on the basis of population and intensity of COVID-19 cases in respective states. Income tax rebate should have been extended to contributions made to chief minister's fund. Most importantly, instead of having informal meetings, forum of Inter State council should have been used by setting up a standing committee to deal with it.

Furthermore, gross fiscal deficits of the states are estimated to be more than 7 percent for the 2020–2021 fiscal year (Reuters 2021). This is very much evident from the fiscal stress that the states have been grappling with, in the current cataclysmic environment. All of the states have been running through the 'scissors effect' incurring both loss of revenue due to economic slowdown and higher expenditure in containing the outbreak. COVID-19 has rendered the old-school backward-looking tax buoyancy forecasting models unreliable thus making the upcoming years for the states cumbersome. And since the growth is likely to be on downhill, tax revenues for the states are likely to be reduced in the coming years as the tax revenue fall sharply in comparison to the GDP. The existing scissors effect would only be prolonged as a result of heavy spending on health. There would also be a shoot in the contingent liabilities (guarantees). The resultant abeyance of future investment projects will eventually bring about growth losses (Mathew 2020). Thus, given the extent of economic damage that the states have already suffered in the last five months, it is more than appropriate *inter alia* for the Center to release past GST compensation dues as part of emergent fiscal stimulus. States' capacity to borrow should be enhanced but unconditionally.

Overall, the experience from the ongoing pandemic has only put forward the systemic importance of federal setup in the neoteric world. While federalism as an operational apparatus has been in place prior to the outbreak, its significance has increased ten-fold in recent times; eventually calling for the efficient coordination between the various levels of the government in order to tackle a cataclysm of current kind. Although there has had been instances of greater centralization with respect to the functioning of center government in containing the pandemic, nonetheless, without the coordination and cooperation between various levels of the government, containment would not have been particularly possible.

Moreover, instructions have been issued by the Center to the state governments to not pursue any secluded plans for vaccination. Such an instruction was extended to ensure effective rollout of the vaccine drive in the entire country. To authorize this, an expert committee on vaccine administration was set up by the central government that would supervise the vaccine rollout. Timely adherence of the directives was expected on the part of state government to ensure the efficacious coordination.

Although it may seem centralizing on the surface however, this was to pave way for proper planning, coordination and cooperation with respect to vaccine roll out. Thereupon, we could gauge another instance of cooperative federalism and cooperation between center and state in containing the outbreak (The Hindu 2020).

In one of meetings with heads of States and UTs, Prime Minister Narendra Modi himself underscored the pertinence of cooperative federalism which according to him would be seen as a hallmark in containing the outbreak in times to come. Thereupon, it is imperative that irrespective of the distribution of roles and responsibilities, all the levels of government are required to work in close coordination with each other in the spirit of cooperative federalism – a *sine qua non* to overcome the current crisis.

Bibliography

Business Standard, 2020. DATA STORY: India's Share of Global Active Covid-19 Cases Shrinks to 1.89% [online]. 10 December. Available from: https://www.business-standard.com/article/current-affairs/data-story-india-s-share-of-global-active-covid-19-cases-shrinks-to-1-89-120121000400_1.html [Accessed 25 March 2021].

Express News Service, 2020. Unlock 3.0: Centre Asks States Not to Put Restrictions on Inter-State Movement of People, Goods [online]. The New Indian Express, 22 August. Available from: https://www.newindianexpress.com/thesundaystandard/2020/aug/22/unlock-30-centre-asks-states-not-to-put-restrictions-on-inter-state-movement-of-people-goods-2186974.html [Accessed 25 March 2021].

Gosh, P., 2020. JEE-NEET: Nationwide Protest, Appeal to Supreme Court [online]. *India.com*, 27 August. Available from: https://www.india.com/news/india/jee-neet-nationwide-protest-appeal-to-supreme-court-ordinance-to-tweak-admission-rules-states-mull-way-out-4123115/ [Accessed 25 March 2021].

Johns Hopkins Coronavirus Resource Center, 2021. COVID-19 Dashboard by the Center for Systems, Science, and Engineering (CSSE) [dataset]. Available from: https://coronavirus.jhu.edu/map.html [Accessed 25 March 2021].

Kaur, B., 2020. At the Heart of Dharavi Model: Basic Public Health, Resolve in Community to Beat COVID-19 [online]. *DownToEarth*, 12 August. Available from: https://www.downtoearth.org.in/news/health/at-the-heart-of-dharavi-model-basic-public-health-resolve-in-community-to-beat-covid-19-72771 [Accessed 25 March 2021].

Mahajan, S., 2020. States Cannot Promote Students without Holding Final Year Exams, May Approach UGC Seeking Extension of Deadline: Supreme Court [online]. Available from: https://www.barandbench.com/news/states-cannot-promote-students-without-holding-final-year-exams-ugc-supreme-court [Accessed 25 March 2021].

Mathew, G., 2020. Explained: How Has Covid-19 Affected Finances of State Governments? [online]. 30 October. Available from: https://indianexpress.com/article/explained/explained-how-covid-19-has-affected-finances-of-state-governments-6906683/ [Accessed 25 March 2021].

NDTV, 2020. States Can Not Confer Degrees Without Exams: UGC to Supreme Court [online]. 19 August. Available from: https://www.ndtv.com/education/ugc-guidelines-news-states-cant-decide-confer-degrees-without-exams-july-6-directive-not-diktat-ugc-sc [Accessed 25 March 2021].

NTA, National Testing Agency, 2021. About NTA. Available from: https://nta.ac.in/about [Accessed 25 March 2021].

PTI, 2020. People, Govts Together Attained Victory Over COVID-19, Fight Not Yet Over: Kejriwal [online]. The Hindu, 25 July. Available from: https://www.thehindu.com/news/cities/Delhi/people-govts-together-attained-victory-over-covid-19-fight-not-yet-over-kejriwal/article32189894.ece [Accessed 25 March 2021].

Reuters, 2021. India's Fiscal Deficit Likely to Be Over 7% in 2020/21. *The Economic Times*, 7 January. Available from: https://economictimes.indiatimes.com/news/economy/indicators/indias-fiscal-deficit-likely-to-be-over-7-in-2020/21/articleshow/80152964.cms?from=mdr#:~:text=The%20final%20fiscal%20deficit%20estimates,for%20the%20next%20financial%20year [Accessed 26 March 2021].

The Hindu, 2020. State Gears Up for Unlock 4.0 [online]. 30 August. Available from: https://www.thehindu.com/news/national/andhra-pradesh/state-gears-up-for-unlock-40/article32482356.ece [Accessed 25 March 2021].

The Hindu Special Correspondent, 2020. Vaccine Distribution: Work in Tandem with Centre, Health Ministry Tells States. *The Hindu*, 3 November. Available from: https://www.thehindu.com/sci-tech/health/vaccine-distribution-work-in-tandem-with-centre-health-ministry-tells-states/article33014514.ece [Accessed 25 March 2021].

The Tribune, 2020. PM Modi Asks Other States to Adopt Punjab's COVID-Combat Model [online]. 16 June. Available from: https://www.tribuneindia.com/news/punjab/pm-modi-asks-other-states-to-adopt-punjabs-covid-combat-model-of-micro-containment-house-to-house-surveillance-100045 [Accessed 25 March 2021].

12 The impact of the pandemic on the Italian regional system

Centralizing or decentralizing effects?

Francesco Palermo

12.1 Introduction

Italy has been severely affected by the COVID-19 pandemic, with a proportionately high number of infections and even bigger mortality rate, due to the large amount of elderly people (22.7 percent of the residents being over 65 years, the highest percentage in Europe). As of 31 December 2020, of a population of about 60 million, slightly more than 2 million people had been infected, with about 75,000 casualties. The impact was extremely uneven among the territories in the 'first wave' (February to June), with the overwhelming majority of the cases being concentrated in just a handful of regions in the north of the country. These areas are the more industrialized parts of the country and hence more exposed to trade with foreign nations. In the 'second wave,' that started in October, the distribution of the infection was far more uniform and affected the whole territory in a similar fashion.

Italy's territorial design comprises 20 Regions, 5 of which have special status and powers (Arban, Martinico and Palermo 2021). Regions are responsible for a wide range of areas including, in particular, organizing and delivering health care (Cicchetti and Gasbarrini 2016). The country's territorial setup has been under discussion since its inception. Its hybrid configuration, in between a full-fledged federal system and a unitary country, has evolved over the last seven decades with a steady expansion of regional powers. When the pandemic reached the country, in early 2020, Italy was facing several transformations in its regional system, which on one hand were put on hold due to the emergency, but on the other raised new concerns and proposals for (counter-) reforms.

The chapter illustrates the legal framework put in place at the national (state) and the subnational (regional) level to face the health emergency and the policy challenges raised or amplified by the pandemic affecting the territorial organization. After a first phase of extreme centralization of powers, the regions (and to some extent the municipalities) gradually resumed their functions. The asymmetric impact of the virus

Table 12.1 Key Statistics on COVID-19 in Italy as of 10 January 2021

Cumulative Cases	Cumulative Cases per 100,000 Population	Cumulative Deaths	Cumulative Deaths per 100,000 Population	Case Fatality Percentage
2,257,866	3,734.4	78,394	129.7	3.5

Source: World Health Organization Weekly epidemiological update – 12 January 2021. Geneva: WHO, 2021. Available from https://www.who.int/publications/m/item/weekly-epidemiological-update

DOI: 10.4324/9781003251217-12

and the equally asymmetric response by the territories revealed both the potential of such an asymmetric territorial governance and the weaknesses of an incomplete, quasi-federal system, especially as far as unclear division of powers and insufficient intergovernmental relations (IGR) are concerned (Table 12.1).

12.2 Facts and legal framework

Italy has been the first European country to be hit by the coronavirus pandemic and to declare the state of emergency, imposing a strict lockdown. After the first, dramatic moments in March and April, it managed to keep the contagion under control until the spread of a new wave of epidemic in the fall and the winter. On 31 January 2020, far ahead of any other European country, the state of emergency was declared by the national government for a period of six months, subsequently prolonged for further periods of six months each.

The constitution does not regulate the state of emergency in detail. It provides however that, "in case of necessity and urgency," the government may adopt "law decrees," that is, "temporary measures having force of law" which are valid for no longer than two months unless they are in the meantime adopted as formal laws by Parliament (art. 77). The state of emergency was declared based on a statutory, not a constitutional provision, the 2018 *Civil Protection Act*, which empowers the government to adopt "any necessary measure" within the limits of the "general principles of the legal system." In the course of 2020, 26 such legislative measures have been enacted, 22 regulations (decrees of the Prime Minister), and several administrative provisions by individual ministries, by the national civil protection and by the commissioner against the COVID-19 emergency (Italian Government, 2021).

What is striking about the legal response to the pandemic is that, in the initial stage, when the emergency was acute, the rules that had been adopted were nearly all national despite the fact that the impact of the virus has been extremely uneven among the regions. Conversely, when the spread of the virus became more uniform as of the fall, the response was more attentive to regional autonomy and to the need to tailor the measures to the socio-economic and health-care conditions of the different regions.

12.2.1 *The initial strong centralization*

Initially, the north was hit much more than the south: until September 2020, Lombardy, which accounts for one sixth of the national population (10 million), had about two fifths of the total number of infections (110,000) and almost half of all casualties (over 17,000). Conversely, some southern regions have been very marginally affected: Calabria (2 million people) had 2,000 cases and 98 deaths and Basilicata (560,000 inhabitants) registered just 920 cases and 28 deaths, as of early October. Despite such differences as well as the fact that health care is a regional power, the early call for the state of emergency massively concentrated the decision-making in the national government. The detailed national provisions applied with no exception on the whole national territory and the margins for the regions were limited to the small niches deliberately left open by the national rules, allowing regions to adopt more restrictive provisions than the national ones, but preventing them to be less strict in any area. The regions were consulted prior to the adoption of national regulations, but consultation was rather a formal exercise, as they cannot oppose measures taken for the overarching sake of protecting public health and national security. As a matter of fact, between March and May 2020, the Standing Conference between the State and the Regions, the prime body for cooperation between the levels of government, which expresses (mostly non-binding) opinions on national legislation when regional interests are affected, met (online) only twice a month, that is, less than in normal times (Cortese 2020).

The regional governors (who are directly elected by the people in all but two Regions or autonomous Provinces and thus bear a significant political weight) were allowed to adopt their own regulations, although only to the extent that was permitted by the national legislation or to introduce stricter rules than the national ones. For example, Regions could determine the distance that people could walk from home, whether walking a dog was allowed, and little more. The national government was adamant in opposing regional attempts to take own initiatives: when in February, the governor of Marche, a region in central Italy that by then had not a single case of infection, declared his intention to close schools, he was called by the Prime Minister during the very press conference. The regional act was immediately challenged before the administrative court and suspended. In general, however, the Regions did not show special interest in being proactive at that stage, as this would have meant conflict with Rome and a degree of responsibility that normally Regions are not ready to take.

Centralization was also conditioned by the heavy hand of the central government on the measures to tackle the devastating economic impact of the pandemic. The 2020 national budget has devoted 179 billion euros (75.3 being additional debt) to tackle the crisis. The lion's share went to subsidies for companies (69.3 billion), followed by support for families (53.3 billion) and for jobs (34.5 billion). Other significant funds were provided for public health system (8.3 billion), regions and municipalities (6.4 billion), public services (5.4 billion), and social subsidies (1.5 billion; Italian Government 2020).

In sum, during the first months, the response to the emergency was characterized by strong centralization of powers both horizontally (from parliament to the government) and vertically (from the Regions to the center). The national regulations formally stressed the need for a better coordination among the levels of government, which in the end meant steering from the top down (Betzu and Ciarlo 2020). Especially in the first phase of the emergency, in March and April, such centralization was generally supported in the political and the public discourse. The main newspapers sharply criticized the attempts by some Regions to introduce small changes, even when this was allowed by national legislation. Conversely, more rigid regional measures were generally applauded, such as in the case of southern Regions further limiting the movement of people returning home from the north.

12.2.2 *Decentralization reappears*

Things started to change at the beginning of May, when the number of new infections dropped, the pressure on the health system was less acute, and the national government eased the lockdown. In that moment, the role of the Regions grew in proportion to the lifting of the national regulations, and subnational actors came back in the picture. Paradoxically, however, more normality did not bring clearer rules, but rather the opposite. This is because the business of government did not fully go back to the constitutional routine, as national emergency rules, while more limited, remained in place. This produced a growing number of conflicts since the Regions started to assert their own constitutional powers and acknowledged that the public health situation was very different across and within the Regions. The Regions sometimes deliberately challenged the national government for political reasons, with the Regions led by center-right parties (two thirds of the total) stronger opposing the center-left majority in Rome, after a short period of political ceasefire. As a matter of fact, while some regional provisions were suspended, others with the same content were not, further increasing legal uncertainty.

A few Regions started to adopt own laws, especially on economic support for companies and for sorting out bureaucratic issues (payments and the like). However, only the autonomous province of Bolzano/Bozen (South Tyrol), the northernmost territory predominantly inhabited by a German-speaking minority and ruled by the party representing such minority, made use of its broader autonomy and passed a law on 8 May, providing the complete restart of activities ahead of the rest of the country. The national government initially challenged part of the law before the constitutional court, but soon withdrew the lawsuit. South Tyrol was also the only Region that engaged in cross-border activities during the closure of borders: thanks to special bonds and institutionalized cooperation with Austria and particularly with the Land Tyrol, it succeeded in negotiating some exceptions to the prohibition of trans-frontier movement and a few people from South Tyrol could be hospitalized in Austria at the peak of the pandemic. It also served as a bridge when it negotiated with Austria the supply of face masks imported from China and distributed a share of them to the rest of Italy, when there was a nation-wide shortage.

While regional legislation remained limited, a flood of regional (over 1,000) and (countless) municipal provisions was passed, raising criticism for adding confusion rather than clarity (Scaccia and D'Orazi 2020). Many regional measures addressed economic activities (re-opening of pubs, restaurants, hotels, and other businesses), sport events (authorization and admission of the public), leisure (in some Regions discos were reopened during the summer, in others they were not), transport (number of persons allowed in regional trains and busses), or public health measures (some Regions introduced obligatory tests for persons travelling from abroad and even from other Regions). The conflict potential was aggravated by a certain confusion in the distribution of emergency powers: when it comes to the adoption of "urgent measures to counter sanitary and public hygiene emergencies," these can be taken by the mayor (art. 50.5 d.lgs. 267/2000), by the regional governor (art. 32.3 law 833/1978), and by the national government under the national state of emergency (d.lgs. 1/2018). This overlap of powers, coupled with the proliferation of "insufficiently coordinated" (Baldini 2020, p. 985) national and regional measures, made it very difficult to clearly understand who was responsible for such measures. A rather dramatic case occurred in Sicily, as the regional governor ordered to evacuate the hotspots for migrants, which were overcrowded due to an influx of migration from Africa in the summer and could not meet the sanitary restrictions. The national government opposed that migration is within exclusive national jurisdiction and suspended the provision, the Region challenged the suspension in the administrative court and eventually lost the case.

12.2.3 Second wave and new conflicts

The picture became more complex when, in October, the second wave of the pandemic hit the country, with even more severe effects in sanitary terms. Unlike in the first phase, the outbreak affected all Regions to a relatively similar degree, exacerbating the problems of some regional health care system (especially in the South) with lower reaction capacity.

Learning from the experience of the first wave, the national government' approach was more open to regional differentiation. The new round of measures was focused especially on the economic consequences of the pandemic, providing for massive financial interventions to support companies, small business, and families, also in view of the funds that were agreed upon at EU level (an impressive total of € 1.8 trillion in the whole Union). When new restrictions were imposed, the different conditions of each territory were considered, and a broader margin of regional intervention was allowed, while keeping the general rule according to which national provisions could be derogated only to adopt stricter but not softer measures.

Within the framework laid down in national legislation, Regions could decide on many significant aspects such as closing of schools, local transport, and freedom of movement within the regional territory. This created a more differentiated normative picture, with at times a patchwork of confusing regulations with a number of paradoxical outcomes. For example, in several Regions (especially in the South), schools remained closed for much longer than in others, due to fears that the weak regional health care system could not sustain a growing number of infections as well as to the inability to reorganize public transportation in a way that could accommodate all students while keeping the social distance. An extreme and somewhat funny example of normative overlap and confusion was the unilateral decision of a regional health authority in September to ban a professional football team of the first division from travelling to another region to play a match because a few players were tested positive, disregarding the special protocol negotiated by the national government and the football league which regulates such cases for the sake of regularly playing the championship.

Unlike in the previous phase, the new national measures were taken in accordance with the Regions. The main body in charge of intergovernmental relations – the Standing Conference between the State and the Regions – was summoned much more frequently and was involved in the adoption of all decisions. In spite of that, neither the degree of political confrontation nor the legal uncertainty decreased. A telling example is the law adopted by the autonomous Region of Aosta Valley in November, indeed very similar to the one of South Tyrol from May. The national government challenged the law in the constitutional court, which first suspended its effects and later (February 2021) struck it down in its entirety simply (and simplistically) arguing that Regions have no power to adopt such laws as the jurisdiction on international prophylaxis belongs exclusively to the State (judgment no. 37/2021).

Similarly, also policy responses at regional level have been subject to volatile political dynamics. No clear pattern as to effective or ineffective strategies in coordination and cooperation can be traced along party politics. Rather, it seems that other factors determine to what extent regional (and local) governing practices are more or less dependent on and affected by the national level. These include the very different fiscal capacities among the Regions, deep differences in health care models (Toth 2014), capacities in regionalized administration, and political personality of regional governors. The regional elections in seven Regions in September 2020 (Veneto, Liguria, Tuscany, Marche, Campania, Puglia, and Aosta Valley) confirmed the mandate of the governors who performed well during the first wave and/or profiled themselves as champions of a clear approach to fight the pandemic, be it advocating stricter rules such as school closure and curfews or supporting the economic sector by calling for more openings of bars, restaurants, and other economic activities.

12.3 Pandemic and reforms: COVID-19 as an accelerator?

When the COVID-19 pandemic hit Italy, the country was about to celebrate the 50th anniversary of the establishment of Regions in the whole territory. Prior to 1970, only five, so-called special Regions existed in its periphery, making Italy the state that has the longest-lasting regional (as opposed to federal) system in place worldwide (since 1948). After several transformations which over more than seven decades enhanced the powers of Regions, time was ripe for reconsidering the territorial structure of the country. Furthermore, three sizeable and economically as well as politically strong Regions in the north, Lombardy, Veneto, and Emilia-Romagna were about to conclude agreements with the national government on the transfer of additional legislative powers (and connected funds) in a long and significant list of areas, from environmental protection to education, from airports to labor security and protection, from foreign trade to disaster management and others. This procedure is provided for by the constitution (art. 116.3) since 2001 but has not been activated thus far. The process was stalled due to the pandemic, and ironically, these regions have been the more affected by the virus, which raised the question as to whether more regional autonomy is desirable or to be opposed (Malo 2020). Finally, a constitutional reform was voted in a national referendum on September 20, which reduced the size of both chambers of the national parliament, this way further limiting the already feeble link between the Senate and the regions and making it politically more difficult to table a reform of the Senate transforming it into a regional representation (Vuolo 2020), a proposal that has been on the agenda for decades but could never be implemented so far.

The pandemic will strongly impact on these ongoing reform processes. Institutional consequences cannot be expected in the short run, as the sanitary and the subsequent economic emergencies are prevailing, and there is no consensus on the territorial design of the country. Proposals have been put forward to include provisions on the state of emergency in the constitution, following the Spanish model (Ceccanti 2020), but the chances for such a reform seem rather limited in the short term. For sure, however, the emergency has revealed the main weaknesses of the Italian regional system: the unclear division of powers between the center and the Regions; the weak intergovernmental relations; and the high degree of asymmetry in powers, administrative capacity, and political strength among the regions (Clementi 2020, who adds the relations between government and parliament at national level).

As to the division of powers, a constitutional reform adopted in 2001 has increased the role of the Regions but has created a number of overlaps and conflict potential (Arban, Martinico and Palermo 2021) and above all has by no means enhanced the "federal spirit" (Burgess 2012), making Italy "a federal country without federalism" (Palermo 2012). Rather, in the political and academic debate, sentiments against regional autonomy are overall on the rise. Like after the economic crisis around 2010 (Valdesalici 2014), the pandemic has confirmed that the division of powers is not sound enough to resist a moment of crisis, and in fact, it amplified the ongoing debate between advocates for more centralization and advocates for more autonomy, with the former being prevalent in the political and also in the academic debate. In particular, the existence of 21 regional healthcare systems, very different as to their effectiveness in service delivery, is sharply criticized and might be subject to pressures for recentralization.

With regard to IGRs, the absence of a territorial chamber and the structural weakness of the existing bodies for intergovernmental cooperation, and notably of the Standing Conference, reduced regional involvement to a mere formality when the center appropriated all powers at the peak of the emergency. In such moments, when stronger coordination is required, the role of mechanisms that effectively represent the voice of the subnational entities becomes crucial. When these mechanisms are ineffective, as in the case of Italy, joint decisions simply become top-down impositions, and the involvement of Regions becomes mere lip service. This happened also when territorial interests were taken into more account, as it was ultimately a national decision to do so. Inefficiency of multilateral IGR mechanisms encourages the more powerful regions to engage in bilateral negotiations thus accentuating the asymmetry inherent in the design of the territorial setup and arousing jealousy among the Regions.

The strong asymmetries, *de jure* and *de facto* (Watts 2008) already existing among the Italian Regions, have become ever more visible and acute with the pandemic. The regional performance in tackling the emergency, especially in the area of health care, has been mixed. Some Regions have done extraordinarily well, despite the severe cuts over the past decade due to the debt-cutting policies, while others made serious mistakes, such as placing COVID-patients in elderly homes (Giarelli and Vicarelli 2020). The differences in performance were reflected in the political sphere, with some regional governors increasing their popular support and others losing it.

In sum, COVID-19 put the existing tensions between calls for further decentralization and for re-centralization under the spotlight and amplified them. At the same time, the ongoing reform processes will be significantly impacted, and their trajectory will not be the same as it would have been without the pandemic. The main pressure is no doubt for a certain degree of re-centralization of public health, which is almost entirely in the hands of the regions and makes up over 80 percent of the regional budgets. Even though most Regions reacted well, the dominant discourse underlines the existing big differences in terms of services, resources, and performance, and it is not likely that the opportunity will be seized to introduce a stronger control by the national government (Ciardo 2020). For some reason, the dominant attitude in both politics and academia on one hand fears that regional differentiation might impair the equal protection of social rights, but on the other hand, it trusts that national legislation is per se better and safer, although comparative practice seems to prove the opposite (Palermo 2020).

Some reforms in the Italian regional system are indeed necessary, and the pandemic made this ever more evident. As to the content of the reforms, however, opinions were all but unanimous before the pandemic and became even more divergent after it. The further diversion of opinions will probably slow down rather than speed up the necessary reforms and increase the conflicts between the center and the territories.

Bibliography

Arban, E., Martinico, G. and Palermo, F. (eds.), 2021. *Federalism and Constitutional Law: The Italian Contribution to Comparative Regionalism*. London: Routledge.

Baldini, V., 2020. Riflessioni sparse sul caso (o sul caos) normativo al tempo dell'emergenza costituzionale. *Dirittifondamentali.it*, 1, 979–985.

Betzu, M. and Ciarlo, P., 2020. Epidemia e differenziazione territoriale. *BioLaw Journal*, Special Issue (1), 201–208.

Burgess, M., 2012. *In Search of the Federal Spirit*. Oxford: Oxford University Press.

Ceccanti, S., 2020. Verso una regolamentazione degli stati di emergenza per il parlamento: proposte a regime e possibili anticipazioni immediate. *BioLaw Journal*, Special Issue (1), 71–78.

Ciardo, C., 2020, Il Servizio Sanitario Nazionale alla prova dell'emergenza COVID-19: il rischio di una sanità diseguale. *BioLaw Journal*, Special Issue (1), 227–238.

Cicchetti, A. and Gasbarrini, A., 2016. The Healthcare Service in Italy: Regional Variability. *European Review for Medical and Pharmacological Sciences* 20 (1 Suppl.), 1–3.

Clementi, F., 2020. Il lascito della gestione normativa dell'emergenza: tre riforme ormai ineludibili. *Osservatorio costituzionale*, 3, 33–47.

Cortese, F., 2020. Stato e Regioni alla prova del coronavirus. *Le Regioni*, XLVIII (1), 3–10.

Giarelli, G. and Vicarelli, G., 2020. Politiche e sistemi sanitari al tempo della pandemia da COVID-19: una lettura sociologica. *Sociologia italiana* 16, 69–86.

Italian Government, 2021. *Coronavirus. La normativa vigente* (Information on the Provisions Adopted to Counter the Virus and Its Effects). Available from: http://www.governo.it/it/coronavirus-normativa

Italian Government, 2020. *Documento di Economia e Finanza 2020*, Sect. III, Programma Nazionale di Riforma. Available from: http://www.dt.mef.gov.it/modules/documenti_it/analisi_programmazione/documenti_programmatici/def_2020/DEF_2020_Programma_Nazionale_di_Riforma.pdf

Malo, M., 2020. Le Regioni e la pandemia. Variazioni sul tema. *Le Regioni*, XLVIII (1), 231–234.

Palermo, F., 2012. "Italy: A Federal Country without Federalism?" *In*: Burgess, M. and Tarr, G.A., eds. *Constitutional Dynamics in Federal Systems. Sub-National Perspectives*. Montreal & Kingston: McGill-Queen's University Press, 237–254.

Palermo, F., 2020. Is There a Space for Federalism in Times of Emergency? *Verfassungsblog* (5) 13. Available from: https://doi.org/10.17176/20200513-133602-0.

Scaccia, G. and D'Orazi, C., 2020. La concorrenza fra Stato e autonomie territoriali nella gestione della crisi sanitaria tra unitarietà e differenziazione. *Forum Quaderni costituzionali*, (3), 108–120.

Toth, F., 2014. How Health Care Regionalisation in Italy Is Widening the North-South Gap. *Health Economics, Policy and Law*, 9 (3), 231–249.

Valdesalici, A., 2014. Features and Trajectories of Fiscal Federalism in Italy. *In:* Lütgenau, S.A., ed. *Fiscal Federalism and Fiscal Decentralization in Europe. Comparative Case Studies on Spain, Austria, the United Kingdom and Italy.* Innsbruck: StudienVerlag, 73–101.

Vuolo, A., 2020. L'insostenibile imperfezione del bicameralismo perfetto. *Diritto Pubblico Europeo – Rassegna Online.* Available from: https://doi.org/10.6092/2421-0528/6718.

Watts, R.L., 2008. *Comparing Federal Systems.* Montreal & Kingston: McGill-Queen's University Press.

13 COVID-19 and first wave response in Kenya

Rose B. Osoro

13.1 Introduction

The COVID-19 pandemic and its containment measures have had tragic impacts on both peoples' lives and their livelihoods, its far-reaching consequences have indelibly disrupted Kenya's economy and businesses. At the beginning of the year, the Kenya National Treasury (NT) had projected the country's economy to grow by 6.1 percent and 7.0 percent for 2020 and 2021 financial years. However, because of the economic impact of COVID-19, these figures have been revised downwards to 2.6 percent and 5.3 percent, respectively. As the situation in Kenya moves with the slow opening of the economy due to the continued indeterminable presence of the corona virus, the NT revised growth rates may just be but wishful thinking.

As of the 2019 Kenya's population and housing census, the country's population stands at 47.5 million consisting of 23.5 million and 24.0 million males and females, respectively, and is mainly composed of youthful populace with 12.1 million households (Kenyan National Bureau of Statistics 2019). Any intervention to mitigate the effects of the pandemic hence must be looked at through the lens of gender equity and youth as the COVID-19 confirmed cases have statistically disproportionately affected males and the youth. As of 27 July 2020, Kenya had registered a total of 17,975 confirmed cases with 285 deaths giving a case fatality rate of 1.6 percent. Of the 17,975 cases, 11,765 (65 percent) were recorded as males and 6,210 (35 percent) as females. Most of the cases, 5,855 (33 percent), were identified in the age group of 30–39 years. Of the total cases, 285 deaths were reported with 213 (75 percent) being males and 72 (25 percent) as females.

The statistics above invalidate previous notions and myths about COVID-19 in Kenya that the virus only affected the elderly; or that it was a "rich man's disease," and the claim that Africans may have a natural immunity against the disease (Table 13.1).

Table 13.1 Key Statistics on COVID-19 in Kenya as of 10 January 2021

Cumulative Cases	Cumulative Cases per 100,000 Population	Cumulative Deaths	Cumulative Deaths per 100,000 Population	Case Fatality Percentage
98,184	182.6	1,704	3.2	1.7

Source: *World Health Organization Weekly epidemiological update* – 12 January 2021. Geneva: WHO, 2021. Available from https://www.who.int/publications/m/item/weekly-epidemiological-update

DOI: 10.4324/9781003251217-13

13.2 Kenya's constitutional framework

Kenya ushered in a new political and economic governance system with the promulgation of a new constitution in 2010. The Constitution introduced a bicameral legislative house, devolved system of government, a constitutionally tenured judiciary, and an independent electoral body among other broad and sweeping changes. The first election under the new constitution was held in 2013. Devolution now in its second term is meant to continue to address governance, economic and development glitches arising from the former 'unitary' system that was viewed as highly centralized, undemocratic, and inequitable. Decentralization, known as *"Ugatuzi,"* remains the centerpiece of reform in Kenya and the most transformative aspect of the country's new constitution. Article 6 of the Constitution provides that the territory of Kenya is divided into the counties and that the governments at the national and county levels are distinct and interdependent and shall conduct their mutual relations on the basis of consultation and cooperation. Each level of government has delimited assignments on expenditures, revenues, and service delivery. The fourth schedule of the Constitution assigns 35 functions to the national government and 14 service delivery functions to the County governments. Constitutionally, functions relating to policy formulation, setting of standards and norms, and any residual functions not fall under the functional jurisdiction of the national government. In order to implement the delimited functions, the two levels of government have been under Article 209 mandated with imposition powers to raise revenues within their jurisdiction (Constitution of Kenya 2010).

Kenya's County governments are relatively autonomous and are represented at the national legislature by the Senate. The Senate's role is to represent and serve to protect the interests of the counties and their governments and to participate in all matters concerning counties; determine the allocation of national revenue among the counties and exercise oversight over national revenues allocated to the counties (Kangu 2015). There are 47 counties forming the territory of Kenya; christened *"48 Governments, 1 Nation."* The Judiciary and independent tribunals are shared functions.

The functions and provision of services of county governments have further been decentralized to the urban areas and cities within the counties (Kenya, G.o. 2012a). There is an existing legal framework that provides for the classification, governance, and management of urban areas and cities. It has been noted that Kenya is still at an early stage of urbanization, but by 2050, about half of the population are expected to be living in cities. Around 27 percent of Kenyans currently live in urban areas. The country is urbanizing at rate of about 4.3 percent per a year. That leaves 73 percent of the population still living in rural areas (World Bank 2015).

13.3 Transfer of functions and Nairobi city county as a decentralized unit

The Country's capital city Nairobi is classified as county number 47. Tensions have arisen with undertones that Nairobi City County ought to be under the jurisdiction of the national government due to the strategic position as the capital city. Recently, the governor under "duress," as he claimed later, signed off transfer of major functions to the national government. The Nairobi county government previously riddled with allegations of corruption and inefficiency has now been left with skeleton functions.

A new body, Nairobi Management Service (NMS) has taken over the running of the capital, and the leader has been given a seat in Cabinet at the national government executive. It is important to note that the national government's role and intervention in the counties' affairs are constitutionally constrained. The constitution dictates that while a function can be transferred from one level of government to the other for clear reasons, the constitutional responsibility for the performance of the functions shall remain with the government to which the functions are assigned by the constitution.

13.4 COVID-19 in Kenya

Africa reported its millionth COVID-19 case early August. It seems that the continent has weathered the pandemic relatively well with less than one confirmed case for every thousand people and 23,000 deaths (Nordling 2020).

Table 13.2 below shows continental confirmed cases of COVID-19 compared to Kenya as follows:

In comparison with world statistics, it was evident in the first wave; the virus had spared the continent of Africa.

In a country of over 40 million people, Kenya has also exceeded expectations. The Country had recorded 743 deaths as of the end of September compared to expert estimates of ominous figures (Ministry of Health Press Release 2020). Following a peak in July, the caseload rapidly abated. Kenyan epidemiologists predict a "long-tailed decline," meaning that the virus is here for the long run.

13.4.1 Emergency and intergovernmental structural interventions response to COVID-19

On 13 March 2020, just a day after the first case of COVID-19 was confirmed in the Country, the government gave directives that have been implemented through policy measures and behavioral protocols aimed at containing the spread of COVID-19. These directives were effected through a special gazette notice by the Cabinet Secretary in charge of health on 6 April 2020. The measures include suspension of learning in all educational institutions; social distancing through minimizing congestion in public transport, shopping malls, entertainment venues, and social gatherings; self-or compulsory quarantine; strict evaluation and monitoring protocol designed to proactively seek out and test persons who may have been exposed; daily nationwide curfew from 11 PM to 4 AM; and Cessation of movement in and out of Nairobi Metropolitan Area. These measures being emergency response were decided and coordinated by the national government with minimal input from the county governments.

Table 13.2 Total Number of Cases, Recoveries, and Deaths in Kenya and in Africa

Cases	Africa	Kenya	% Share
Confirmed cases	1,632,634	44,196	2.7
Recoveries	1,343,479	31,725	2.3
Deaths	39,357	825	2.1

Source: WHO, 16 October 2020

It is believed that support and compliance of county governments of the measures undertaken prevented widespread infections and averted the misery feared by specialist health leaders. The system, as fragile as it is, has not broken yet (Fielder 2020). That notwithstanding, other groups (Law society of Kenya, religious groups, and business-people) regarded the measures as punitive even to an extent of seeking judicial intervention to block execution.

One of the intergovernmental structural measures put in place to respond and cushion Kenyans from the adverse effects of the pandemic was the establishment of a National Coordination Committee on the Response to the Corona Virus Pandemic (NCCRCP). The committee, chaired by the Cabinet Secretary for the Ministry of Interior and Coordination of National Government with its several working groups including the National Economic and Business Response (NEBR), had the responsibility of availing information to facilitate formulation of appropriate strategies for intervention on socio-economic effects of the disease. The Committee's membership included Cabinet Secretaries in charge of Health, National Treasury, Foreign Affairs, Information and Communication Technology, Public Service, Defense, Agriculture, Attorney-General, Head of Public Service, the Council of Governors (CoG) chairperson, Principal secretary in charge of Interior, Chief of Staff Office of President, Chief of Defense Forces, Director-General National Intelligence Service, and Deputy Chief of Staff for Policy and Strategy.

Through its structure and composition, the NCCRCP was being spearheaded by the national government with a majority in membership with an assumption that County governments were adequately consulted and represented by including the CoG's chairperson to the committee. There has not been any overt complaint of under-representation or lack of consultation of county governments although many decisions of this committee were directly communicated by the national government.

The NCCRCP was established to provide a coherent national framework to respond to the pandemic, provide leadership, and policy guidance on the overall response to the pandemic among other functions. It has been the main coordinating agency on COVID-19 and has had support structures and coordination mechanisms in form of working groups namely:

- National Emergency Response;
- National Economic and Business Response;
- County Coordination and Food Security Committee;
- National Security Preparedness and Response Working Groups.

The NCCRCP together with its various working groups have jointly been able to improve coordination of reporting from the county level, provide daily media briefings, and impact assessment of public health interventions, train 91,557 health Care workers, sensitize 64,000 community health volunteers, validate 38 laboratories from an initial two, enhance resource mobilization, develop interim human resources for health protocols, and recruitment of additional staff for COVID-19 response.

In our view, the pandemic has strengthened the intergovernmental relations between the two levels of government in a cross-sectoral manner. For instance, the statutory intergovernmental apex body, the National and County Governments Coordinating Summit, comprising the president and the 47 governors has convened three Extra-Ordinary Sessions within six months of the pandemic unlike a once-a-year session previously. The first session was convened on 10 June 2020 by the president with all the governors to: Review effectiveness of the containment measure; Commit county governments to deliver isolation facilities with at least 300-bed capacity; and develop protocols for progressive reopening of the economy.

13.4.2 *Managing the COVID-19 crisis – fiscal measures*

The government has made a raft of fiscal measures to cushion citizens and businesses from the adverse effects of COVID-19 pandemic. This is through the implementation of a range of fiscal measures in the context of the Finance Act 2020. The fiscal measures were announced by the President on 25 March 2020 and later tabled in Parliament through the Finance Bill on 6 May 2020 for debate and approval. Most members for the first time attended the proceedings virtually in compliance with COVID-19 rules and regulations. It is worth noting that county governments did not introduce any new legislation on the revenue raising powers as a response to COVID-19.

The fiscal measures contained in the Finance Act 2020 were targeted to provide in the medium term the much-needed relief to the economy and necessitate additional disposable income to the people and businesses. These measures included: 100 percent Tax Relief for low-income earners; Reduction of both Income Tax Rate and Corporation Tax from 30 percent to 25 percent; Reduction of the turnover tax rate from the current 3 percent to 1 percent for all Micro, Small, and Medium Enterprises (MSMEs), and Appropriation of an additional cash transfer allocation to the elderly, orphans, and other vulnerable members of the society. The paradox of the government's tax relief measures is that some sectors of the economy have not been able to directly benefit as aspired.

The government further initiated an eight-Point Economic Stimulus Programme (ESP) which is currently under implementation in all the 47 counties (National Treasury 2020b). The eight-Point ESP is intended to stimulate growth and cushion families and companies during the COVID-19 pandemic. They include allocating additional resources to:

1 Hire local labor for rehabilitation of access roads and footbridges to alleviate the effect on the youth;
2 Ministry of Education to hire 10,000 teachers and 1,000 Information and Communication Technology interns to support digital learning and acquisition of 250,000 fabricated desks in preparation for reopening of learning institutions;
3 Fast track payment of outstanding VAT refunds and other pending payments to SMEs and provide seed capital for SME Credit Guarantee Scheme;
4 Hire additional 5,000 healthcare workers and expand bed capacity in public hospitals;
5 Supply of firm inputs through e-vouchers, targeting 200,000 small-scale farmers to alleviate food security and assist flower and horticultural producers to access international markets;
6 Soft loans to hotels and related establishments through Tourism Finance Corporation (TFC) and to engage 5,500 community scouts and to preserve 160 community conservancies;
7 Rehabilitate wells, water pans, and underground tanks in the Arid & Semi-Arid Areas. Additional allocation for flood control measures;

8   Enforce the "Buy Kenya Build Kenya" Policy through an allocation to purchase locally manufactured vehicles.

While the actual number of beneficiaries of the above interventions cannot be ascertained, there is optimism among citizens that something is actually being done.

13.4.3 *Social economic impact of COVID-19*

One of the notable outputs from the NCCRCP was the commissioning of a survey that was conducted by the National Bureau of Statistics (KNBS) to provide information on the effects of COVID-19 on interactions between social and economic factors. Interestingly, the survey showed a somewhat rosy picture of the state of the economic status of the citizens. Nationally, 78.1 percent of households reported to be food secure about 77.6 percent of the households reported having no challenges in accessing market/grocery store to purchase food items (Statistics 2020b). In normal circumstances, abundance of food means reduced prices. However, this was not the case. The survey found out that about four out of five (78.8 percent) of the households indicated having experienced an increase in food prices attributable to COVID-19 pandemic. Moreover, the fall in world oil prices and favorable weather conditions have contributed to the stability.

On the flipside, 59.2 percent of the respondents reported a change in their cost of travel due to the pandemic. Further, we observed that 14.4 percent of the respondents changed their main means of transport out of which 62.2 percent opted to walk while 19.4 percent opted to use "Boda Boda" (motorcycle taxis). There have been at least 1,716,706 job losses among the working population aged between 16 and 64 years between April and June 2020. The unemployment rate increased to 10.4 percent in the second quarter of 2020 compared to 5.2 percent recorded in the first quarter of 2020 (Statistics KNBS 2020a).

13.4.4 *Regional collaboration*

While there have been elaborate steps taken by the government to contain the spread of the virus, some of the initiatives taken have threatened to derail regional trade. Stringent measures adopted by Kenya do not tally with those of the neighbors leading to retaliatory actions. Regional trade has been paralyzed. The stand-off escalated when the Kenyan government announced the closure of its borders affecting negatively on regional trade. The borders are slowly opening up but possession of COVID-19 Free Certificate is still a requirement irrespective of the cost implications.

13.4.5 *Easing of the measures and a threat of the second wave*

As we write this toward the end of October 2020, some of the government measures have been lifted with partial reopening of learning institutions being the greatest leap. Interestingly, there is an unsettling trend emerging in the last week of October. There is an increase in the number of new infections eliciting feelings of a second wave. Hospitals have announced full capacity, and the field hospitals that had been established and not used before are being reopened. This is a worrying trend, and both levels of governments are on high alert (Figure 13.1).

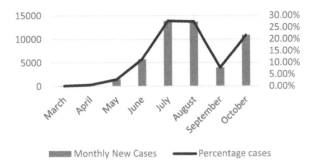

Figure 13.1 Monthly COVID-19 Cases from March until October 2020 in Kenya
Source: Cumulated weekly WHO numbers.

13.5 COVID-19 and devolution in Kenya

13.5.1 Coordination challenges and successes during the pandemic

As highlighted earlier, Kenya is a devolved state with two distinct and interdependent levels of government – national and county – that are required to conduct their mutual relations in a consultative and cooperative manner. The Constitution equally provides for a system of intergovernmental relations, including dispute resolution between and among the governments.

Other than 'The Summit,' legislation further provides for sectoral working groups and Committees to enable consultations between the national government line ministries and the county departments (Kenya, G.o. 2020c). Horizontal coordination, the Constitution provides for cooperation and relations amongst the 47 counties hence creating the CoG to provide a platform for consultations and sharing of information among the county governments (Kenya, G.o. 2020c). For instance, on vertical fiscal relations, the national Public Finance Management Act establishes the Intergovernmental Budget and Economic Council to provide a forum for intergovernmental consultations on financial matters (Kenya, G.o. 2012b). Despite the presence of an elaborate intergovernmental framework, during the pandemic, the system had largely been unresponsive, prompting re-emergence of other avenues of engagement such as NCCRP.

Health is a devolved function. There are however particulars of the function that are concurrent in nature as the two levels of governments have shared jurisdiction, collaboration, and joint tasks. The effective implementation of the health functions squarely therefore lies in the mutual collaborative and cooperative approach by the two levels of government. The national government is constitutionally allowed to legislate on health policy and national referral health facilities while counties are restricted to legislating in respect of county health facilities and pharmacies; ambulance services; promotion of primary health care; licensing and control of undertakings that sale food to the public; veterinary services excluding regulation of the profession. The public health system in Kenya is characterized by 0.04 doctors; 0.1 nurses and midwives; 0.8 beds per 1,000 inhabitants. The emergence of COVID-19 and the eminent spread has therefore decorously caused trepidation in both levels of government.

13.5.2 *County government initiatives and coordination*

The CoG on its own has equally held nine sittings and convened a virtual COVID-19 Conference, eight governors representing the CoG have through the intergovernmental processes been co-opted into committees of the NCCRCP just for the purposes of coordinating mitigating efforts toward COVID-19. The CoG through its leadership embraced the newly established intergovernmental structures established.

While the vertical intergovernmental structures have been coordinated through the national government, Counties through the CoG have equally established their own horizontal frameworks for engagement. All Counties have established Emergency Operation Committees co-chaired by Governors and County Commissioners (a representative of the National Government at County level) to enable effective coordination of County response.

The CoG similarly developed a model regulation to necessitate the establishment of a County Emergency Fund, to be adopted by county governments and facilitate mobilization of resources toward COVID-19 mitigation. The fund consists of all monies donated toward COVID-19 emergency response at the county level. As of 29 April 2020, all the counties had committed a percentage of their resources.

13.5.3 *Procurement of COVID-19 supplies and fiscal transfers' conflict*

Public procurement processes during this pandemic have come with their own complexities. County governments through legislation are required to procure medical supplies from the State-Owned Agency for economies of scale and effective regulation and standard control. There have been numerous calls for transparency in the procurement of COVID-19-related supplies without much success. Allegations of corruption through overpriced supplies are rampant, and concerned officers have appeared before parliamentary committees (Presidency 2018). Claims of high-level misappropriation of COVID-19 funds have been rife.

Remarkably, while there have been strengthened intergovernmental relations between the two levels of government in terms of coordination of processes and communication during the period, the greatest missing link has been resourcing of county governments.

As at the end of the 2019/2020 fiscal year in June, county governments had not received 9.4 percent worth of their equitable share of allocation which is in complete violation of the Constitution, and the Statutory Cash Disbursement Schedule approved by parliament (National Treasury 2020d). This amount was in addition to an extra allocation to the Counties as part of COVID-19 pandemic emergency response measures. Complexity in funding for the counties further arose out of the Senate's inability to pass the basis for revenue sharing among county governments. The Senate had a protracted dispute that eventually was brokered by the president and opposition leader. By the time the Senate approved the basis, it was two months into the new fiscal year (National Treasury 2020a). In October, three months into the new fiscal year, 50 percent of the expected quarterly allocation was disbursed. It is clear that delayed disbursement to county governments will muddle county capacity to address the pandemic adequately.

Notwithstanding the absence of intergovernmental transfers, the CoG has made significant strides toward the support of the most vulnerable in select counties through partnership with development partners. As of 15 October 2020, some of the notable efforts to mitigate the pandemic include: establishment of active quarantine facilities and testing in 34 counties; 43 counties have trained and sensitized 4,860 health care workers and 8,602 community health volunteers; implementation of home-based care in 34 counties for a total of 6,665 persons under the care in the month of September have recovered from the virus (Council of Governors 2020c). The development partners key support through the CoG included: Provision of dignity hygiene products for women in the reproductive age within quarantine/isolation facilities; supported six tele-counsellors for manning hotlines in three counties, and strengthened and enhance women, youth, and PWD participation and influence in COVID-19 response coordination at the County level. Of greater importance is the development of the COVID-19 County Socio-Economic Re-Engineering and Recovery Strategy (CCSERS). The strategy is expected to guide County Governments to jump-start their economies through targeted planning and budgeting for steady growth (Council of Governors 2020a). We believe that the CCSERS will provide a link with the national government through its entities hence strengthening the already visible intergovernmental relations. CCSERS offers an opportunity to assess the cross-sectoral relations beyond the health function which has been occasioned by the pandemic. While we might not draw a conclusion of the sustainability of the current strengthened intergovernmental relations between the two levels of governments, we believe that enhanced intergovernmental relations enables greater governments' outputs.

We note that both levels of government have the realization that efficient and timely testing is a vital prerequisite for early identification and reporting. This coupled with adequate contact tracing, isolation and quarantine of contacts are critical prevention measures in slowing down the spread of the pandemic. Mass testing has however not been implemented due to high costs involved, inadequate technology, and expertise required to conduct the tests. As of June 2020, the government reported that there were 25 laboratories readily available in the country with capacity to conduct the tests.

As of 18 October 2020, the Ministry of Health reported cumulated tests numbers at 621,976. It is our view that, with that level of testing, the national government can only gain traction in testing if county governments are capacitated and effectively resourced to assist in the process.

We have observed that COVID-19 has exposed weaknesses in the healthcare system that must be addressed going forward. Kenya's health system is made up of several systems notably, private, public, and faith based. The Public system is further divided into County and national government facilities. This calls for effective coordination between the two levels of government. These systems manifest a mismatch between available care and needs especially in critical specialist care. Kenya has only 537 intensive care beds and 265 ventilators to a population of 49 million. Further due to the pandemic routine activities have reduced such as antenatal care, deliveries, and immunization programs whose detrimental effects will be felt much later. The cost of managing COVID-19 is beyond the reach of average Kenyans who are economically poor and uninsured.

13.6 Conclusion

In conclusion, although no one yet knows the future for COVID-19, most experts agree that it is not going away anytime soon. COVID-19 crisis management has shown in some cases intergovernmental relations stood firm. Instances where there was national government obstruction, counties have innately responded horizontally by coming together and proactively standing up as governments. The role of each level of government therefore cannot be underscored. Intergovernmental relations both vertical and horizontal are of great consequence going forward. A collaborative and consultative environment between the two levels of government and among the 47 county governments is thus paramount.

Bibliography

Constitution of Kenya, 2010. *Constitution of Kenya*. Kenya Law. Available from: http://www.kenyalaw.org:8181/exist/kenyalex/actview.xql?actid=Const2010

Council of Governors, K., 2020a. *County COVID-19 Social Economic Re-Engineering Recovery Strategy, 2020/21–2022/23*. Available from: https://cog.go.ke/component/k2/item/211-county-covid-19-re-engineering-and-recovery-strategy-2020-21-2022-23

Council of Governors, K., 2020b. Statement on Preparedness of County Governments on COVID-19. Available from: https://www.cog.go.ke/cog-reports/category/109-covid-19; file:///C:/Users/user/Downloads/Press%20statement%20on%20preparedness%20of%20County%20Governments%20on%20COVID-19%20-%203rd%20September%202020.pdf

Council of Governors, K., 2020c. *Statement on COVID-19 Mitigation*. Council of Governors. Available from: https://www.cog.go.ke/media-multimedia/statements/category/109-covid-19?download=434:press-statement-on-preparedness-of-county-governments-on-covid-19-15th-october-2020-2020

Fielder, J., 2020. COVID-19 in Africa: Ground-Level View from a Clinician in Kenya-Why Are Cases Lower in Africa. *MedPage Today*. Available from: https://www.medpagetoday.com/infectiousdisease/covid19/89246

Judiciary, K., 2020. Milimani Law Courts Operations during COVID-19 Pandemic. Judiciary. Available from: https://www.judiciary.go.ke/download/public-notice-milimani-law-courts-operations-during-covid-19-pandemic/

Kangu, J.M., 2015. *Constitutional Law of Kenya on Devolution*. Nairobi: Strathmore University Press. Available from: https://press.strathmore.edu/uploads/journals/strathmore-law-journal/2SLJ1/2SLJ1_13Ke-Const-law-on-devolution-Kangu-TKabau.pdf

Kenya, G.o., 2012a. *County Government Act*. Kenya Law. Available from: http://www.parliament.go.ke/sites/default/files/2017-05/CountyGovernmentsAct_No17of2012_1.pdf

Kenya, G.o., 2012b. *Public Finance Management Act*. Kenya Law. Available from: http://kenyalaw.org:8181/exist/kenyalex/actview.xql?actid=No.%2018%20of%202012

Kenya, G.o., 2020c. *Intergovernmental Relations Act*. Kenya Law. Available from: http://kenyalaw.org:8181/exist/kenyalex/actview.xql?actid=No.%202%20of%202012

Kenyan National Bureau of Statistics (KNBS), 2019. *Kenya Population and Housing Census (KPHC)*. Available from: https://www.knbs.or.ke/?wpdmpro=2019-kenya-population-and-housing-census-volume-i-population-by-county-and-sub-county

Ministry of Heath, 2020. *Ministry of Health Press Releases*. Nairobi. Available from: https://www.health.go.ke/press-releases/

Mininstry of Health Kenya, 2020. *Targeted Testing Strategy for Corona Virus Disease 2019 (COVID-19) in Kenya*. Nairobi. Available from: https://www.hcalth.go.ke/wp-content/uploads/2020/07/Targeted-Testing-Strategy-for-COVID-19-in-Kenya.pdf

National Treasury, K., 2020a. *County Governments Cash Disbursement Schedule for FY 2020–21*. National Treasury. Available from: http://www.parliament.go.ke/sites/default/files/2021-08/schedule%20of%20cash%20disbursements%20to%20counties%20FY%202021-2022.pdf

National Treasury, K., 2020b. *Draft 2020 Budget Review and Outlook Paper*. National Treasury. Available from: - http://ntnt.treasury.go.ke/wp-content/uploads/2020/11/Press-Release-on_Draft-2020-BROP.pdf

National Treasury, K., 2020c. *Explanatory Memorandum for the Public Finance Management COVID-19 Emergency Response Fund Regulations, 2020*. National Treasury. Available from: http://ntnt.treasury.go.ke/wp-content/uploads/2020/11/PFM-COVID-19-Regulations-2020-Final-Regulations.pdf

National Treasury, K., 2020d. *Public Statement on the Status of Payments to County Governments'*. National Treasury. Available from: https://www.treasury.go.ke/media-centre/general-press-releases.html?download=1150:public-statement-on-the-status-of-payments-to-county-governments

Nordling, L., 2020. Africa's Pandemic Puzzle: Why So Few Cases and Deaths. *Science*, 369 (6505), 756–757.

Presidency, K., 2018. *Executive Order No.2 of 2018 on the Procurement of Public Goods, Works and Services by Public Entities*. Presidency. Available from: https://www.president.go.ke/2018/06/13/executive-order-on-procurement-of-public-goods-works-and-services-by-public-entities/

Presidency, K., 2020a. *7th Presidential Address on the Corona Virus Pandemic: 8 Point Economic Stimulus Programme*. Available from: https://www.president.go.ke/2020/05/23/the-seventh-presidential-address-on-the-coronavirus-pandemic-the-8-point-economic-stimulus-programme-saturday-23rd-may-2020/

Presidency, K., 2020b. *National Emergency Response Committee Review Report*. Presidency. Available from: https://www.president.go.ke/2020/03/12/17428/

Presidency, K., 2020c. *Presidential Address on the State's Interventions to Cushion Kenyans agaisnt Economic Effects of Covid-19 Pandemic*. Presidency. Available from: https://www.president.go.ke/2020/03/25/presidential-address-on-the-state-interventions-to-cushion-kenyans-against-economic-effects-of-covid-19-pandemic-on-25th-march-2020/

Statistics (KNBS), K.N., 2020a. *Quarterly Labour Force Report*. Nairobi: Kenya National Bureau of Statistics (KNBS). Available from: https://www.knbs.or.ke/?page_id=3142

Statistics (KNBS), K.N., 2020b. *Survey on Socio Economic Impact of COVID-19 on Households Report*. Kenya National of Statistics (KNBS). Available from: http://dc.sourceafrica.net/documents/119956-COVID-19-Survey-Key-Indicators-Report.html

World Bank. 2016. *Kenya Urbanization Review*. World Bank, Washington, DC. © World Bank. https://openknowledge.worldbank.org/handle/10986/23753 License: CC BY 3.0 IGO.

14 Federalism and the COVID-19 crisis

Trends, tensions, and testing innovations in Malaysia

Tricia Yeoh

14.1 Introduction

The COVID-19 pandemic took place at a time when Malaysia was undergoing a significant political transition, as a leadership crisis caused the government to collapse and be replaced by a new administration altogether in early March 2020. The newly formed Perikatan Nasional (PN) government had to very quickly grapple with the public health crisis that was thrust into its hands.

Already a highly centralized federal system, the twin pandemic and political developments led the country's federal government to adopt top-down approaches to managing COVID-19 through the implementation of federal laws and regulations. As a result of the highly centralized response, tensions between the federal government and several state governments in Malaysia inevitably arose. This was especially the case since many states engaged in their own pandemic response and stood their ground in the face of instructions issued by the federal government without meaningful prior consultation.

The pandemic thus offered a useful opportunity to test the robustness and practicality of the country's existing federal structure. While public health is in the 1957 Federal Constitution's Concurrent List (under which both the federal and state levels of government have joint jurisdiction), the 1988 Prevention and Control of Infectious Disease Act (the law that was used to enforce Malaysia's Movement Control Order [MCO]) is a federal law. Further, the related 2020 Prevention and Control of Infectious Diseases (Declaration of Infected Local Areas) Order defined the "infected area" to include all states and three federal territories in Malaysia. This became a point of legal contention when the federal government chose to open the economy more quickly, whereas states wanted to retain stricter lockdown measures. Other related laws and policies that were significant in the COVID-19 response included the Ministry of Health Disaster Management Plan and the Malaysia Strategy for Emerging Diseases and Public Health Emergencies (MySED) II Workplan (2017–2021) (Ministry of Health 2020), all of which fall under the purview of the federal government.

Although the federal government's decision was ultimately adhered to by all states, this was an interesting case study on whether the states could exercise their joint rights over public health. Further, the third layer of government – local government – has been largely ignored in Malaysia since local government elections were first suspended and then abolished in 1976. Local government falls under state government purview, but it is important to note that there also exists the National Council on Local Governments (NCLG), which is chaired by the Prime Minister, a further sign

DOI: 10.4324/9781003251217-14

Table 14.1 Key Statistics on COVID-19 in Malaysia as of 10 January 2021

Cumulative Cases	Cumulative Cases per 100,000 Population	Cumulative Deaths	Cumulative Deaths per 100,000 Population	Case Fatality Percentage
133,559	412.7	542	1.7	0.4

Source: *World Health Organization Weekly epidemiological update* – 12 January 2021. Geneva: WHO, 2021. Available from https://www.who.int/publications/m/item/weekly-epidemiological-update

of centralization tendencies. Despite these trends, the 1976 Local Government Act does empower local governments and grants them amongst other powers, the ability to preserve public health and prevent the outbreak and spread of diseases, and to regulate and enforce quarantine, the disinfection of persons, and the disinfection of places and things.

COVID-19 has placed increasing fiscal pressure on all levels of government. The federal government's economic stimulus packages have led to higher national debt-to-GDP ratio and fiscal deficit figures, exceeding original targets. As an oil-producing country, 19 percent of Malaysia's annual revenues are financed via oil and gas resources, an unsustainable dependence on the country's national oil producing company Petronas. The oil-producing states of East Malaysia's Sabah and Sarawak are demanding greater oil royalty, sales tax on oil and gas products, and a bigger say over their own natural resources. All of this will invariably impact upon the federal government's fiscal flexibility, and in turn, its ability to cushion the economic blows that the pandemic will continue to wreak on the nation (Table 14.1).

14.2 COVID-19 in Malaysia

The first Malaysian case of COVID-19 was confirmed on 4 February 2020, after a Malaysian had returned from Singapore (Elengoe 2020). Thus began the first wave of COVID-19 cases, but this ended fairly quickly with very low numbers. The second wave of infections broke out in late February and grew rapidly in the following three weeks. Up to the end of this second wave, which is estimated to have concluded at the end of September, there were a total of 10,167 people who tested positive (Malaysiakini 2020). Between February and September, the number of cases reached a peak on 4 June, when a total of 277 new cases were recorded in a single day. The first – and still the deadliest to date – cluster was that of the *tabligh* cluster, infecting 3,375 people, or more than a third of all infection cases in the country. Held over a period of four days from 27 February to 1 March at a mosque in the heart of the country's capital Kuala Lumpur, the *tabligh* was an Islamic missionary event organized by the Tablighi Jama'at movement and was attended by 16,000 people, including 1,500 foreigners (Reuters 2020).

After having been sworn in as the new Prime Minister on 1 March, Muhyiddin Yassin publicly banned mass gatherings on 13 March. To this effect, the federal National Security Council (NSC) mobilized a national response with technical guidance from the Ministry of Health (Ministry of Health 2020). The national testing capacity was increased from 1,000 tests per day in January 2020 to over 38,000 tests per day in September 2020; several government hospitals were converted into "full or partial COVID-19 hospitals," and quarantine centers such as training institutes and nursing dormitories were made available (Ministry of Health 2020). In addition, public communication was carried out through regular press briefings and government platforms including websites, social media, and messaging applications.

The government implemented a MCO which began on 18 March 2020 and which was initially tightened as the numbers of cases rose steadily. Under the MCO, only industries within a strictly defined list of "essential goods and services" would be permitted to operate, and even those would have to apply and receive confirmation from the Ministry of International Trade and Industry (MITI). Cross-state travel was allowed only upon police approval, and individuals were not allowed to travel beyond 10 km of their residence. These rules were eventually gradually loosened, as the public health risks fell alongside the number of daily new infections. A Controlled Movement Control Order (CMCO) was thus implemented on 4 May, followed by a Recovery Movement Control Order (RMCO) on 10 June.

Although Malaysia has a robust public healthcare system with universal access to healthcare, private citizens and communities contributed to the control and prevention of the virus spread. A "Whole of Government, Whole of Society" approach was adopted to respond to the crisis (Ministry of Health 2020). Communities rallied together under a #*kitajagakita* tagline, which is also the name used for a website that connects non-governmental organizations (NGOs) with communities in need to raise funds and provide food, goods, and services. Some fundamental problems included the shortage of medical equipment: In an online survey conducted by a group of Malaysian doctors, of the respondents working in Ministry of Health hospitals, 77 percent of respondents said that they had experienced shortage of personal protective equipment (PPEs), and 58 percent said they had to resort to "do-it-yourself" (DIY) PPEs and make their own non-medical masks and other protective equipment (Lim 2020). As a result of these shortcomings throughout the MCO period, private citizens were roped into donating funds and even assembling PPEs.

Although Malaysia successfully flattened its curve between late June and July, the MCO on the whole has had devastating effects particularly on business owners and low-income communities in Malaysia, costing the economy RM2.4 billion a day. Because of the strict lockdown measures that the government chose to adopt in which businesses were forced to close for almost three months, many small and medium enterprises (SMEs) have been particularly badly hit. A survey conducted by SME Malaysia in April 2020, an association of SMEs, found that almost 60 percent of firms surveyed reported zero revenue during the MCO, with almost 30 percent saying that they would give unpaid leave to their staff. The unemployment rate reached a record high of 5.3 percent in May 2020, recording an additional 47,300 people unemployed between April and May (Department of Statistics Malaysia 2020). The tourism, retail, and food and beverage (F&B) sectors have been particularly affected; for instance, 15 percent of hotels were reported as possibly having to shut down operations (Ying 2020). The government chose not to carry out large-scale lockdowns in the proceeding months, but instead used targeted enhanced MCOs (TEMCO) to isolate specific affected areas, such as certain locations in Kedah.

Malaysia underwent a rapid third wave of COVID-19 infections starting from late September to early October, following the return of politicians to Peninsular Malaysia who had travelled to the state of Sabah in East Malaysia for their campaigns in the run-up to the Sabah state election on 26 September. Although numerous experts cautioned against repeating a nationwide lockdown, for fear that the economy would not be able to withstand the additional shock, this third wave has been the most severe since the beginning of the pandemic. Escalating rapidly and exponentially from an average of 400 new daily cases in early October to a peak of 2,525 new daily cases on 31 December 2020,[1] the COVID-19 situation was further exacerbated by the fact that state borders were opened throughout December, resulting in many Malaysians travelling across the country for the holidays and to visit their relatives in their respective hometowns. The Malaysian government's relaxed measures may also be attributed to pressure from players within the tourism industry, and more generally, to economic pressure. As a result of the third wave, the number of confirmed cases in the country reached a cumulative number of infections of 113,010 by the end of December 2020 (The Star 2020). In this respect, the government resorted to announcing a CMCO in Sabah, Selangor, Kuala Lumpur, and Putrajaya in October, which was later extended to January 2021.

While the government emerged with an array of economic stimulus packages totaling USD68.7 billion in the initial outlay, including, among other programs in its PENJANA Short-Term Economic Recovery Plan, a six-month loan moratorium and wage subsidies, small businesses may yet not be able to weather the storm. Low-wage earners were already vulnerable; a large proportion of those living in low-cost flats work as informal laborers such as petty traders, tailors, and freelancers and therefore lack the social security that formal workers enjoy (Puteri and Kunasekaran 2020). Since many of the poorest households are not equipped with the necessary infrastructure to work from home, not going to work would have meant a significant loss of income (Puteri and Kunasekaran 2020). The 2021 Budget that was tabled and passed in Parliament in November also contained an array of offerings, including tax relief measures, cash aid programs, extension of existing wage subsidy programs, and other handouts aimed at assisting the economy. It is expected that the government will be forced to emerge with new measures in the coming year, given that more lockdowns have been imposed following the third wave of COVID-19 cases, and that the economy has not been able to recover.

14.3 COVID-19 and federalism in Malaysia

14.3.1 *Constitutional framework of the different levels of government*

Article 1 of the 1957 Federal Constitution of Malaysia describes the country as a federation of 13 states and three territories. However, state powers have gradually eroded, giving rise to greater central powers within the federal government. That process began when local council elections were abolished in 1965. Federal emergency measures were further introduced in 1969 and state economic development corporations (SEDCs) were used to spearhead the nationwide New Economic Policy in 1971. Over the following decades, other institutional mechanisms were introduced that further strengthened the federal government's hold over states.

On the surface, there appears to be a clear demarcation of powers between the federal and state governments. The Ninth Schedule of the Federal Constitution recognizes the semi-autonomous nature of states, which have some "constitutionally entrenched division of powers in the legislative, executive, judicial and financial fields" (Shad 2019, p. 74).

In practice, there has been ample scope for the solidification of a powerful central government. For example, Article 71(3) allows the federal government to amend a state constitution if there is non-compliance by a state with the federal constitution. Article 75 provides that the federal law shall prevail when any state law is inconsistent with a federal law, while Article 76 allows the federal government to make laws pertaining to state matters if it promotes the uniformity of laws or if it is requested to do so by states. Article 76A permits parliament to delegate its powers to the states. Article 81 of the Federal Constitution states that the executive authority of every state is to be exercised to ensure compliance with federal law and should not impede or prejudice the exercise of the federal government.

The Federal Constitution recognizes three levels of government: federal, state, and local. Article 150 of the Federal Constitution provides authority to the King to proclaim emergency measures (the King acts upon the advice of the Prime Minister). The federal government can also utilize emergency provisions to suspend state rights under the same Article. The Ninth Schedule, which spells out the jurisdiction of the federal and state governments, identifies "public health, sanitation and prevention of infectious diseases" in the Concurrent List, where both federal and state governments have joint control. However, "medicine and health" fall under the Federal List, therefore assigning the federal government ultimate control over the funding and administration of the Ministry of Health, alongside all state health departments, public hospitals, and community clinics throughout the country.

14.3.2 COVID-19 management and intergovernmental relations

Although state governments have official representation within the National Action Council,[2] in its very first meeting in March on the COVID-19 mitigation plans, the federal government excluded the heads of state governments controlled by the opposition coalition. The federal government later reversed this decision and invited the subnational leaders to subsequent meetings. In May, the federal government abruptly announced that the MCO would ease, giving only three days' notice. Nine state governments in total reacted immediately by saying they were either not following (Kedah, Sabah, Pahang, Penang, Kelantan, and Sarawak) or not fully complying (Selangor, Perak, and Negeri Sembilan) with the easing of the COVID-19 control measures concerning economic activity, otherwise known as the CMCO. They believed that the reopening of all sectors and industries was too abrupt, arguing that buffer time was needed to allow state governments and companies to adopt new standard operating procedures (SOPs) to ensure hygiene and public health. Interestingly, four out of these nine states were politically aligned with the federal government, where previously, federally aligned states would typically adhere to the center's instructions without protest. Many of the states' Chief Ministers felt that there should have been proper consultation with the states beforehand, stating that they would have been the ones implementing the decisions, and that the federal government should have assessed the situation and capacity of the states prior to making decisions (Fong 2020).

Some experts cited Article 81 to argue that states must adhere to the federal law of the 1988 Prevention and Control of Infectious Diseases Act, since all states had in 1989 agreed to promulgate a uniform law to prevent and control infectious diseases in Malaysia, enforceable throughout the country. There is, however, an alternative, and equally compelling, view advanced by other experts that states have the right to defy the federal government's law on the grounds that the Federal Constitution places "public health, sanitation, and prevention of infectious diseases" within the Concurrent List in the Ninth Schedule. It is also bolstered by the provisions of the Local Government Act as described above. Since all laws must adhere to the supremacy of the Federal Constitution, this means that both federal and state governments are to jointly decide on issues pertaining to these areas with equal weight.

Because the Constitution is vague on how "joint decisions" are to be made, it has never been clear whether state legislative assemblies need to vote on a particular matter of concurrent interest – and further, pass state-level legislation to that end – or whether mere 'consultation' is all that is required. At a meeting held on 28 April between the federal and state governments, the gradual reopening of the economy was apparently raised by the Prime Minister.

However, one state government chief executive (the Chief Minister of opposition-led Penang) claimed that the following approach was agreed upon at the meeting: first, the "District Risk Reduction Programme" proposal by the federal Ministry of Health was to target the reopening of "green zones" only; second, the official SOPs were to be shared with all states prior to any reopening; and third, the states were to be given time to strategize. However, the federal government proceeded on 1 May to announce that all zones – green, orange, red – would simultaneously reopen on 4 May, without informing the states or sending them the SOPs (Astro Awani 2020). The federal government responded harshly with a statement saying that companies may possibly sue state governments if they refused to reopen. This was rebutted by the Penang state government, which stated that it was prepared to face legal challenges from industry players if that is the repercussion for protecting its people from the pandemic.

Although seemingly contentious, all state governments eventually adhered to the federal government decision to reopen the economy. First, it would not have been possible for the states to enforce a stricter lockdown, since enforcement bodies like the police are controlled by federal authority. Second, although state governments may have been able to employ local government officers to enforce local government policy on licensing requirements, which it controls, this was not contested in the court of law since no businesses eventually sued state governments. Restaurants, eateries, and other retail outlets were not reopening all that rapidly in any case, given there was very poor foot traffic at the time the MCO was relaxed.

As previously pointed out, the federal government announced a CMCO in several states following the third wave of COVID-19 in the last quarter of the year, namely in Sabah, Selangor, Kuala Lumpur, and Putrajaya. However, this announcement was not well-received by the Selangor state government, who claimed that the federal government had not consulted Selangor beforehand. The Selangor Chief Minister was "shocked by the announcement" but was not surprised as this had happened previously. In fact, a few days prior to that, the federal government had announced a CMCO for Klang, a district within Selangor that was more severely affected by COVID-19, without consulting the state government (Free Malaysia Today 2020). It was only after the state government expressed dismay at not having been consulted that the NSC met with the Selangor Chief Minister, and the latter announced that the NSC would provide the CMCO details of Klang, and that the state government would work with all agencies accordingly.

Sabah, Penang and Selangor were the only state governments that expressed disappointment over not having been consulted on various occasions, including when the federal government first decided to open up the economy in May 2020, and later when it unilaterally implemented the CMCO in Selangor. These public expressions took place within the states led by opposition coalitions. In short, the political coalitions that are not aligned with the center made their views publicly and vehemently known. The other states that chose not to comply with the opening of the economy also expressed their disappointment but were less vocal about their decisions and actions. By the time the October CMCO was announced, the Sabah state government had already changed hands from an opposition-aligned coalition to one that was supportive and aligned with the ruling coalition at the center.

Such were the political polemics that played out nationally. However, the reality on the ground was that intergovernmental health coordination took place relatively smoothly. For instance, state health directors worked in a professional and coordinated fashion with state executive council members in charge of health, whether in government-aligned or opposition-controlled states (Welsh 2020). These state health directors are employed by and seconded to the states, and technically do not report to the state governments. There was therefore an increase in vertical interaction between these federal appointees and state government representatives, in ways that were novel and previously unnecessary.

14.3.3 State government innovations on COVID-19 and federalism in Malaysia

Despite the pre-existing centralization of Malaysia's institutions, it is crucial to note that some states exercised their constitutional powers to guide the emergency response within their borders, including Sabah and Sarawak (the two states of East Malaysia that have greater autonomy relative to their Peninsular Malaysia counterparts under the Federal Constitution). Sarawak issued their own circulars on regulatory compliance such as on the closing of premises, and both states created their own immigration regulations (Welsh 2020).

Apart from federal government assistance, all state governments also contributed their own economic stimulus packages, with the wealthier, more well-resourced states emerging with larger packages. Welsh's (2020) research provides a detailed breakdown of the state-level special assistance funds, in which state allocations specific to the COVID-19 response ranged between USD583,300 in Perlis to USD551.7 million in Sarawak. Taken together, including the Federal Territory of Kuala Lumpur, subnational governments provided a total of USD980 million of COVID-19 targeted assistance, which included cash transfers and food aid for vulnerable communities, the purchase of additional medical equipment, the waiver of fees and bills, among others (Institute for Democracy and Economic Affairs 2020). States have therefore provided additional funds throughout the COVID-19 crisis. However, these funds only represent about 1.5 percent of what the federal government has spent, which clearly indicates that it is the federal government that is ultimately in charge of managing the country's economy and the subsequent fiscal impact of the COVID-19 crisis.

Further, several state governments used their own resources to conduct their respective testing and contract tracing. Selangor and Penang both provided funds for additional testing, and many states developed their own tracing applications, for instance Johor (Jejak Johor), Selangor (SELangkah), and Sarawak (CovidTrace and Qmunity).[3] Notably, Penang and Sarawak did an excellent job of providing public communication to their constituents by having regular briefings on Facebook. Penang created 24-hour hotlines and its own COVID-19 website. Sarawak formed its own State Disaster Management Committee, which launched three different applications including to monitor travelling into and within Sarawak, and a general information dashboard. Finally, the states of Sarawak, Sabah, Selangor, and Penang collaborated with civil society and charity networks to coordinate donations and medical assistance (Welsh 2020).

The fact that all states took the initiative to emerge with their own unique innovations to respond to COVID-19, whether through contact tracing applications or website launches, has transformed the way public health is managed in Malaysia. Although in constitution and in policy a matter of the federal government, in practice the management of public health has become much more decentralized. This period has been especially interesting for the East Malaysian states of Sabah and Sarawak to exercise their autonomy to impose strict preventive measures. Until August 2020, the two states even required Malaysians entering from the peninsula (West Malaysia) to undergo quarantine upon arrival. It is equally important to understand that these measures took place as the two states have become increasingly politically significant, amidst national political instability and contestation.

However, in assessing state-level innovations, incidents of federal-state conflict can be noted. Although in the first half of the year, there was apparently close cooperation and data sharing between the federal Health Ministry and NSC with the operation centers of the Selangor state government, this practice was stopped in the latter half of the year (Dzulkefly, 20 October 2020).While the Selangor state government was allowing the Minister of Health's personnel access to its application SeLangkah, the state had further requested to obtain data from the federal government to enable integration between its application and the federal government's application MySejahtera.

Obtaining data from MySejahtera would assist the Selangor Health Department in predicting where future infections might break out in the state. However, the federal government's Ministry of Health declined to share the raw data, citing "past incidents" where data was wrongly interpreted and caused panic among Malaysians (Malay Mail, 4 November 2020). As a result, the state government had to rely on publicly available data from press conferences and other "random sources" instead of having a meaningful information exchange with the federal government.

14.4 Conclusion

Although in the sum of things there have not been any major changes in law or policy – there have been no formal reassignments of responsibilities, and intergovernmental structures remain very much as they were prior to the pandemic – the experience of COVID-19 has provided interesting lessons on how states can innovate around the system. While the federal government continues to run all public hospitals and community clinics, state governments also have executive councillors (Exco members) mandated to provide financial assistance and coordination over health. Private hospitals have also played a prominent role in managing the pandemic by providing COVID-19 tests at a fee; several state governments have in fact started their own private hospital chains, and continue to have a share in how they are run.[4]

Further, the federal government seems to recognize state rights to some degree. In announcing the Conditional Movement Control Order, Defense Minister Ismail Sabri said that Sarawak was exempt from Act 342, as the state has its own 1999 Protection of Public Health Ordinance which allows the state minister responsible for public health to regulate movement in and out of the infected local area (Malay Mail, 8 June 2020). When announcing that in principle all non-Muslim places of worship can operate, Minister Ismail Sabri also said this was subject to approval by state governments, which would issue their own guidelines (Chung 2020).

Has federalism helped or hindered the management of the pandemic in Malaysia? In some ways, it possibly hindered efficiency on the ground, especially with respect to managing the logistical and economic complexities of the supply chain needed to run businesses and provide food security, as well as providing charitable aid and financial assistance to vulnerable communities. However, the legal and policy systems did not necessarily prevent states from activating their own response mechanisms, and the federal government did not intervene in this respect considering the positive outcomes of these responses.

The pandemic has certainly raised some interesting questions as to what states can do to assert their constitutionally established authority. Although in the end – after several days of resistance – all states complied with federal instructions in the case of the CMCO, states with a larger independent resource base took pandemic management into their own hands in a number of interesting ways as outlined above. This indicates that if local governance autonomy is to deepen and decentralize further in Malaysia, this will most likely emerge through a bottom-up approach rather than being devolved from a top-down process. COVID-19 has also shown that sharing public policy between different levels of government can result in positive outcomes. The federal government will not necessarily resist the initiative of state governments if they do not conflict with the center's goals, and if both parties agree on a common shared outcome (Yeoh 2020).

However, in the final analysis, it also seems clear that political position-taking remains the order of the day. Regardless of constitutional framework, the federal government could have much more meaningfully worked with all state governments – government or opposition-aligned – in order to obtain more efficient results and fulfil the objective of better managing the pandemic overall. Through the end of the year, the third wave of infections continued to rise significantly. To manage the pandemic and emerge with solutions that do not simultaneously damage the economy, a clearer and more rules-based system of managing federal-state relations would bring benefits to all.

Notes

1 The cases have continued to climb steadily to reaching daily averages of between 3,000 and 4,000 new cases at the end of January 2021.
2 State governments also have official representation in many other national-level councils, such as the National Council on Local Government (NCLG), National Land Council (NLC) and National Finance Council (NFC). However, one critique is that these national councils are ultimately chaired and controlled by the Prime Minister, who has the discretion to select any other federal Cabinet member as member of the councils.
3 For a full list of states that emerged with their own applications, see Welsh (2020).
4 The Johor state government founded Kumpulan Perangsang Johor, which started the first KPJ Specialist Centre in the state of Johor in 1981. Today, KPJ Healthcare Berhad is a publicly listed company, whose network has more than 28 private hospitals in Malaysia, 2 hospitals in Indonesia, a sizeable share in a hospital in Bangkok and a hospital in Bangladesh

(KPJ 2020). Separately, the Selangor state government through its State Economic Development Corporation (PKNS) subsidiary SELGATE Corporation lists 12 private hospitals on its website (SELGATE 2020).

Bibliography

Astro Awani, 5 May 2020. Consider This: CMCO (Part 1) – What Wrong in the Consultation Process? [Video]. Available from: https://www.youtube.com/watch?v=pxyt3Lkf6Ac [Accessed 10 May 2020].

Chung, N., 2020. Churches, Temples Can Open at 1/3 Capacity. *Free Malaysia Today*, 15 June. Available from: https://www.freemalaysiatoday.com/category/nation/2020/06/15/restrictions-loosened-for-non-muslim-houses-of-worship/ [Accessed 6 September 2020].

Department of Statistics Malaysia, 14 July 2020. *Key Statistics of Labour Force in Malaysia*, May 2020 [online]. Available from: https://smemalaysia.org/survey-results-on-smes-sustainability-and-survival-during-mco/ [Accessed 19 September 2020].

Dzulkefly A., 20 October 2020. Data Sharing Key to Combating Covid-19. *Malaysiakini* [online]. Available from: https://www.malaysiakini.com/news/547265 [Accessed 26 January 2021].

Elengoe, A., 2020. COVID-19 Outbreak in Malaysia. *Osong Public Health and Research Perspectives*, 11 (3), 93–100. Available from: https://www.ncbi.nlm.nih.gov/pmc/articles/PMC7258884/ [Accessed 17 September 2020].

Free Malaysia Today, 8 October 2020. Putrajaya Did Not Consult State Govt over Klang CMCO, Claims Selangor Exco [online]. Available from: https://www.freemalaysiatoday.com/category/nation/2020/10/13/selangor-rep-slams-putrajayas-unprofessional-cmco-announcement/ [Accessed 26 January 2021].

Fong, D.R., 2020. Nothing Personal, Sabah CM Tells Putrajaya on Non-Compliance with CMCO. *Free Malaysia Today*, 5 May. Available from: https://www.freemalaysiatoday.com/category/nation/2020/05/05/nothing-personal-sabah-cm-tells-putrajaya-on-non-compliance-with-cmco/ [Accessed 26 January 2021].

Institute for Democracy and Economic Affairs, 2020. State-Level Stimulus Packages. Available from: http://www.ideas.org.my/state-level-stimulus-packages/ [Accessed 17 July 2020].

KPJ Healthcare Berhad, 2020. Who We Are. Available from: http://kpj.listedcompany.com/profile.html [Accessed 20 September 2020].

Lim, I., 2020. Malaysia's PPE Shortage, Supply Issues: Doctors Propose National Stockpile, Centralised Unit for Better Distribution [online]. *Malay Mail*, 16 May. Available from: https://www.malaymail.com/news/malaysia/2020/05/16/malaysias-ppe-shortage-supply-issues-doctors-propose-national-stockpile-cen/1866801 [Accessed 20 September 2020].

Malay Mail, 8 June 2020. RMCO: Act 342 Applicable to All States Except Sarawak, Says Ismail Sabri [online]. Available from: https://www.malaymail.com/news/malaysia/2020/06/08/rmco-act-342-applicable-to-all-states-except-sarawak-says-ismail-sabri/1873518 [Accessed 8 September 2020].

Malay Mail, 4 November 2020. Selangor Exco Claims State 'Blindsided' without Detailed Covid-19 Data, Has to Play Guessing Game [online]. Available from: https://www.malaymail.com/news/malaysia/2020/11/04/selangor-exco-claims-state-blindsided-without-detailed-covid-19-data-has-to/1919185 [Accessed 26 January 2021].

Malaysiakini, 20 September 2020. Covid-19 in Malaysia [online]. Available from: https://newslab.malaysiakini.com/covid-19/en [Accessed 20 September 2020].

Ministry of Health, September 2020. Universal Health Coverage and COVID-19 Preparedness & Response. Kuala Lumpur: Institute for Health Systems Research, Ministry of Health. Available from: http://www.ihsr.moh.gov.my/images/publication_material/techreport/wpro-covid_final.pdf [Accessed 20 September 2020].

Puteri, M.M. and Kunasekaran, T., 27 March 2020. The Impact of Covid-19 on the Urban Poor: Three Major Threats – Money, Food and Living Conditions. Kuala Lumpur: Khazanah Research Institute. Available from: http://www.krinstitute.org/assets/contentMS/img/template/editor/The%20Impact%20of%20Covid-19%20on%20the%20Urban%20Poor.pdf [Accessed 19 September 2020].

Reuters, 2020. Coronavirus: How Malaysia's Sri Petaling Mosque Became a Covid-19 Hotspot [online]. *South China Morning Post*, 18 March. Available from: https://www.scmp.com/news/asia/southeast-asia/article/3075654/how-malaysias-sri-petaling-mosque-became-coronavirus [Accessed 11 September 2020].

SELGATE, 2020. SELGATE Group of Hospitals. Available from: https://selgatehealthcare.com/selgate-group-of-hospitals/ [Accessed 20 September 2020].

Shad S. F., 2019. *Our Constitution*. Subang Jaya: Sweet and Maxwell.

Survey Results on SMEs Sustainability and Survival during MCO. *SME Malaysia*, 19 May. Subang Jaya: Thomson Reuters Asia Sdn Bhd. Available from: https://smemalaysia.org/survey-results-on-smes-sustainability-and-survival-during-mco/ [Accessed 19 September 2020].

The Star, 31 December 2020. Covid-19: Record High of 2,525 Cases on New Year's Eve, Eight Deaths [online]. Available from: https://www.thestar.com.my/news/nation/2020/12/31/covid-19-record-high-of-2525-cases-on-new-year039s-eve-eight-deaths [Accessed 26 January 2021].

Welsh, B., 2020. The Unsung Role of State Govt's in Battling Covid. *Malaysiakini*, 3 July. Available from: https://www.malaysiakini.com/columns/532836 [Accessed 20 September 2020].

Yeoh, T., 2020. Federal-State Friction Amid Malaysia's Dual Political and Pandemic Plight. *New Mandala, Australian National University.* Available from: https://www.newmandala.org/wp-content/uploads/2020/08/Federal-state-friction_Tricia-Yeoh2.pdf [Accessed 2 September 2020].

Ying, T.P., 2020. 15 per cent of Hotels in Malaysia May Have to Close Operations [online]. *New Straits Times*, 26 April. Available from: https://www.nst.com.my/news/nation/2020/04/587662/15-cent-hotels-malaysia-may-have-close-operations [Accessed 19 September 2020].

15 COVID-19 in the Mexican federation

Managing the health and economic crises

Laura Flamand, Monica Naime and Juan C. Olmeda

15.1 Introduction

The federal system in Mexico has responded in a relatively uncoordinated fashion to the health and economic crises caused by the spread of COVID-19. There are two significant structural reasons for this: the centralized, asymmetrical nature of the federal system, and the fragmentation of healthcare services.

Mexico is facing a dire crisis in its healthcare system and its economy during the pandemic. The case fatality rate of Mexico has been the highest in the region since May 2020 and the world's second highest since October 2020 (Roser et al. 2020). In economic terms, the GDP contracted around 9.1 percent in 2020 (BBVA Research 2021). Mexico's three orders of government implemented uncoordinated policies to fight these crises between March and December 2020. These actions led to growing tensions in the Mexican federation after the first ten months of the pandemic.

Without clear federal guidelines and standards to manage the crisis, state governments have reacted unevenly, deepening social inequalities. Because relatively affluent states have more capable governments and more robust health systems, their populations have been protected more effectively than those of the poorest states (Table 15.1).

15.2 COVID-19 in Mexico

The first case of COVID-19 in Mexico was confirmed on 27 February 2020, and the first two deaths occurred on March 18. Since then and until 31 December 2020, according to government statistics, COVID-19 has taken more than 131,190 lives, with more than 1,486,313 confirmed cases (CONACYT 2020). This means 975 deaths and 11,060 cases per 1 million inhabitants. The observed case-fatality ratio in Mexico more than triples that of the United States, Argentina, and Brazil (Roser et al.

Table 15.1 Key Statistics on COVID-19 in Mexico as of 10 January 2021

Cumulative Cases	Cumulative Cases per 100,000 Population	Cumulative Deaths	Cumulative Deaths per 100,000 Population	Case Fatality Percentage
1,507,931	1,169.5	132,069	102.4	8.8

Source: World Health Organization Weekly epidemiological update – 12 January 2021. Geneva: WHO, 2021. Available from https://www.who.int/publications/m/item/weekly-epidemiological-update

DOI: 10.4324/9781003251217-15

2020).[1] The general situation deteriorated further by the beginning of 2021, when the daily number of new cases and deaths set new records and reached higher figures than those observed during 2020.

The accuracy of these figures has been questioned considering the rather low number of tests completed in the country. Worldwide, Mexico is the country testing the least, with two or fewer tests performed for every confirmed case (JHU 2020). Healthcare workers have been especially vulnerable during the pandemic: 13 percent of the confirmed cases are nurses and physicians, and Mexico leads the world statistics with the highest death toll among healthcare workers with 2,400 (Amnesty International 2020; Montes 2021).

The severe effects of COVID-19 in Mexico must be set into the context of a fragile health system when compared with other countries for many reasons. First, the public health system is fragmented in two large and deeply unequal subsystems. One system protects people with contributory social security protection. The second system takes care of those lacking such coverage, approximately six out of ten people. The per capita public health expenditure is 39 percent higher for the group of insured people compared to those uninsured (SS 2019). Second, public health expenditure is extremely low in Mexico, amounting to approximately 2.8 percent of GDP compared to 6.6 percent in Argentina and 4.0 percent in Brazil. Third, the proportion of out-of-pocket expenditures in Mexico (41 percent) is considerably larger than in other countries of the region such as Argentina (15 percent) and Brazil (28 percent). Fourth, the Mexican health system operates with an enormous deficit in human resources. In order to reach the median of the OECD countries, 120,000 additional physicians would need to graduate and enter the health care system (Flamand 2020).

Apart from the health toll, the pandemic has also severely affected the highly open Mexican economy. The GDP dropped in the second quarter of 2020 by 17.1 percent compared to the previous quarter (INEGI 2020a), making this shock twice as strong as the economic crisis of 2009 and the tequila crisis of 1994 (see Figure 15.1).

This general slowdown of the economy resulting from restrictions on mobility was accompanied by major drops in three crucial productive sectors: exports, tourism,

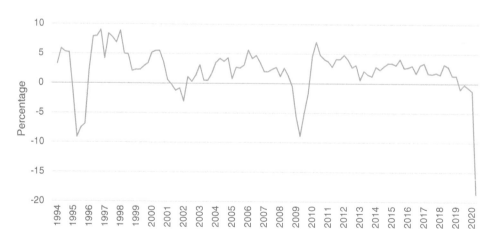

Figure 15.1 Annual Variation of the Quarterly GDP in Mexico.
Source: Prepared by the authors with information from INEGI 2020a.

and oil. First, due to the abrupt slowdown in the American and Chinese economies, the demand for exports has diminished considerably (World Bank 2020; IMF 2020). Second, the tourism sector has plummeted with severe consequences in terms of employment. This sector accounts for nearly 16 percent of both jobs and GDP (Mooney and Zegarra 2020). Third, with borders closed and travel restricted, the price of the Mexican oil blend dropped 57 percent in April 2020 compared to the prices in December 2019 (Bank of Mexico 2020).

These disturbances have meant that the peso depreciated 15 percent from January to August 2020 (IMF 2020). Also, 4.4 million people have lost their jobs during the second quarter of the year (INEGI 2020b). This increase in unemployment is significantly above the levels of the 2008 financial crisis and is not expected to return to pre-crisis levels until the middle of 2021 (OECD 2020). Of those who have lost their jobs due to this unprecedented crisis, 71 percent worked in the tertiary sector, and 92 percent do not have access to the health care system (INEGI 2020c).

The pandemic is likely to deepen inequalities around the world, as predicted in several studies. This is especially relevant in a country as unequal as Mexico. The economic and health costs of the pandemic are differentiated, not only by economic sector but also by geography, income, and gender. Metropolitan areas have been more extensively impacted than rural areas for two reasons. First, the density of the population allows easier transmission of the infection. Second, mobility restrictions have lasted longer in metropolitan areas. In terms of income, the case-fatality ratio is twice as high in the poorest municipalities than in the richest ones (CONEVAL 2020a), and it is estimated that up to 10.7 million people will fall below the extreme poverty line (CONEVAL 2020b). Finally, in terms of gender, compared to the same period in 2019, the number of violent deaths of women has increased 12 percent and that of emergency calls for domestic violence 53 percent (INMUJERES 2020). In addition, according to official estimates, close to 150,000 unwanted pregnancies are to be expected and at least 21,500 additional teenage pregnancies (CONAPO 2020). This brief account highlights the deep and long-lasting impact that COVID-19 will have on the economic and health crisis in Mexico.

15.3 COVID-19 and federalism in Mexico

Mexico is a federal republic composed of the central government and 32 subnational units: 31 states and Mexico City. Federalism was formally proclaimed as a form of government in 1824 when the first Mexican Constitution was enacted after independence. However, federalism was later abandoned because of internal fights for the control of power during most of the 19th century. It was not until 1917, after the Mexican Revolution, that a new Constitution was adopted, and federalism became again the *de jure* form of organization.[2]

Nevertheless, the evolution of Mexican federalism was not linear during the 20th century. Until the 1980s, the country remained highly *de facto* centralized given that the political system was dominated by a single political party which controlled almost all elected positions. The situation began to change in the last decades of the 20th century because of both democratization and decentralization. Democratization happened when opposition parties began to win electoral contests at the local level. Decentralization took place when the federal government devolved responsibilities to states and municipalities. Several recentralizing measures have been implemented since the beginning of the 21st century, mainly as an attempt to solve coordination problems that emerged in the post-decentralization scenario (Olmeda and Armesto 2017).

Mexican subnational governments enjoy a certain level of autonomy since constitutionally they can enact their own norms and legal regulations and have responsibility over several policy areas. Fiscally, however, they are highly dependent on federal transfers: on average, only 10 percent of the total income of subnational governments results from local taxes. This fact is crucial for understanding how the characteristics of the Mexican federal system have permeated the response of both the national and subnational governments to the COVID-19 crisis.

As per the federal Constitution, public health is a shared responsibility of federal, state, and municipal governments. In addition, as we have already mentioned, the health care system is *de facto* deeply fragmented. There are several subsystems providing care for formal sector workers, government employees, oil workers, and the armed forces. Furthermore, since the beginning of 2020, the National Institute of Health for Wellness (INSABI) had pledged to provide complete coverage for an ample list of health interventions and medicines to those in the informal economy (six out of ten workers). Unfortunately, when COVID-19 arrived in Mexico, the Institute was operating without formal rules and with insufficient funds for such a large and ambitious task. Mexico has traditionally spent rather meagerly on health care, 5.5 percent of GDP compared to the average in the OECD countries of 8.8 percent including both private and public expenditures. Furthermore, the quantity and quality of health care facilities in Mexico vary enormously across the states. Thus, poor uninsured people in the states with weak health care structures are exposed to the highest risk.

The Mexican Constitution provides for extraordinary public health actions in the case of emergencies. The Ministry of Health is mandated to immediately take the necessary measures with the agreement of the President to prevent and control risks in specific parts of the territory for definite periods in such cases. These federal measures include the assignment of tasks to federal, state, or municipal authorities as well as to health professionals, including measures related to public gatherings; air traffic and maritime and land transit; free use of telephonic, telegraphic, and mail media as well as radio and television transmissions; and any other determined by the Ministry. This, however, does not imply that subnational governments relinquish their legal powers regarding the implementation of health security measures. Rather, when facing health emergencies, the responsibilities of state governments in Mexico are determined by the legal regulations regarding local public health in their territory, those assigned by the Ministry of Health given the extraordinary public health actions and, finally, those established by the National Public Health Council.

Three weeks after the first case was confirmed in Mexico, on 19 March 2020, the National Public Health Council met and declared the pandemic a health emergency. This declaration is not equivalent to a state of emergency in the sense that it gives special powers to the executive, but rather provides a mandate for prioritizing its attention to the matter. The declaration of the health emergency allowed for the adoption of health, economic, and fiscal measures. At the federal level, up to August 14, the government had adopted 53 measures to respond to the sanitary, economic, and social impact of the pandemic (CEPAL 2020). The first measure was for the President to approve the reallocation of up to 0.7 percent of the GDP to an emergency fund to face the pandemic. The federal government also adopted specific measures strengthening the health system to control the disease, including adapting public hospitals toward COVID-19 services, expanding the public network with the inclusion of private hospitals, and importing the essential equipment required to care for patients effectively.

The federal government has argued that caution was needed when halting the economy because poor people needed to be protected, mainly those living on a daily subsistence income. This is especially relevant as close to 60 percent of people work in the informal economy and thus are excluded from contributory social security. The federal government has not expanded social assistance, nor deferred or reduced taxes (Lustig et al. 2020). Consequently, people in the informal economy continued working, thus increasing the probability of getting infected by the virus, while they only had access to poorly equipped and resourced health facilities, that is, those available via the newly created INSABI.

On 23 March 2020, the National Public Health Council declared a "National Campaign of Healthy Distancing" which suspended in-person education activities. The campaign also recommended vulnerable employees to stay away from their workplaces and strongly encouraged the population overall to stay at home (SS 2020). However, no mandatory mobility restrictions were imposed across the country, and flights were not cancelled, although the US–Mexico border was closed for any nonessential travel. On March 23, the federal Ministry of Education decided to cancel in-person instruction for the entire education system across the country (SEP 2020). By that time, however, 10 out of the 31 state governments plus Mexico City had already canceled school activities in their territories (Excelsior 2020).

A general trend from the beginning of the crisis was that the state governments adopted their own measures to face the pandemic because the federal authorities were not acting fast enough. In addition to cancelling classes, approximately 10 out of the 32 states closed bars, restaurants, museums, and beaches earlier than these closures were proposed by the federal authorities. Yucatán went as far as to impose fines for people not following confinement regulations; Chihuahua suggested that people who had tested positive for COVID-19 may even face jail time if they failed to abide by the confinement requirements. In Jalisco, state authorities pushed for adopting their own testing policies, arguing that the federal government was not performing enough tests.

This proactive approach by state governments was consistent in the early months. At the state level, responses were quicker, more numerous and rather heterogenous. Between March 1 and 31 July 2020, 629 measures were adopted by state governments to manage the dire health and economic consequences of the pandemic (Cejudo et al. 2020). All states adopted measures restricting work and movement, and most of them implemented food support programs. The economic relief programs devised by state governments ranged from wage subsidies plus cash transfers to deferrals and discounts on taxes for both individuals and businesses. In addition, tax inspections have been postponed (OECD 2020). Almost half of these measures were fully financed with resources from state governments coffers (Cejudo et al. 2020).[3] States governed by parties in opposition to the President have been the most active in adopting measures to deal with the crisis.

At the municipal level, a much lower number of measures have been adopted: 159 municipalities in 25 out of 32 states have adopted specific initiatives (CONAMER 2020). Although the legal framework limits the role of municipal governments in health and sanitary services, and they cannot impose preventive health measures, cities and towns found other ways to act. Municipalities do have legal competences for regulating public spaces (i.e., markets, parks, and graveyards), water provision and treatment as well as waste management. With these legal mandates, municipalities have adopted 371 measures ranging from fiscal stimuli to prohibition of massive events combined with mandatory lockdowns of questionable legality.

There is an emerging consensus that the lack of coordination is the defining characteristic of the actions and emergency plans adopted by different levels of government in Mexico. Coordination is absent both in vertical relations (among federal, state, and municipal governments) and in horizontal ones (i.e., agreements across ministries at the same level of government). Intergovernmental cooperation was reached only partially in specific areas; for example, 7 out of 32 state governments announced the adoption of a common scheme for the reopening of their economies on May 29 (Najar 2020).

15.4 Is the Mexican federal system different because of the COVID-19 pandemic?

Considering the general situation described in the previous sections, three points should be stressed regarding the effects of the COVID-19 pandemic in the Mexican federal system. First, there are key differences between the actions adopted by the federal government and those promoted by state authorities. These differences emerged in the types of instruments used, and the population targeted, especially when addressing the economic consequences of the pandemic. The federal government used existing social programs and focused on individuals who were already receiving social benefits. State governments, however, created new instruments overnight and attempted to care for a more heterogeneous group of citizens.

Second, the lack of coordination slowly evolved into an open political conflict between federal authorities and several governors from parties in opposition to President López Obrador and his political party, Morena. The governor of Jalisco, Enrique Alfaro, accused federal authorities of mismanaging the COVID-19 crisis and of blocking the massive implementation of fast testing devised by his own state government. Later, Governor Alfaro accused the federal Ministry of Health of manipulating the COVID-19 statistics so the ministry could extend social distancing measures, thus punishing Jalisco by slowing down the reopening of the state economy. The governor of Chihuahua, Javier Corral, became a vocal actor in opposition to the federal economic recovery plan, arguing that financial aid was not sufficient. In a more dramatic move in the same vein, at the end of July, nine governors signed an open letter asking for the resignation of Hugo López-Gatell, the federal Vice-Minister of Health and the leading tactician of the federal government plans to fight the pandemic, accusing him of failing to control the disease.

In addition, and as a response to the uncertainty faced by state governments given the severe decrease in national and subnational tax collection, a group of governors called for a revision of the fiscal pact, in place since 1978. States currently have limited fiscal alternatives to obtain additional resources, as the amount of debt they may accrue is capped by federal regulations (CIEP 2020). The ultimate crisis in the Mexican federation occurred at the beginning of September when ten governors left the National Conference of Governors, an organization created in the early 21st century to coordinate state governments' actions when negotiating with the federal authorities on a variety of policy issues (Flamand 2010).

Third, the uneven reaction of state governments to the pandemic may be explained by their asymmetric nature (i.e., in terms of financial resources and bureaucratic capabilities) and thus appears to have deepened social inequalities. That is, relatively affluent states tend to have more capable governments and more robust health systems and therefore have been able to deal with the crisis in a more effective manner than the poorest subnational units. This may explain the much higher fatality rate in poorer municipalities than in richer ones.

On May 14, the federal government announced the "New Normality," a plan presenting state and municipal level reopening scenarios. It included the opening of 324 "municipalities of hope" the following week (SE 2020). Three weeks after the announcement, only 60 municipalities remained open, as the pandemic continued to spread (Ariadna Ortega 2020). By the beginning of September, Mexico was already returning to pre-pandemic levels of mobility. In fact, at the beginning of that month, one quarter of states had reopened all activities, except for in-person education. At the same time, the number of tests remained low in the country: while the World Health Organization recommends performing at least 20 tests for every positive case before relaxing social distancing measures (WHO 2020), in September, the number for Mexico was 2.4 tests for every positive case (Hasell et al. 2020).

In Mexico, there have been complex and close interactions between electoral politics on one hand, and the policies developed to contain contagions and to alleviate the economic effects of the pandemic on the other. A prime example is the policy differences between the federal government of president López Obrador and the government of Mexico City headed by Claudia Sheinbaum. They were both elected under the banner of the same political party, Morena.[4]

Since the beginning of the pandemic, the government of Mexico City has implemented policies to safeguard the incomes of workers and businesses, in contrast to the lackluster stimulus packages advanced by the federal government. This was a bold move considering the massive financial dependence of the states on federal grants.

Regarding the closing of nonessential activities in mid-March and mid-December of 2020, several news articles have reported clashes between López Obrador and Governor Sheinbaum in private despite a show of unity in public. Governor Sheinbaum apparently insisted on closing earlier to prevent further contagions on both occasions. Given the importance of the activity of the city for the economic performance of Mexico overall, federal officials strongly opposed early closures, apparently causing the highest levels of occupation of hospitals beds and of deaths associated with COVID-19 in late January 2021.

The federal system in Mexico has responded in a somewhat uncoordinated fashion to the health and economic crises caused by the spread of COVID-19. There are two significant structural reasons for this. The first is the centralized and asymmetrical nature of the federal system. The second is the fragmentation of the healthcare system. However, without clear federal guidelines and standards to manage the crisis, state governments have reacted unevenly, deepening social inequalities. The result was that isolated decision-making, disconnected fluxes of information, and uncoordinated actions all deepened public uncertainty. The Mexican federal government has failed to take a vigorous leadership during this crisis. The result is that resources have been used inefficiently, and severe problems have arisen in implementing the policies designed to protect the Mexican population from COVID-19.

Notes

1 According to data collected by the Coronavirus Resource Center of Johns Hopkins University & Medicine (2020), the case-fatality ratio for Mexico is the second highest in the world, reaching 8.5 percent and only surpassed by Yemen. The value for Brazil and Argentina is 2.5 percent and for the US 1.7 percent.
2 Three further constitutions were enacted by Mexico in 1835, 1843 and 1857. In the first two cases, they imposed a centralized form of government.
3 According to data collected by Cejudo et al. (2020): 47 percent of the state actions to combat Covid-19 were completely state funded; 10 percent were financed by the state government in cooperation with the federal or municipal orders, civil society organizations or private funding; 3 percent do not have state funding; and for 39 percent the source of funding is unknown.
4 Sheinbaum is also one of the forerunners for the next presidential election in 2024. In Mexico, after serving one term neither the president nor any governor may be reelected.

Bibliography

Amnesty International, 2020. Exposed, Silenced, Attacked: Failures to Protect Health and Essential Workers during the COVID-19 Pandemic. London: Amnesty International. Available from: https://www.amnesty.org/en/documents/pol40/2572/2020/en/ [Accessed 7 February 2021].

Ariadna Ortega, 2020. Mapa COVID: en tres semanas, los municipios de la esperanza bajaron de 300 a 60. Ciudad de México: Expansion, 14 June. Available from: https://politica.expansion.mx/estados/2020/06/14/mapa-covid-en-tres-semanas-los-municipios-de-la-esperanza-bajaron-de-300-a-60 [Accessed 7 February 2021].

Bank of Mexico, 2020. Precio de la mezcla mexicana de petróleo [online]. Mexico City: Bank of Mexico Available from: https://www.banxico.org.mx/apps/gc/precios-spot-del-petroleo-gra.html [Accessed 3 September 2020].

BBVA Research, 2021. Mexico Economic Outlook. First Quarter 2021. Mexico City: Banco Bilbao Vizcaya Argentaria (BBVA). Available from: https://www.bbvaresearch.com/en/publicaciones/mexico-economic-outlook-first-quarter-2021/ [Accessed 7 February 2021].

Cejudo, G.M., Gómez-Álvarez, D., Michel, C.L., Lugo, D., Trujillo, H., Pimienta, C. and Campos, J., 2020. Federalismo en COVID: ¿Cómo responden los gobiernos estatales a la pandemia? Versión 4. Ciudad de México: Centro de Investigación y Docencia Económicas (CIDE). Available from: https://www.researchgate.net/publication/341680758_Federalismo_en_COVID_Como_responden_los_gobiernos_estatales_a_la_pandemia_version_4 [Accessed 7 February 2021].

CEPAL, 2020. COVID-19 Observatory for Latin America and the Caribbean: Measures by Country. Santiago de Chile: Comisión Económica para América Latina y el Caribe (CEPAL). Available from: https://www.cepal.org/en/topics/covid-19 [Accessed 7 February 2021].

CIEP, 2020. Deuda subnacional. Endeudamiento en los estados frente al COVID-19. Cuauhtémoc, Mexico City: Centro de Investigación Económica y Presupuestaria (CIEP). Available from: https://ciep.mx/deuda-subnacional-endeudamiento-en-los-estados-frente-al-covid-19/ [Accessed 7 February 2021].

CONACYT, 2020. COVID-19 Tablero México [online]. Ciudad de México: Consejo Nacional de Ciencio y Technologia (CONACYT). Available from: https://coronavirus.gob.mx/datos/ [Accessed 7 February 2021].

CONAMER, 2020. Respuestas regulatorias a la epidemia COVID-19 [online]. Ciudad de México: Comisión Nacional de Mejora Regulatoria (CONAMER). Available from: https://conamer.gob.mx/respuestas-regulatorias-covid-19/EstadosMunicipios/Index [Accessed 7 February 2021].

CONAPO, 2020. Impacto de la contingencia sanitaria de Covid-19: Día Internacional de la Planificación Familiar. Ciudad de México: Consejo Nacional de Población (CONAPO). Available from: https://www.gob.mx/presidencia/es/articulos/version-estenografica-conferencia-de-prensa-informe-diario-sobre-coronavirus-covid-19-en-mexico-249441?idiom=es [Accessed 7 February 2021].

CONEVAL, 2020a. Visor geoespacial de la pobreza y la COVID-19 en los municipios de México [online]. Ciudad de México: Consejo Nacional de Evaluacion de la Politica de Desarrollo Social (CONEVAL) Available from: https://coneval.maps.arcgis.com/apps/dashboards/db5c233bb31f4c4189ded7d0edcacf92 [Accessed 7 February 2021].

CONEVAL, 2020b. La política social en el contexto de la pandemia por el virus SARS-CoV-2 (COVID-19) en México. Ciudad de México: Consejo Nacional de Evaluacion de la Politica de Desarrollo Social (CONEVAL). Available from: https://www.coneval.org.mx/Evaluacion/IEPSM/Paginas/Politica_Social_COVID-19.aspx [Accessed 7 February 2021].

Excelsior, 2020. Desde hoy, suspenden clases en 10 estados [online]. Mexico City: Excelsior. 17 March 2020. Available from: https://www.excelsior.com.mx/nacional/desde-hoy-suspenden-clases-en-10-estados-ante-pandemia/1370186 [Accessed 7 February 2021].

Flamand, L., 2010. Sistema federal y autonomía de los gobiernos estatales: avances y retrocesos. In: Méndez, J.L., ed. *Los grandes problemas de México*. Ciudad de México: El Colegio de México, 495–522.

Flamand, L., 2020. Federalism and COVID: Managing the Health and Economic Crisis in the Mexican Federation. Ottawa: Forum of Federations. Available from: http://www.forumfed.org/2020/04/laura-flamand-federalism-and-covid-19/ [Accessed 7 February 2021].

Hasell, J., Mathieu, E., Beltekian, D., Macdonald, B., Giattino, C., Ortiz-Ospina, E., Roser, M. and Ritchie, H., 2020. A Cross-Country Database of COVID-19 Testing. *Scientific Data*, 7 (1), 345. doi: 10.1038/s41597-020-00688-8.

IMF, 2020. Policy Responses to COVID19 [online]. Washington, DC: International Monetary Fund (IMF). Available from: https://www.imf.org/en/Topics/imf-and-covid19/Policy-Responses-to-COVID-19#M [Accessed 8 February 2021].

INEGI, 2020a. Estimacion oportuna del Producto Interno Bruto durante el cuarto trimestre de 2020. Auguascalientes City: Instituto Nacional de Estadística y Geografía (INEGI). Available from: https://www.inegi.org.mx/contenidos/saladeprensa/boletines/2021/pib_eo/pib_eo2021_01.pdf [Accessed 8 February 2021].

INEGI, 2020b. Encuesta Telefónica de Ocupación y Empleo 2020. Aguascalientes, Mexico: Instituto Nacional de Estadística y Geografía (INEGI). Available from: https://www.inegi.org.mx/investigacion/etoe/ [Accessed 8 February 2021].

INEGI, 2020c. Encuestra Telefónica sobre COVID-19 y Mercado Laboral. Aguascalientes, Mexico: Instituto Nacional de Estadística y Geografía (INEGI). Available from: https://www.inegi.org.mx/investigacion/etoe/ [Accessed 8 February 2021].

INMUJERES, 2020. Violencia contra las mujeres: Indicadores básicos en tiempos de pandemia. Ciudad de México: Instituto Nacional de las Mujeres (INMUJERES). Available from: https://www.gob.mx/inmujeres/documentos/violencia-contra-las-mujeres-indicadores-en-tiempos-de-pandemia [Accessed 8 February 2021].

JHU, 2020. How Does Testing in the U.S. Compare to Other Countries? Baltimore: Johns Hopins University of Medicine (JHU), 2020. Available from: https://coronavirus.jhu.edu/testing/international-comparison [Accessed 8 February 2021].

Lustig, N., Martínez-Pabon, V., Sanz, F. and Younger, S.D., 2020.The Impact of COVID-19 Lockdowns and Expanded Social Assistance on Inequality, Poverty and Mobility in Argentina, Brazil, Colombia and Mexico. Washington, DC: Center for Global Development. Available from: https://www.cgdev.org/sites/default/files/impact-covid-19-lockdowns-and-expanded-social-assistance.pdf [Accessed 8 February 2021].

Montes, J., 2021. Covid-19 Takes Outsize Toll on Mexican Health Workers; The Country Is among those with the Highest Mortality among Health Workers; 'It's Been Carnage' [online]. New York: *Wall Street Journal*, 9 January.

Mooney, H. and Zegarra, M.A., 2020. Extreme Outlier: The Pandemic's Unprecedented Shock to Tourism in Latin America and the Caribbean. In: Djankov, S. and Panizza, U. eds. *COVID-19 in Developing Economies*. London: CEPR Press, 112–126.

Najar, A., 2020. *Coronavirus en México: ¿por qué AMLO enfrenta una rebelión de gobernadores en la etapa crítica de la pandemia de covid-19?* London: BBC News Mundo.

OECD, 2020. OECD Employment Outlook 2020: Worker Security and the COVID-19 Crisis. Paris: Organisation for Economic Cooperation and Development (OECD). doi: 10.1787/1686c758-en Available from: https://www.oecd-ilibrary.org/employment/oecd-employment-outlook-2020_1686c758-en [Accessed 8 February 2021].

Olmeda, J.C. and Armesto, A., 2017. La Recentralización y los Gobernadores: ¿Por Qué no Siempre se Oponen? Analizando el Caso de México. *Ciudad de México: Foro Internacional*, 227 (1), 109–148. Available from: http://www.scielo.org.mx/scielo.php?script=sci_arttext&pid=S0185-013X2017000100109 [Accessed 8 February 2021].

Roser, M., Ritchie, H., Ortiz-Ospina, E. and Hasell, J., 2020. Coronavirus Pandemic (COVID-19) [online]. OurWorldInData.org. Available from: https://ourworldindata.org/coronavirus?fbclid=IwAR0GhhnIBw7H_0pKWOb4ubsuTYX52bf9O3nk6wz75w8hOjD9SgvSO5lOs7U [Accessed 8 February 2021].

SE, 2020. La nueva normalidad: Estrategia de reapertura de las actividades sociales, educativas y económicas. Ciudad de México. Available from: https://www.cmic.org/la-nueva-normalidad/ [Accessed 8 February 2021].

SEP, 2020. Acuerdo número 02/03/20 por el que se suspenden las clases en las escuelas de educación preescolar, primaria, secundaria, normal y demás para la formación de maestros de educación básica del Sistema Educativo Nacional, así como aquellas de los tipos medio superior y superior dependientes de la Secretaría de Educación Pública. [online]. Official Journal of the Federation. Secretaría de Educación Publica (SEP): Mexico City, 2020. Available from: https://www.dof.gob.mx/nota_detalle.php?codigo=5589479&fecha=16/03/2020 [Accessed 8 February 2021].

SS, 2019. *Indicadores de Gasto Público en Salud 2003–2017*. Mexico City: Secretaria de Salud(SS).

SS, 2020. Acuerdo por el que se establecen las medidas preventivas que se deberán implementar para la mitigación y control de los riesgos para la salud que implica la enfermedad por el virus SARS-CoV2 (COVID-19) [online]. Mexico City: Secretaria de Salud(SS), 2020. Official Journal of the Federation. Available from: https://www.dof.gob.mx/nota_detalle.php?codigo=5590339&fecha=24/03/2020 [Accessed 8 February 2021].

WHO, 2020. Public Health Criteria to Adjust Public Health and Social Measures in the Context of COVID-19. World Health Organization (WHO): Geneva, 2020. Available from: https://apps.who.int/iris/handle/10665/332073 [Accessed 8 February 2021].

World Bank, 2020. Pandemic, Recession: The Global Economy in Crisis. In: *Global Economic Prospects, June 2020*. Washington DC: The World Bank. doi: 10.1596/978-1-4648-1553-9.

World Health Organization Weekly epidemiological update – 12 January 2021. Geneva: WHO, 2021. Available from https://www.who.int/publications/m/item/weekly-epidemiological-update

16 COVID-19

The first wave response from Nepal

Puspa Raj Kadel

16.1 Introduction

Nepal's new federal system had to provide healthcare services for COVID-19 from the start of the pandemic. At the same time, the new federal system provided economic relief to sectors that were hardest hit.

The capital region of the Kathmandu Valley was particularly affected. Initially, the national government had to impose a complete lockdown for four months beginning on 24 March 2020. During this period, cases of COVID-19 were minimal compared to the economic impact of the virus. Daily wage earners were among many segments of the community dramatically affected. As a result, there was pressure from the business community and workers to ease the lockdown. The national government gradually eased the lockdown. However, afterward, the number of cases of COVID-19 increased significantly.

Nepal's federal system of governance performed well in the critical management of its COVID-19 pandemic response.

Challenges to governance during the pandemic were the needs to provide the following:

- Strengthened relationships among the three tiers of government;
- Needs-based funding to the local government by the provincial and federal governments according to the caseloads;
- Favorable economic and development policies in response to affected sectors, including agriculture, tourism, industry, returning migrants, and informal workers; and
- Effective mobilization against COVID-19 by community support organizations and cooperatives.

Nepal has endured a great deal in the first wave of the COVID-19 pandemic. The new federal country had little experience in coordinating either the economy or the health

Table 16.1 Key Statistics on COVID-19 in Nepal as of 10 January 2021

Cumulative Cases	Cumulative Cases per 100,000 Population	Cumulative Deaths	Cumulative Deaths per 100,000 Population	Case Fatality Percentage
264,521	907.9	1,912	6.6	0.7

Source: World Health Organization Weekly epidemiological update – 12 January 2021. Geneva: WHO, 2021. Available from https://www.who.int/publications/m/item/weekly-epidemiological-update

DOI: 10.4324/9781003251217-16

system of the land. The country had to face the collision of an unprecedented health crisis with its new democracy and its fledgling federal system (Table 16.1).

16.2 COVID-19 in Nepal

The first COVID-19 case in Nepal was confirmed on 23 January 2020 in a 32-year-old male who had returned from China on January 9. The second case was confirmed on March 23 in a young female who had flown to Kathmandu from France via Qatar. With a fear of infections from the pandemic, a noticeable number of people departed from the Kathmandu Valley. In the third week of March, Nepal began to see a significant entry of people from India as there was a huge increase in the number of new cases in that country as well. India's decision to implement a lockdown hastened the decision of many to return to Nepal.

To prevent the spread of the disease, Nepal focused its efforts on planning, prevention, and preparation. As prevention measures, the government prepared health guidelines and took safety measures as specified by WHO with the formation of the COVID-19 Crisis Management Centre (CCMC) in June 2020.

Additionally, to prevent spread of COVID-19, the government imposed a nationwide lockdown from March 24 to 15 July 2020 including travel restrictions to and from international destinations immediately, followed by restrictions on domestic flights later.

The first COVID-19 death in Nepal occurred on 14 May 2020, that of a 29-year-old woman, eight days after having given birth. Despite the significant efforts of the government to prevent the spread of COVID-19, the number of cases has been increasing, and until the end of 2020, more than 200,000 people had been affected and 1,337 had died. The situation of COVID-19 in Nepal, as of 31 December 2020, is given in Table 16.2.

As of 23 November 2020, Bagmati province had the highest number of fatalities of all seven provinces (657), followed by Lumbini Province (185). The lowest number of fatalities was seen in Karnali Province (23), followed by Sudurpaschim Province (37). The largest number of active cases occurred in Bagmati province (12,355), followed by Lumbini province (1,840) and Gandaki province (1,827). The lowest number of active cases was in Karnali province (136), followed by Province 2 (343). The details can be seen in Figure 16.1 below:

The situation in Kathmandu Valley is alarming. By 23 November 2020, out of the total affected, 46.66 percent cases had occurred there. Similarly, the fatalities in the valley were 37.47 percent of the total 1,337 fatalities in the entire country up to that date (Figure 16.2).

Table 16.2 Impact of COVID-19 on the Human Sector in Nepal

Total RT-PCR Tests	Total Positive Cases	Total Deaths	Total Recovered Cases	Recovery Rate (%)	Total Active Cases	Death Rate (%)
1,957,454[a]	260,593[a]	1,856[a]	233,624[b]	89.7[b]	6,378[a]	0.71[b]

Sources: [a] Ministry of Health and Population, Situation Update #38, as of 5 January 2021; [b] Calculations by Carl Stieren from sources: Worldometers.info. Available from: https://www.worldometers.info/coronavirus/country/nepal/;
Note: COVID-19 situation as of 31 December 2020

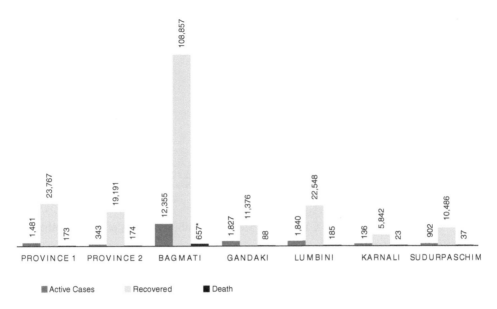

Figure 16.1 Provincial Distribution of COVID-19 cases in Nepal.

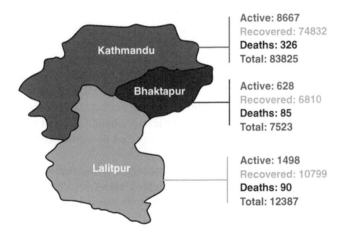

Figure 16.2 COVID-19 Cases in Kathmandu Valley in Nepal.

Similarly, if we compare the COVID-19 situation of Nepal with countries in the South Asian Association for Regional Cooperation (SAARC), the fatality rate of Nepal up to 23 November 2020 was higher (0.6 percent) than Bhutan, Sri Lanka, and Maldives. However, the rate was lower than in the other countries. Nepal's active case rate is 11.4 percent lower than Sri Lanka (30.8 percent), Bangladesh (17.7 percent), and Afghanistan (16.7 percent). However, Nepal's active case rate was higher than those in Bhutan, India, Maldives, and Pakistan. The recovery rate is highest in Bhutan (94.7 percent), followed by India (93.7 percent) and Maldives (91.6 percent). Nepal's recovery rate was 88 percent up to 23 November 2020, which was higher than the rates in Sri Lanka, Afghanistan, and Bangladesh (Figure 16.3).

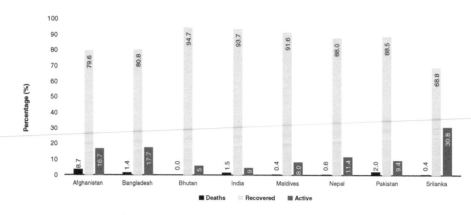

Figure 16.3 COVID-19 Cases in the SAARC Member States as of 21 November 2020.

16.3 Impact of COVID-19 on the economic sectors

COVID-19 has had a significant negative impact on the Nepalese economy. The impact has occurred in many sectors of economy. Particularly affected were external trade, capital spending by the government and credit expansion of the bank and financial institutions (BFIs). Due to the reduction in revenue, Nepal's federal budget has decreased by about 12 percent from the projected amount. The GDP growth rate that had been projected at 8.5 percent for the last financial year has decreased to about 2 percent. Government expenditures are slowing down, the investment environment has been disrupted, and private investment has also been decreasing. The liquidity position in the economy is increasing, and therefore, the market interest rate has decreased by half from the previous year. Moreover, the tourism sector, which provides about 3 percent of GDP, is completely closed. The earnings of informal sector of the economy have declined, and income of marginalized people has decreased.

The tourism, education, manufacturing, and infrastructure construction sectors have been heavily impacted. The Nepalese economy, which relies heavily on remittances, is affected due to the increase in returnee migrant workers. In response, the national government has formed a team to study the overall impact of COVID-19 on the economy (Table 16.3).

Similarly, the import of industrial supplies, fuel, capital goods, transport equipment, parts, and accessories has decreased owing to the impact of COVID-19. Table 16.4 below demonstrates the trend of imports of major goods during the same period.

Other major areas had losses due to the COVID-19 pandemic:

- **Infrastructure spending decreased:** At the end of the Fiscal Year 2019/2020, the financial and physical progress in the infrastructure development sector decreased 54.6 percent and 18 percent, respectively.
- **Job losses:** Employment declined and restricted economic activity affected livelihoods and income. The road and transport sector, which was estimated to provide 45,000 jobs, could not achieve so. COVID-19 directly affected around 315,000 porters, passenger service, and taxi providers in the tourism sector.

Table 16.3 Monthly Situation of Major Economic Indicators in Nepal (Amounts Rs. Billion)

Particulars	2019					2020				
	Mid-Month									
	March to April	April to May	May to June	June to July	July to August	March to April	April to May	May to June	June to July	July to August
Consumer inflation (Y-O-Y)	4.44	5.29	6.16	6.02	6.95	6.74	5.83	4.54	4.78	3.49
Consumer inflation (compared to previous month)	0.58	1.19	1.14	0.64	2.58	0.62	0.34	−0.10	0.86	1.33
Food and beverage	1.35	1.54	2.52	1.40	3.10	1.68	0.59	−0.55	1.71	2.76
Non-food and service	−0.02	0.93	0.06	0.04	2.18	−0.21	0.14	0.26	0.20	0.22
Exports	8.6	8.7	9.3	9.3	8.8	3.9	3.3	5.9	9.7	9.6
Imports	112.5	116.5	121.7	118.7	106.7	58.3	42.6	75.7	96.0	85.8
Travel income	7.1	9.1	5.4	5.1	4.4	1.7	0.9	1.2	3.0	0.6
Travel spending	6.4	5.7	6.8	9.1	7.0	1.3	0.6	1.0	1.3	1.6
Remittance inflows	71.0	72.1	73.7	80.3	75.4	34.5	53.9	94.0	101.4	92.7
Government expenditure	81.1	86.2	–	–	4.3	64.6	85.8	122.3	210.5	2.0
Current expenditure	57.7	65.3	–	–	3.6	44.6	76.7	98.4	116.0	1.7
Capital expenditure	19.2	19.4	–	–	0.6	8.7	9.1	11.9	65.2	0.1
Revenue	81.0	59.1	–	–	66.8	43.9	16.1	41.0	146.0	58.8
Deposit mobilization	24.9	29.2	43.0	129.3	−14.2	53.4	44.8	74.1	173.1	−5.4
Private-sector credit	46.5	15.6	24.8	30.1	14.7	40.0	−13.3	−10.4	36.8	−17.3
Weighted average deposit rate	6.7	6.7	6.6	6.6	6.8	6.7	6.4	6.2	6.0	5.8
Weighted average lending rate	12.3	12.2	12.2	12.1	12.1	11.8	11.0	10.4	10.1	10.5
Base rate of commercial banks	9.64	9.59	9.48	9.57	9.45	9.36	8.96	8.66	8.50	8.08

Source: Nepal Rastra Bank and FCGO

Table 16.4 Trend of Imports[a] in Nepal (Amounts in Rs. Billion)

S.N.	Classification of Goods	2019					2020				
		Mid-Month					Mid-Month				
		March to April	April to May	May to June	June to July	July to August	March to April	April to May	May to June	June to July	July to August
1	Foods and beverages	16.9	16.2	16.8	14.7	15.1	13.4	16.7	19.9	18.2	19.5
2	Industrial supplies	39.3	41.2	44.2	43.8	39.0	19.1	10.4	26.2	35.2	28.2
3	Fuels and lubricants	22.1	22.6	24.6	21.1	15.7	10.9	8.3	7.9	15.0	8.5
4	Capital goods, parts and accessories	15.6	16.5	17.2	20.6	17.1	8.0	2.8	10.2	15.3	14.2
5	Transport equipment, parts and accessories	8.7	10.5	9.3	9.0	9.6	2.5	0.6	3.4	4.0	6.0

Source: Nepal Rastra Bank.
a Major commodities based on UN trade statistics' classification by broad economic categories (revision 4).

- **Power project shortfalls:** COVID-19 also affected the power projects, especially electricity production; only 149 MW (15 percent) was produced, against the target of 1,000 MW. This was combined with a low demand of electricity especially during lockdown, as the industry sector has almost ground to a halt.
- **Schools closed:** The significant impact of COVID-19 has also seen in the education sector. With the increase in infected cases, the national government decided to close all teaching institutions and halt regular teaching and exams. A total of 35,520 schools, 1,425 higher education institutions, and 1,349 vocational schools have been impacted. The teaching of 8.1 million children of pre-primary to secondary level has been disrupted as well as that of 143,000 students of vocational training and 423,946 students of higher-level education (National Planning Commission 2020).
- **Healthcare services declined:** In the health sector, because of the fear of transmission of COVID-19 viruses, people rarely visited the Out Patient Departments of hospitals. As a result, the outpatient services have decreased by 90 percent during the 4 months of lockdown. It has also impacted the services for pregnant and new mothers, children, senior citizens, and persons with disabilities. Moreover, regular checkups, vaccine service, treatment of malnourished children, and family planning services have also been disrupted.
- **Tourism hardest hit:** The tourism sector has been perhaps hardest hit by the pandemic. In fiscal year 2019/2020, travel income decreased by 19.2 percent to Nepal Rupees (NPR) 60.89 billion from NPR 75.37 billion in the previous year. In the first month of fiscal year 2020/2021, this had decreased by 86.1 percent to NPR 605.6 million from a height of NPR 4.36 billion in the same period of the previous year (Central Bureau of Statistics, Government of Nepal 2020).

However, there were some beneficial economic impacts. The first economic boost was the reduction in the cases of black-market currency exchanges for remittances, known as *hundi* transactions in Nepal. Despite the decrease in migrant workers, the total amount of remittances has not reduced significantly. The second economic boost was the increase of agricultural production due to the inflow of returnee migrants going back to their villages. The third was the reduction in imports causing increases in foreign currency reserves. The fourth was the necessary and increased attraction to online information and services in all levels of government, causing growth in the digital economy.

16.4 COVID-19 and federalism in Nepal

16.4.1 *General features of Nepal's federal system*

Nepal is a country of geographical diversity. The country has had a unitary form of government since 1768. In that year, Prithvi Narayan Shah of the Kingdom of Gorkha, after his conquest of neighboring kingdoms, moved his capital to Kathmandu. The Shah dynasty then ruled a unified Nepal from 1769 to 2008.

However, under a centralized monarchy, Nepal was not able to achieve the development goals of the country and, with only a limited democracy, had excluded many from participation in government. As a way forward that united almost all political parties in Nepal, federalism was chosen as the system of state. A central federal government and seven provinces, federal constituent units of government, were created. Federalism was an inclusive practice for Nepal. So, with the addition of proportional development in all the parts of the country, the mobilization of resources and reducing economic, social and religious discrimination, the monarchy was abolished, and Nepal was transformed into a democratic federal republic.

The Constitution of Nepal, adopted in 2015, affirms Nepal as a secular federal parliamentary republic. The constitution provides three main structures: federal, province, and local levels which exercise the power of the state of Nepal pursuant to the constitution and relevant laws. Nepal has 7 provinces, each province composed of 8–14 districts. The districts, in turn, comprise local governments known as urban and rural municipalities. There are a total of 753 local governments which include 6 metropolitan municipalities, 11 sub-metropolitan municipalities and 276 municipalities (a total of 293 urban municipalities), and 460 rural municipalities. Each local government is composed of wards. There is a minimum number of wards in a local government – at one point, it was 11 wards – and in total, there are 6,743 wards in 753 local governments.

Local governments enjoy executive and legislative as well as limited judicial powers in their local jurisdiction. The provinces have a unicameral parliament based on a Westminster system of governance. Local and provincial governments exercise some exclusive powers and some concurrent powers, shared with provincial and/or federal governments. The Supreme Court is the highest authority to interpret the laws, and it can direct the parliament to amend or enact new laws as required.

The constitution assigned a larger functional, semi-judicial, and fiscal authority to elected local governments. There are also greater responsibilities for effective service delivery and accountability to citizens. The executive power of the local level was devolved to the village assembly and municipal assembly, according to the constitution and federal laws. Those powers provide functions, roles, and responsibilities of village and municipal assemblies. Residual powers – those powers not specified in the constitution – are governed by federal laws. Local levels can formulate periodic plans and annual budgets as well as collecting taxes and exercising other revenue raising powers.

However, tax and revenue collection on matters that fall within the concurrent list and on matters that are not included on any list, are carried out by the federal government. In addition, the constitution states that all revenues received by the Government of Nepal must be deposited into the Federal Consolidated Fund. This fund is then shared among the state and local governments, according to the formula recommended by the National Natural Resources and Fiscal Commission.

There are four mechanisms of fiscal transfers:

1   Equalization grants;
2   Conditional grants;
3   Matching grants; and
4   Special grants.

Special grants exist to transfer financial resources from the federal government to provincial and local governments and similarly from the provincial governments to their respective local governments. Moreover, there are also resource sharing and revenue sharing mechanisms among the federal, provincial, and local governments.

Table 16.5 Geographical Area, Population, GDP, MPI, and HDI of Provinces of Nepal

Name of the Province	Area	Population (2011)	GDP (%)	M`PI	HDI
Province 1	25,905 km²	4,534,943	15	0.085	0.553
Province 2	9,661 km²	5,404,145	13	0.217	0.485
Bagmati Province	20,300 km²	5,529,452	41	0.051	0.560
Gandaki Province	21,504 km²	2,403,757	8	0.061	0.567
Lumbini Province	22,288 km²	4,741,716	13	0.133	0.519
Karnali Province	27,984 km²	1,327,957	4	0.230	0.469
Sudurpaschim Province	19,915 km²	2,552,517	6	0.146	0.478

16.4.2 Provinces: new entities in Nepal's federal structure

Table 16.5 below contains several key indices that detail the situation in the provinces. Gandaki Province and Bagmati Province have almost the same Human Development Index (HDI) value: (0.567 and 0.560) followed by Province 1 (0.553). Similarly, for the Multidimensional Poverty Index (MPI) values of the provinces, the incidence of poverty is highest in Karnali province (0.230) followed by Province 2 (0.217).

Bagmati province and Gandaki province are the provinces having the least poverty (0.051 and 0.061, respectively). Regarding the Gross Domestic Product (GDP), out of the total GDP (at the producers' price) of NPR 3,464.31 billion, the contribution of Bagmati Province is estimated to stand at the highest with 41 percent, and that of Karnali Province is estimated to stand at the lowest with 4 percent in FY 2018/2019. In the case of population, Bagmati province is densely populated (5,529,452) with the geographical coverage of 20,300 km² whereas Karnali Province has lowest number of population (1,327,957) although has covered highest geographical area (27,984 km²).

16.5 Managing emergencies and the delivery of healthcare

With these new governance structures, accountability has also been shared among the three tiers of government. At the federal level, the Ministry of Health and Population is the central organization for the formulation of health-related policies. Budgetary decisions and program implementation have been divided up; the local level is responsible for a large part of the responsibilities. The 753 local governments oversee more than 4,000 health facilities and are responsible for providing the health facilities at the local level. Nepal's federal structure delegates many administrative decisions to the local level. Public health is a shared responsibility across governmental spheres, but primary healthcare and sanitation are exclusively local government functions. The main institutions that deliver basic health services are public hospitals, private hospitals, primary health care centers (PHCCs), and health posts.

Recently, all the central hospitals, provincial hospitals, medical colleges, academic institutions, and hub-hospitals have been designated to provide treatment care for COVID-19 cases. So far, more than 2,000 hospital beds across the country are allocated for isolation of suspected and confirmed cases (Ministry of Health and Population 2020).

16.6 Healthcare mechanisms established by all three levels of government

After the pandemic hit Nepal, new *ad hoc* mechanisms were established by executive decisions to respond to the crisis. An 11-member COVID-19 Prevention and Control High Level Coordination Committee (HLCC) was set up as the main mechanism to respond to COVID-19, reporting to the Deputy Prime Minister. The Committee was "formed under Prime Minister K.P. Oli to carve out precautionary measures against the possible outbreak of COVID-19. The committee comprises ministers from major ministries including Home, Defense, Finance, Health, Tourism, Foreign, Industry, Education, and Agriculture" (The Diplomat 2020). The HLCC was given a sweeping mandate to carry out necessary functions relating to prevention and control of COVID-19. Within less than a month of the formation of the HLCC, the Council of Ministers formed another CCMC with detailed and clear terms of reference, which eventually replaced the HLCC. At the top of the CCMC was a directorate led by the Deputy Prime Minister and five other senior Minsters from the Federal Council of Ministers, which steered the overall response to pandemic. A Facilitation Committee to support the CCMC's functions was formed under the leadership of the Chief Secretary, which included the Secretary of the Federal Ministry of Home Affairs and the Chiefs of four security forces (Nepal Army, Nepal Police, Armed Police Force, and National Investigation Department).

Four different operations were set up under the Facilitation Committee to deal with the following:

1   Health services and treatment (Medical Ops);
2   Supply medicine and equipment (Logistic Ops);
3   Maintenance of law and order (Security Ops); and
4   Information and technology support (Media & IT Ops) (Karki, 2020).

Similarly, at the provincial level as well, CCMCs – a replication of the Federal CCMC – were established in each province, led by the Chief Minister. As part of their roles, the federal government was concentrated on formulating policies, coordinating with the provincial governments and management of necessary human resources and medical equipment and medicines.

The provincial governments focused on establishing isolation centers and testing labs and managed medicines and other essential services as well as functioning as a bridge between federal and local governments.

Similar structures were established in each local government, led by its Chairperson or Mayor. As the coronavirus began to spread, local governments took the lead in establishing help desks, prohibiting public gatherings, establishing information centers, setting up hand-washing facilities, allocating isolation beds, instituting quarantine procedures at public and private hospitals, and relief distribution including food items for the most needy people and implementing testing and tracking schemes.

All the central hospitals, provincial hospitals, medical colleges, academic institutions, and hub-hospitals have been designated for the treatment and care of COVID-19 cases. So far, more than 2,000 hospital beds across the country are allocated for isolation of suspected and confirmed cases (Ministry of Health and Population 2020).

The government has decided to provide a hospital facility in each local body. Priority has been given to the strengthening of health facilities in all subnational levels.

16.7 How intergovernmental relations worked in response to COVID-19

Local governments have been at the forefront of managing and monitoring activities related to the delivery of basic healthcare services and preventing the spread of the COVID-19 virus. Their responsibilities have been critical to the pandemic response effort. The federal and provincial governments have provided local governments with additional standards, directives, and procedures for the prevention and management of COVID-19 infections. Local governments have been initiating and conducting various activities on their own for the prevention and control of COVID-19. Local governments have carried out awareness-raising programs, operated health desks at their main entry points, and have run fever clinics. Elected representatives, officials, and health workers have been active in establishing and managing quarantine facilities and health check-ups. They also played an important role in initiating contact-tracing where infections were identified. They also facilitated the taking of Rapid Diagnostic Tests (RDT) and polymerase chain reaction (PCR) tests (Democracy Resource Center Nepal 2020). The roles of local governments were focused around establishing and managing quarantine facilities and distributing relief material to needy people.

Even though all three levels of government worked together, a systematic but centralized approach was adopted which did not provide much space for subnational governments to influence the response to the pandemic, except for carrying out routine responsibilities with their limited resources.

Furthermore, District Level CCMCs were also eventually set up in all districts with Chief District Officers given greater authority and leadership over the COVID-19 response, which further compromised the roles of provincial and local government.

During the crisis, there was good vertical intergovernmental cooperation as well as horizontal coordination and collaboration among the provincial governments, between the provincial and local governments, and among the local governments. This has significantly helped in managing the quarantines and isolation centers and in sharing the best practices to stop the spread of COVID-19 at the community level.

16.7.1 Managing the fiscal impact and response to COVID-19

The lockdown affected economic activities in Nepal in a significant way. Many workers and laborers were severely affected.

The Government of Nepal has tried to respond to the COVID-19 crisis through fiscal and monetary measures.

Fiscal measures targeted by the government fall into three broad categories:

1. **Instituting immediate health measures**. These measures were aimed at increasing access to testing for COVID-19 infections and the establishment of quarantine facilities as well as a waiver on customs duties for medical items related to COVID-19 such as masks, sanitizer, and surgical gloves.
2. **Reducing the impact on livelihoods**. The federal government implemented food distribution programs, extended eligibility for the Prime Minister's Employment Program and provided discounts on utility bills.
3. **Providing economic support to firms**. The national government had deferred the payment of taxes and provided concessional loan facilities to severely affected

businesses. The cumulative cost of these programs is estimated at 5 percent of the GDP. Measures taken by Nepal Rastra Bank, that is, Central Bank, were aimed at providing liquidity support to banks and facilitating the provision of credit to the private sector. The key measures announced by the central bank included a relaxation of regulatory requirements for banks and financial institutions and a reduction of targeted interest rates as part of the country's interest rate corridor (World Bank 2020).

Additionally, to address fiscal issues, the Federal Government established a COVID-19 Prevention, Control, and Treatment fund (COVID-19 fund) at the federal level. Similar funds were also replicated at the provincial and local level at the direction of the national government. The purpose of the COVID-19 fund was to support prevention, control, and treatment of COVID-19 patients, to provide relief to the poor and vulnerable, and to cover the expenses of infrastructure and human resources. A seven-member committee led by the Vice-Chairperson of the National Planning Commission was also formed to operate the Federal COVID-19 fund, with the Secretaries of relevant ministries as members. The provincial and local level funds were each operated by a committee led by Chief Minister and Chairpersons/Mayors, respectively.

In the provincial budgets for Fiscal Year 2020/2021, all the provinces have allocated a significant budget in response to the COVID-19 pandemic. They have allocated budgets mainly on COVID-19 control, relief and rehabilitation, employment generation, and education. They intend to upgrade the quality of hospitals, capacity building of health professionals, special agriculture programs, and subsidized loans to the industries affected by COVID-19.

16.8 The federal system and the management of the pandemic in Nepal

The nationally led response by the federal government was relatively successful in preventing the spread of the pandemic in its early phase. However, once the pandemic started to spread across India, it prompted the mass migration of thousands of Nepali workers back to Nepal. At this stage, governments began focusing on expanding the quarantine and isolation centers in public places. With the increased caseloads, the federal government established nationwide testing labs to the extent possible. Since the first incidence of COVID-19 in Nepal, more than 60 testing labs have been established and equipped, almost from scratch. In all provinces, COVID-19 hub hospitals were established and equipped with testing kits, PPE, gloves, and trained staff at all levels of government.

Quarantine and isolation facilities were also established throughout the country in coordination with provincial and local governments. The federal government slowly increased daily RT-PCR testing from a few hundred tests to over 10,000 per day by October.

Similarly, the role of provincial governments in controlling the pandemic has been praiseworthy. Provinces established isolation centers, their own testing labs, and managed the distribution of medicines and other essential services.

The elected political representatives have been instrumental in managing COVID-19 at the local level.

Within the new federal system in Nepal, local governments have been useful in dealing with COVID-19. The federal structure placed elected governments in decision-making roles and devolved authority. This step has been beneficial in the control of the spread of the virus. It has also increased the response to the pandemic with accountability. However, some unclear roles and responsibilities need to be clarified among the three tiers of government. Also, the capacity of sub-national governments needs be increased. Institutions need to be created, and human resources and funding need to be found to respond to such crises.

16.9 Innovations and lessons learned during the first wave in Nepal

The experience of dealing with the pandemic had provided some significant positive signs for Nepal's new federal setup:

- **Provinces and municipal governments acted.** The COVID-19 pandemic has proved as an opportunity for the subnational governments, especially local governments, to reach out to people and demonstrate the real essence and benefits of federalism for the local community.
- **Local governments stepped in.** The performance of the local governments in response to the pandemic at the community level has helped federalism gain wider prominence in the country.
- **Roles and responsibilities were clarified for all governments.** Local government, as well as the federal government, found greater clarity regarding their roles and responsibilities and the need for a coordinated approach in this type of pandemic for future.
- **Villages welcomed back Nepalis returning from abroad.** This influx also provided the opportunity for local governments to facilitate and motivate the returnee migrants to stay in their villages and start productive activities or their own work at their residential places to earn income.
- **The health sector will be getting investments.** The health sector, a relatively low priority sector, has risen in prominence. Heavy investments are going to be made in this sector. Service here will be a priority at all levels of government.

16.10 Conclusion and recommendations

The impact of the four-month-long lockdown in response to the coronavirus has affected Nepal's economy significantly. The lockdown was responsible for the halt in revenue collection, reduction in remittance inflows, closure of industries and markets, restrictions in travels, loss of jobs by the Nepalese migrant workers abroad and in domestic labor markets. With the ease of the lockdown, economic activities are gradually returning. However, we are also witnessing an increase in COVID-19 cases which poses further challenges. There are 107,755 cases throughout the country of which 39 percent are in the Kathmandu Valley.

COVID-19 has entered the community transmission stage following a surge in infection and death rates.

As a least developed country, Nepal is facing serious challenges in managing health facilities including testing, tracing, and treatment in isolation. Nobody knows how long this pandemic will prevail. It might continue for months or even years.

With the current state of resources and the ongoing needs, the government could benefit from implementing these recommendations:

- **Build provincial and local capacity.** Nepal is still in the transitional federalism stage regarding transferring powers and responsibilities. The provincial and local governments lack resources and depend heavily on the federal government fiscal transfers for health infrastructure and human resource. Efforts should focus on building the capacity of provincial and local governments to better respond.
- **Create a needs-based model for health financing.** Current and anticipated COVID-19 caseloads require additional budget allocations to local governments. Provincial and federal governments need to develop a transparent and justifiable criterion for allocating funds across different levels.
- **Learn to manage rapidly changing healthcare needs.** Nepal is still facing challenges in managing quarantines/isolations, technical capacity (labs, technologies, and stock of medical supplies) to respond caseloads which should be taken care of.
- **Clarify the roles and responsibilities of each level of government.** More work is needed in strengthening intergovernmental coordination.
- **Focus on testing, tracing, and treatment.** There are already more patients requiring treatment than the absorptive capacity of hospitals, including those in Kathmandu. So, resources need to be directed to where it is needed. To achieve this, health financing needs to be evidence-based and not just one-size-fits-all.
- **Help civil society organizations, private sectors, and nongovernment organizations to mobilize strategically.** These groups are active at different levels. Mobilizing more strategically helps to create awareness and support the revival of economic activities.
- **Help returning migrants.** Provide them with enterprise creation opportunities targeting their current skills to increase their contribution to the national development.
- **Formulate policy to revive each affected industrial sector.** Incentives should provide subsidized loans and reduction of tax/VAT rates.
- **Prioritize the agricultural sector.** Loans with extremely low interest rates to the real farmers need to be provided.
- **Control the border with India according to the COVID-19 case load in both countries.** The major cause of transmission was the open and unregulated border with India. One of the major lessons is how the border between two independent countries should be regulated to control the pandemic.
- **Increase social sector expenditures, especially in healthcare.** More funding for this sector is an urgent requirement for all levels of government.
- **Digitalize all levels of government.** Growth in the digital economy would be spurred by this action. It would help fulfill the government slogan of "Digital Nepal."

Bibliography

Central Bureau of Statistics, Government of Nepal, 2020. *Current Macroeconomic and Financial Situation of Nepal* (Based on Annual Data of 2019/20 and first month of 2020/21). Available from: https://www.nrb.org.np/contents/uploads/2020/08/Current-Macroeconomic-and-Financial-Situation.-English.-Based-on-Annual-data-of-2019.20-1.pdf [Accessed 23 February 2021].

Democracy Resource Centre, Nepal, 2020. *Role of Local Governments in COVID-19 Prevention and Quarantine Management*, Update 2. Available from: https://www.democracy resource.org/wp-content/uploads/2020/05/COVID-19_Update-2_1June2020-Second.pdf [Accessed 23 February 2021].

Government of Nepal, Ministry of Health and Population. 2020. *Health Sector Emergency Response Plan, COVID 10 Pandemic*. Kathmandu: Ministry of Health and Population, 2020. Available from: https://publichealthupdate.com/health-sector-emergency-response-plan-mohp-nepal/ [Accessed 23 February 2021].

Karki, B., 2020. *Multi-Level Government and COVID-19: Nepal as a Case Study*, Melbourne Forum on Constitutional Building. Melbourne: University of Melbourne, 2020. Available from: https://law.unimelb.edu.au/__data/assets/pdf_file/0009/3475818/MF20-Web3-Nepal-Karki-FINAL.pdf [Accessed 23 February 2021].

Ministry of Finance. 2018/2019. *Economic Survey*. Government of Nepal. Available from: https://www.mof.gov.np/uploads/document/file/compiled%20economic%20Survey%20 english%207-25_20191111101758.pdf [Accessed 21 September 2021].

Ministry of Health and Population, 2020. Available from: https://mohp.gov.np/en [Accessed 23 February 2021].

Ministry of Health and Population, 2021. Situation Update #38, as of-5 Jan 2021. Available from: https://mohp.gov.np/en [Accessed 23 February 2021].

Multidimensional Poverty Index, Nepal, 2020. Government of Nepal: National Planning Commission. Singha Durbar, Kathmandu. Available from: https://ophi.org.uk/wp-content/uploads/Nepal_MPI-22-12-2017.pdf [Accessed 23 February 2021]. National Planning Commission, 2020. *Impact of COVID-19 Pandemic on the Economy*, draft report.

Nepal Rastra Bank, 2020. *Current Macroeconomic and Financial Situation of Nepal* (Based on One Month's Data Ending Mid-August 2020).

Pandey, S., 2020. *Federalism and the COVID-19 Crisis: Nepal's Condition and Efforts*. Ottawa: Forum of Federations, 2020. Available from: http://www.forumfed.org/publications/ federalism-and-the-covid-19-crisis-federalism-and-the-covid-19-crisis-nepals-condition-and-efforts/ [Accessed 23 February 2021].

Shrestha, R. Development Asia, 2020. How Nepal Is Facing the Challenges of a Federal System, Asia Development Bank: Metro Manila, Philippines, 2020. Available from: https:// development.asia/policy-brief/how-nepal-facing-challenges-federal-system [Accessed 23 February 2021].

Singhania, D., Pokharel, T., Pandey, R. and Callen M., 2020. *COVID-19 Funding in Federal Systems: Lessons from Nepal*, International Growth Centre, 2020. Available from: https:// www.theigc.org/blog/covid-19-funding-in-federal-systems-lessons-from-nepal/   [Accessed 23 February 2021].

United Nations Nepal, 2020. *COVID-19 Nepal: Preparedness and Response Plan (NPRP)*. Available by downloading from this page of Reliefweb. Available from: https://reliefweb.int/ report/nepal/covid-19-nepal-preparedness-and-response-plan [Accessed 23 February 2021].

Wikipedia, 2020. Provinces of Nepal. Wikipedia, 20 September 2015. Available from: https:// en.wikipedia.org/wiki/Provinces_of_Nepal [Accessed 23 February 2021].

World Bank, 2020. *Nepal Development Update Post-Pandemic Nepal – Charting a Resilient Recovery and Future Growth Directions*, World Bank Group. Available from: https:// openknowledge.worldbank.org/handle/10986/34178 [Accessed 23 February 2021].

17 COVID-19 and Nigerian federalism

Julius O. Ihonvbere

17.1 Introduction

The political geography of Nigeria has always been complicated, unsteady, and uncertain. Novel issues are introduced daily, and these are often shaped by class, regional, party, and other primordial interests. A largely mono-economy dependent on crude oil sales, with weak institutions that are bedeviled by corruption and inefficiencies, its largest achievement since 1999 has been the sustenance of liberal democratic practice (Babalola 2019; Ihonvbere 2020). Though the return to liberal democratic rule in 1999 has opened the country's political space to mass political actions, the alignment and realignment of socio-political forces and careful explorations of elite interests often show by how much the limits of the Constitution can be stretched. Nigerians know that there remains a lot of work to be done to ensure and assure democratization, positive pluralism, accountability, the rule of law, and social justice.

Political discourses before and since redemocratization, while calling for different forms of confederation, federalism, and other political arrangements have been unanimous on the acceptance of a federal political arrangement (Ibiam 2016). The debate has been on resource control and the structure and division of powers between the center and the constituent units: the 36 States and Federal Capital Territory (FCT). Today, there is substantial agreement that the Central government is way too powerful for the good of Nigeria's federal structure (Yagboyaju and Akinola 2019). Yet, the extant structure, aside from revenue collection and resource control, has not prevented the States from providing good governance and investing available resources in the promotion of the common good (Table 17.1).

17.2 COVID-19 in Nigeria

The Federal Government has done well in its response to COVID-19, mounting a public education campaign, shutting the borders, closing all schools, limiting travels

Table 17.1 Key Statistics on COVID-19 in Nigeria as of 10 January 2021

Cumulative Cases	Cumulative Cases per 100,000 Population	Cumulative Deaths	Cumulative Deaths per 100,000 Population	Case Fatality Percentage
97,478	47.3	1,342	0.7	1.4

Source: *World Health Organization Weekly epidemiological update* – 12 January 2021. Geneva: WHO, 2021. Available from https://www.who.int/publications/m/item/weekly-epidemiological-update

DOI: 10.4324/9781003251217-17

within the country, shutting the airports markets, places of worship and entertainment, setting up a COVID-19 Presidential Task Force (PTF), a National Monitoring Committee, and activation and expansion of its social development programs to support the "poorest of the poor" particularly through the Conditional Cash Transfer Initiative (Abdulrauf 2020; Federal Republic of Nigeria 2020). The country's National Centre for Disease Control (NCDC) works with other stakeholders including the Presidency and the Ministry of Health and gives daily briefings to the nation. The officers of the NCDC and PTF have visited most of the states in the country to inspect isolation centers, laboratories, and hospitals to establish the levels of preparedness and capacity to engage the COVID-19 challenge (Babalola 2020; NCDC 2020a). The visits were equally opportunities to review public campaign and awareness initiatives. Though the country had only two centers for testing for infectious diseases, the Government has provided funds to upgrade existing facilities, procure equipment and ambulances, establish more testing centers, and isolation centers (Dixit, Ogundeji and Onwujekwe 2020). On 8 October 2020, the PTF announced that all the 36 States and FCT now have facilities for Digital Surveillance of COVID-19 as well as functional laboratories for testing and made the usual appeal that Nigerians should patronize them (NCDC 2020b). Interestingly, while the NCDC and PTF are engaged in daily updates about COVID-19, aside from Lagos State, the other states are not following in similar direction. It is yet to be seen if the state governments will maintain these facilities.

The COVID-19 infection case figures have been relatively low: 58,848 confirmed cases, 50,385 discharged, and 1,112 deaths as of 1 October 2020 (NCDC 2021a). This is a rather low figure for a country of over 200 million. Aside from the top four epicenters of the pandemic, Lagos (19,461), The FCT (5,709), Plateau (3,450), Oyo (3,261), Edo (2,626), Rivers (2,432), and Kaduna (2,419), the infection figures are almost evenly distributed across the other states with some states recording almost insignificant infections (NCDC 2021a). Lagos is high because of its population, and it also serves as the commercial and transport hub of the country. The Governor of the State, Babajide Sanwo-Olu, has been surprisingly proactive and creative, and the intense campaign and investment in contact tracing and a relatively effective initiative of house-to-house testing are yielding results (Government of Lagos State 2020). Lagos has also established Testing Centers in all its local government and Community Development Areas with a public campaign encouraging citizens to see them as help centers and not death centers. Overall, testing in the country remains low at under 500,000 at the end of September 2020 (Onuah 2020).

The low casualty figures in Nigeria have contradicted all permutations and forecasts. The assumption was that, due to very poor health infrastructure, high concentration of population at the peri-urban centers and shanties, and the very poor attention to rural communities in terms of social infrastructure, the pandemic was going to hit Nigeria very hard. The difficulty in communication between capital cities and rural communities also promoted fears as to how to communicate messages on COVID-19 protocols to poor rural dwellers. All calculations and predictions, even for Lagos with its over 20 million population, failed to come true.

17.3 Low cases of infection and policy limitations

Nigeria must, however, not be carried away with the low cases of infection and casualties. As pointed out earlier, testing has been very slow, and community spread may only just be around the corner. This is where the big bang will occur if serious and urgent steps are not adopted at the state and local government as well as community levels. All the cities have very crowded slums with no health facilities (African Center for Strategic Studies 2020). Most communities still lack access to water and electricity. Though the National Orientation Agency (NOA) has offices all over the country, it has failed woefully to make itself relevant in the campaign against COVID-19. While its leaders complain about funding, the truth is that they have been unable to come up with innovative ways to raise funds, package the COVID-19 protocol message, and reach out to under-served communities. Similarly, the low reading culture in the country has meant that newspapers and magazines circulate very poorly in the cities and not at all in the rural areas.

The levels of unemployment, ignorance, and poverty are also high. With the lockdown or border closures in most states, the poor began to get desperate and ready to challenge control policies (Kalu 2020). Indeed, several such challenges occurred in cities like Lagos, Warri, and Abuja. With poor monitoring, existing disconnection between the people and their communities from the custodians of state power at all levels, the official structures of power have not been able to effectively convey appropriate information to the populace. The truth is that door-to-door testing is haphazard and few and far between, people are not volunteering, it costs a fortune to use private facilities, and the bureaucracy at public facilities are not encouraging. The stigmatization of post-COVID-19 patients, general beliefs in informal treatment options, and the well-known poor relationship between patients and healthcare managers have also discouraged voluntary testing (AFP 2020). The low figures may therefore not actually reflect the true state of coronavirus infections in Nigeria.

17.4 Ignorance, superstition, and COVID-19

With the traditional neglect of the rural areas and inner cities and closure of markets, offices, and businesses, the palliatives distributed by governments did not resolve the problem of hunger and anxiety in society. Some State governments did not bother to distribute palliatives, and this generated ever more anger and opposition to the COVID-19 protocols. In some cases, items sent by the Federal Government were hoarded by officials for future use during political campaigns. This was confirmed during the recent massive protest code-named #ENDSARS by youths fed up with the system and political leadership where several warehouses loaded with palliatives were raided and looted all over the country (Obiezu 2020). There have also been accusations and counter accusations about the quality of the distributed materials as well as the extent of distribution. At the local government areas (LGAs), some chairmen politicized the distribution only favoring their political factions or political party members.

Interestingly and unfortunately, there is still a lot of superstition, ignorance, and misperception among the populace. This is amazing given the global campaign and increasing local efforts at promoting public education on the coronavirus. Many have quickly bought into all sorts of conspiracy theories especially those propounded by hundreds of online videos and write-ups condemning the World Health Organization, Bill and Melinda Gates, and the great political powers of the global system that the virus was designed for everywhere but Africa and aimed to recreate the world in a particular fashion, concluding that COVID-19 is a hoax. The poor, even educated persons argue publicly that the "Hunger Virus" is more dangerous than the Coronavirus! Many will argue that they were yet to know or see anyone infected or killed by the disease. Some contend that COVID-19 does not kill Africans and in comfortable ignorance of the devastating effects of COVID-19 in countries like South Africa, Egypt, and Ghana, they proceed to spread this misinformation to the public. There is also the erroneous view held in the rural areas that the local gin or concoctions (usually a cocktail of herbs and roots immersed in alcohol) can eliminate the virus from the system (Onyemelukwe 2020).

Some Nigerians have continued to buy into arguments made elsewhere that the summer heat would end the spread of the virus in Europe and America, that the hot African sun will "melt" the virus. An even more widely held view, privately supported by some health practitioners, is that Nigerians, like most Africans, have natural immunity from access to fresh foods produced without chemicals, and the traditional use of several malaria, yellow fever, and other medicines such as Nivaquine and Camoquine. Most of these drugs are available without prescription and in a country where self-medication is very rampant; abuse of drugs without prescription has precipitated several tales of woe. The churches were not left out. Many corrupt and poorly informed church leaders used the opportunity to make ludicrous claims about their ability to prevent the virus through the power of the Holy Spirit through "special" prayers. They sold "special" anointing oils, Holy water, and perfumes to their ignorant followers who continue to wallow in ignorance about the dangers of the coronavirus.

Given the rather high profile of the early cases of infection among governors, top government officials, politicians, top academics, and businessmen, some Nigerians have contended that the virus only "catches" the rich and powerful that travel round the world and stay in big hotels, not poor people (CBC News 2020). This perspective arose from the fact that only prominent deaths from COVID-19 made the news and it therefore began to appear that other lower segments of society were not being infected. Clearly, these views, while reflecting the extent of ignorance and hunger in the land, also expose the poor level of public education. To some extent, you have numerous communities in the country without a single case of coronavirus where business has remained as normal as possible. During political campaigns as witnessed in the gubernatorial elections in Edo and Ondo States in late 2020, only "visiting" politicians and dignitaries wore face masks at meetings and rallies. The people mingled and rubbed shoulders as always and amazingly, there was no spike in the rate of infection, contrary to widespread fears. The Independent Electoral Commission (INEC) made it mandatory that wearing a face mask was a precondition to vote. Political party leaders complied by distributing masks. Those in the voting queues wearing masks took them off as soon as they had voted.

17.5 Power structures and responses to COVID-19

The coronavirus pandemic was, if nothing else, a true test of the *hardened* nature of Nigeria's federal structure and practice. When the Index case was reported on 27 February 2020 in Lagos, it quickly became obvious that the country had made no preparations. It took a little while to settle down and put in place some agencies to tackle the challenge. In large measure, the Federal government took it as a national challenge, rose to the occasion, and has managed, with a variety of intervening factors and forces, to keep the rate of infection to a manageable level and the discharge rate very high with the death rate relatively low. Since that date, the Federal Government has not relaxed in its efforts to educate the public, provide social palliatives to poor segments of society, establish institutions, interface with herbal medicine practitioners, encourage scientific research, partner with civil society, engage regional leaders in the fight against COVID-19, and continue to provide daily updates using all available media at its disposal (NCDC 2021b).

If the Federal Government had a fairly quick reaction time, the states and local governments were caught napping. Lagos state was the only exception, not just because the Index case was in Lagos but the government quickly appreciated the possible impact of the virus on its huge population. Some state governors, such as in Cross River, claimed that they were not doing any "lockdown" but were "locking out" the coronavirus. In others, as in Kogi, the existence of the virus in the state was denied. Kogi people were described as very "strong" and naturally protected from the virus. Many states especially in the northern part of the country simply remained silent, pretending that it was best to adopt that position until an outbreak was reported. In Kano, the report of hundreds of deaths was quickly attributed to "Meningitis" though the dead, in compliance with Muslim rites, were buried without autopsy. It took the intervention of the President of Nigeria and the dispatch of a team from the NCDC and Federal Ministry of Health to confirm that some of the deaths were COVID-19-related. Many states built ramshackle structures that they called isolation centers with little or no facilities just rickety beds and tables. Others simply whitewashed some old facilities and commissioned them with fanfare. In sum, most did not take the pandemic seriously enough, did not engage in holistic enlightenment campaign, provided no succor for the poor, imposed no lockdown, and provided little or no leadership to the people and their communities (Okeke 2020). Interestingly, the only lockdown respected by Nigerians was the federal lockdown. As for the local governments, they showed no initiative and only waited for instructions from the state governors before engaging in minor assignments. They could not fumigate markets and schools, distributed very few face masks and sanitizers, and waged almost no public campaign. Aside from Lagos State where state government assistance and policies pushed the local governments and Development Centers into action, there is no record of any autonomously generated initiative or programs by a local government in response to the pandemic.

In terms of responses to COVID-19, the Nigerian system operated more like a unitary rather than a federal system. The states and local governments largely sat back and waited for federal leadership. Each state and the FCT received a COVID-19 financial assistance of N1 billion but most did not deploy the funds to the fight against COVID-19 (KPMG 2020). This did not come as a surprise because what has been described as "feeding bottle" federalism where the states rely heavily on monthly revenue sharing with the federal government has continued to distort and weaken the country's federal arrangement. Save for a handful of states, the majority of the 36 states and FCT do not generate significant resources internally. This leaves them dependent on federal allocations, grants, and bailouts.

The Central government was fully in charge of funds, ideas, programs, and policies. The states were prepared to follow the lead of the federal government, and such disposition only allowed the center to get stronger and bolder in its dealings with the constituent units. It was not uncommon to see federal officials visiting states, inspecting facilities, issuing directives, commissioning projects, and promising support. The federal and interstate lockdown periods were enforced by the federal police and army. States like Imo recruited professionals like Professor Maurice Iwu to lead the effort against COVID-19 while others left the initiative in the hands of politicians. It is instructive to note that the responses to the COVID-19 pandemic did not generate any new political issues around the structure of the Nigerian federation. Though opposition, pro-democracy, and regional pressure groups continued to raise the need for restructuring or "true federalism" – essentially to carry out far-reaching constitutional reforms aimed to devolving more powers, responsibilities, and control over resources to the constituent units – the President of Nigeria announced that his government would not be intimidated or pressured into any form of political rearrangement.

The COVID-19 pandemic empowered the federal government to take charge, define policies, establish institutions, and bring the states under its "control" especially in the areas of health, education, social investment, security, and general propaganda. In the 2021 federal budget, several items, policies, and programs have been provided that would continue these federal opportunities (Budget Office of the Federation 2021).

17.6 Institutional responses to COVID-19

The Nigerian Legislature was not left out of the response to COVID-19. The issues of public response, expansion of health facilities, training and insurance for healthcare workers, compensation for frontline workers, and deepening of the emergency response system were tabled and discussed before the National Assembly was compelled to shut down (National Assembly 2020). The 109 Senators donated 50 percent of their salaries to the National COVID-19 Relief Fund, while the 360-member House of Representatives donated 100 percent of the salaries for March and April. With the shutdown, the Speaker and principal officers continued to interface with the Presidency and Ministers on the provision of palliatives to the most affected communities. The Speaker of the House of Representatives held meetings with the Chinese Ambassador to Nigeria on the ill-treatment of Nigerians in China as well as with stakeholders with a view to providing free electricity service for two months to all Nigerians. As well, all representatives were encouraged to go to their constituencies and provide palliatives, sanitizers, public education, and other forms of support in response to COVID-19.

There were, however, no clear strategies to engage other sectors or institutions to collaborate on mapping a grassroots-based or bottom-up strategy to the pandemic. There was no sustained conversation with trade unions, students' organizations, farmers associations, traditional, and religious leaders, civil society, the media, and the medical community, especially at the state level. While this was largely the result of the general unpreparedness, it was equally a reflection of the historical suspicions and absence of common grounds on any issue in the country.

17.7 The second wave of COVID-19

Given the comparatively low rates of infection, deaths, and dislocations in the economy occasioned by the first wave of the pandemic, the Nigerian government, following recommendations from the PTF and NCDC, gradually relaxed the lockdown in the country (NCDC 2021c). However, to the government's credit, it continued to insist on public adherence to COVID-19 protocols. In some states, structures earlier set up for testing, contact-tracing, and public enlightenment were abandoned or dismantled. Nigerians steadily went back to their old ways. Many that had face masks put them in their pockets on wore them under the chin. Hotels, night clubs, places of worship, supermarkets, and public places were opened. While the relaxation of the lockdown saw many private concerns and offices install sanitizer-dispensing equipment at their entrances and within the establishments, as soon as initial supplies ran out they were not refilled. Nigerians were engaging in handshakes and long hugs in public while they did everything against established protocols. The anti-COVID-19 pandemic group resumed their arguments that it was not COVID-19 that killed people but other diseases. Facebook and WhatsApp platforms were filled by European and American videos striving to convince the uninformed that COVID-19 was deliberately invented to reduce world population, and the vaccinations were meant to reduce global population by 3 billion. The Nigerian media remained active in cautioning Nigerians that the pandemic was not over. Then the second wave came and panic set in.

The daily infection figures quadrupled moving from between 400 and 500 to 900 to over 1,000 infections daily. For instance, on 10 January 2021, the infection figure was 1,585 with Lagos, FCT, Kaduna, Plateau, and Oyo states taking the lead. The national infection rate was 99,063, death rate stood at 1,350 with 79,417 recoveries. As of 12 January 2021, only 1,033,858 samples had been tested in the country which is embarrassingly low (NCDC 2021a). The death rates were up, isolation centers are once again filling up, and this time, government was caught unawares. What is strange in the Nigerian second wave experience is the attitude of the Federal Government. While some countries with rising infections were shutting their airports and borders, Nigeria has not done that. In fact, the country introduced a policy requiring all Nigerians to obtain National Identity Numbers (NIN) and link these with their phone numbers. Those that failed to so do within two weeks, later extended by another four weeks, would have their phone lines disconnected (Nigerian Communications Commission 2020). This precipitated a mad rush to the few and far offices of the National Identity Management Commission (NIMC). Senior public officials were horrified to witness hundreds of people without facemasks struggling and crushing each other to gain access to the NIMC offices to obtain the NIN. No doubt a super-spreader opportunity, this was a direct creation of government. To make matters worse, the Federal Road Safety Commission (FRSC) announced that the NIN was now a requirement for obtaining a drivers' license.

With the second wave, members of the Nigerian power elite continued to hold large lavish weddings and parties where COVID-19 protocols took a back seat. The markets remain very crowded with very few people wearing face masks and no evidence of public enlightenment in place. The Federal Government directed the reopening of schools on the 18 January though the Minister of Education has announced that this date would be reviewed following widespread condemnation by academic unions and civil society groups (Xinhua 2021). This, again, if not properly handled, would be dangerous for the country: over 90 percent of schools have no running water, and adequate plans have not been made to provide water for hand washing, face masks and sanitizers are not available, and seating arrangements in compliance with social distancing regulations have not been made. Most primary and secondary schools have no basic emergency health facilities.

So far, the most state and local governments are not acting as if they are aware of the second wave. It is business as usual. Though the Federal Government has directed that all Isolation Centers be re-opened, many states have not taken decisive actions. The airports have not been shut, and over 100 persons have escaped the COVID-19 arrival tests forcing the government to publish their passport numbers and threaten a six-month travel ban for non-compliance. Contact tracing is not effective, and the general irresponsibility of the public in their ignorance and/or arrogance has simply refused to comply with COVID-19 protocols. Nigeria has failed to expend its testing facilities to enable it to get a fairly good picture of infection rates. Since many states are not conducting tests, it means that the infection rate is much higher than declared. Unless urgent steps are taken to rev up testing, contact tracing, public enlightenment, and treatment, a disaster could still be in the offing in Nigeria.

17.8 Responses and lessons in Nigeria

Nigerian political and social science discourse has always bemoaned the fragility, weakness, and limited hegemony of the Nigerian state. This is largely due to its inability to dominate civil society. It relies more of political domination especially through the legal monopoly of the structures of coercion. The state has failed in virtually every sector, and since political independence in 1960, the state and its custodians have not resolved a single challenge – from education, health, and transportation, through security, agriculture, and power to social services, industrialization, and building public confidence (Ihonvbere 2020). With no dependable and replicable data for planning, contact tracing, and distribution of palliatives remains complicated. The COVID-19 pandemic has exposed its weaknesses and incapacity to respond to the needs of the people. Suffering an underlying popularity deficit in terms of state-civil society relations, its efforts in responding to the pandemic have not yielded appreciable results. By some stroke of luck, unlike in India or South Africa and Brazil, the infection and morbidity rates have been comparatively low.

The first observation is that Nigeria's response to the COVID-19 clearly exposes the fault lines in the country's federal arrangement and practice. It also confirms the position of critics over the years that the Center was too powerful, too intrusive, too large, and too costly to manage. The Legislative Exclusive List in the 1999 Constitution contains 68 items while the Concurrent list contains 30 items. This gives excessive responsibilities and powers to the federal government. Of course, where there is a clash, the Federal interest prevails. Second, the response also exhibited the weaknesses of the 36 states and FCT and the 774 LGAs save for Lagos State, the country's business, and former political capital, the other tiers were not prepared and found it difficult to coordinate responses and align them with national initiatives where necessary. Third, the LGAs have remained silent, as if non-existent. With poor administrative structures, overstaffing, poor infrastructure, excessive political control, and intrusion by the State Governments, they lack the ability to respond adequately, even if only on preventive grounds. Fourth, it took time for the media to kick into the response. This slow response can be attributed to initial poor communication between government and media practitioners and weak public education. Fifth, civil society has been slow in fully appreciating the impact and implications of COVID-19. Hampered by the constant badgering from the state and sections of the Legislature, lacking resources as external funding has been dwindling and lacking effective institutional capacity, it has been very slow in reaching out to, and educating the populace.

The private sector, with time, kicked in with donations of cash to support the fight against COVID-19 (GBC Health 2020). They have also recently announced a plan to distribute food items to the 774 local governments through the state governments to support the poor. The government has announced that the cash donations received from the sector would not be distributed but deployed to post-COVID-19 restructuring and rehabilitation of the health sector. Even then, the private sector has not done enough in the areas of public education and support for underserved communities and constituencies.

The long-standing calls for the establishment and development of Primary Health Care Centers (PHCs) in the 8,804 Wards of the country to bring healthcare closer to the people have been largely ignored or treated with levity. Now the chicken has come home to roost and everything is top down. All ideas, financing, initiatives, supervision, and policies are top down. Lagos state is perhaps the only state to have remained upbeat and proactive in the federation. The state governor, a two-time COVID-19 survivor, has been leading by example and being very creative in designing strategies to contain the pandemic. The pandemic has confirmed the value of a decentralized political system and the importance of democratized decision-making processes to encourage innovation and accountability.

Clearly, Nigeria's federation will no longer remain the same after the pandemic. If a section of the power elite appears to be finding accommodation in a federally dominated arrangement, that, in itself, is generating new political pressures from below that can be expected to challenge the status quo. The growing strength of the regional ethnic groups, the "Revolution Now" protests, the "#End SARS" agitations, the numerous strike actions in virtually all sectors are pointers to this trend. From economic and social arrangements, institution building, and relations between and within constituent units and the Centre, it is expected that the permutation would experience a substantial shift. The federal government is realizing that it cannot do it all alone and that a strengthened state and local structure would consistently ease its own burdens.

Bibliography

Abdulrauf, L., 2020. Nigeria's Emergency (Legal) Response to Covid-19: A Worthy Sacrifice for Public Health? [online]. *Verfassungsblog*, May 18. Available from: https://verfassungsblog.de/nigerias-emergency-legal-response-to-covid-19-a-worthy-sacrifice-for-public-health/ [Accessed 22 January 2021].

AFP, 2020. Virus Stigma Weighs Heavily in Sub-Saharan Africa [online]. *Bangkok Post*, May 20. Available from: https://www.bangkokpost.com/world/1921320/virus-stigma-weighs-heavily-in-sub-saharan-africa [Accessed 22 January 2021].

African Center for Strategic Studies, 2020. Mapping Risk Factors for the Spread of COVID-19 in Africa [online]. May 13. Available from: https://africacenter.org/spotlight/mapping-risk-factors-spread-covid-19-africa/ [Accessed 22 January 2021].

Babalola, D., 2019. The Political Economy of Federalism in Nigeria. Switzerland: *Palgrave Macmillan*. Available from: https://doi.org/10.1007/978-3-030-05493-9 [Accessed 22 January 2021].

Babalola, D., 2020. Federalism and the Covid-19 Pandemic: The Nigerian Experience [online]. *UACES Territorial Politics*, May 22. Available from: https://uacesterrpol.wordpress.com/2020/05/22/federalism-and-the-covid-19-pandemic-the-nigerian-experience/ [Accessed 22 January 2021].

Budget Office of the Federation, 2021. 2021 Budget Documents [online]. *Federal Republic of Nigeria*. Available from: https://www.budgetoffice.gov.ng/index.php/resources/internal-resources/budget-documents/2021-budget [Accessed 22 January 2021].

CBC News, 2020. Coronavirus: Why Some Nigerians Are Gloating about COVID-19 [online]. April 22. Available from: https://www.bbc.com/news/world-africa-52372737 [Accessed 22 January 2021].

Dixit, S., Ogundeji, Y.K. and Onwujekwe, O., 2020. How Well Has Nigeria Responded to COVID-19? [online]. *Future Development*, July 2. Available from: https://www.brookings.edu/blog/future-development/2020/07/02/how-well-has-nigeria-responded-to-covid-19/ [Accessed 22 January 2021].

Federal Republic of Nigeria, 2020. COVID-19 Regulations, 2020 [online]. March 30. Available from: https://pwcnigeria.typepad.com/files/fg-covid-19-regualtions.pdf

GBC Health, 2020. Nigerian Private Sector Supporting Government Efforts to Fight COVID-19 [online]. March. Available from: https://gbchealth.org/nigerian-private-sector-supporting-government-efforts-to-fight-covid-19/ [Accessed 22 January 2021].

Government of Lagos State, 2020. Lagos State Infectious Diseases (Emergency Prevention) Regulations 2020 [online]. March 27. Available from: https://pwcnigeria.typepad.com/files/infectious-diseases-regulations-2020.pdf [Accessed 22 January 2021].

Ibiam, A.E., 2016. Federalism, Democracy and Constitutionalism: The Nigerian Experience. *Journal of Law, Policy and Globalization*, 53, 1–14. Available from: https://core.ac.uk/download/pdf/234650754.pdf [Accessed 22 January 2021].

Ihonvbere, J.O., 2020. Federalism and the COVID-19 Crisis: Nigerian Federalism [online]. Forum of Federations. Available from: http://www.forumfed.org/publications/federalism-and-the-covid-19-crisis-federalism-and-the-covid-19-crisis-nigerian-federalism/ [Accessed 22 January 2021].

Kalu, B., 2020. COVID-19 in Nigeria: A Disease of Hunger. *The Lancet Respiratory Medicine*, 8 (6), 556–557. Available from: https://www.ncbi.nlm.nih.gov/pmc/articles/PMC7190300/ [Accessed 22 January 2021].

KPMG, 2020. Nigeria: Government and Institution Measures in Response to COVID-19 [online]. October. Available from: https://home.kpmg/xx/en/home/insights/2020/04/nigeria-government-and-institution-measures-in-response-to-covid.html [Accessed 22 January 2021].

National Assembly, 2020. COVID-19: Senate Considers Bill to Boost Advanced Healthcare in Nigeria [online]. Available from: https://nass.gov.ng/news/item/1513 [Accessed 22 January 2021].Nigeria Centre for Disease Control (NCDC), 2020a. COVID-19 Outbreak in Nigeria: Situation Reports [online]. Available from: https://ncdc.gov.ng/diseases/sitreps/?cat=14&name=An%20update%20of%20COVID-19%20outbreak%20in%20Nigeria [Accessed 22 January 2021].

Nigeria Centre for Disease Control (NCDC), 2020b. Public Health Advisory on COVID-19 [online]. Available from: https://covid19.ncdc.gov.ng/advisory/ [Accessed 22 January 2021].

Nigeria Centre for Disease Control (NCDC), 2021a. Confirmed Cased by State [online]. Available from: https://covid19.ncdc.gov.ng/ [Accessed 22 January 2021].

Nigeria Centre for Disease Control (NCDC), 2021b. Guidelines [online]. Available from: https://covid19.ncdc.gov.ng/guideline/ [Accessed 22 January 2021].

Nigeria Centre for Disease Control (NCDC), 2021c. Implementation Guideline for Eased Lockdown [online]. *Official Updates from NCDC*. Available from: https://statehouse.gov.ng/covid19/guides-protocols/ [Accessed 22 January 2021].

Nigerian Communications Commission, 2020. Press Statement: Implementation of New SIM Registration Rules [online]. *Federal Republic of Nigeria*, December 15. Available from: https://www.ncc.gov.ng/media-centre/news-headlines/928-press-statement-implementation-of-new-sim-registration-rules [Accessed 22 January 2021].

Obiezu, T., 2020. Nigerians Justify Massive Looting of COVID-19 Supplies [online]. *Voice of America (VOA)*, October 27. Available from: https://www.voanews.com/covid-19-pandemic/nigerians-justify-massive-looting-covid-19-supplies [Accessed 22 January 2021].

Okeke, R., 2020. COVID-19 Pandemic, Federalism and Nigeria's Leadership Challenges. *Advance*, 1–12. Available from: https://advance.sagepub.com/articles/preprint/COVID-19_PANDEMIC_FEDERALISM_AND_NIGERIA_S_LEADERSHIP_CHALLENGES/12127038 [Accessed 22 January 2021].

Onuah, F., 2020. Nigerian Authorities Cite Need for More COVID-19 Test Sample Collections [online]. *Reuters*, September 3. Available from: https://www.reuters.com/article/us-health-coronavirus-nigeria/nigerian-authorities-cite-need-for-more-covid-19-test-sample-collections-idUSKBN25U2MQ?edition-redirect=ca [Accessed 22 January 2021].

Onyemelukwe, C., 2020. COVID-19, Misinformation, and the Law in Nigeria [online]. *Bill of Health*, August 19. Available from: https://blog.petrieflom.law.harvard.edu/2020/08/19/misinformation-disinformation-covid19-nigeria-law/ [Accessed 22 January 2021].

Xinhua, 2021. Nigeria to Reopen Schools Despite Spike in COVID-19 Cases [online]. *CGTN Africa*, January 15. Available from: https://africa.cgtn.com/2021/01/15/nigeria-to-reopen-schools-despite-spike-in-covid-19-cases/ [Accessed 22 January 2021].

Yagboyaju, D.A. and Akinola, A.O., 2019. Nigerian State and the Crisis of Governance: A Critical Exposition. *Sage Journals*, 9 (3), 1–10. Available from: https://doi.org/10.1177/2158244019865810 [Accessed 22 January 2021].

18 Pakistan

COVID-19, federalism and the first wave response

Sameen A. Mohsin Ali

18.1 Introduction

By the end of 2020, Pakistan had recorded over 475,000 confirmed cases of novel coronavirus, with over 10,000 lives lost. At the end of the first wave, in July, lockdowns were lifted, and businesses, public transport, restaurants, and educational institutions re-opened. There was no doubt that the spread of the virus had slowed, and the consensus is that Pakistan managed to avert disaster in the first wave of the pandemic. However, there are no clear explanations as to why or how this happened, the government and medical professionals continued to remind people to remain vigilant of a second wave (Hussain 2020; Mahmood 2020; Mirza 2020).

This chapter divides the first wave of the pandemic in Pakistan into two phases. In the first phase, the pandemic response was confused as the federal government seemed unable to put together a coherent strategy or provide provincial governments with any direction. At this stage, Pakistan's federal structure saved lives as the provinces stepped up and put in place mitigation and control measures to contain the virus. By April, in the second phase, the federal government had shifted gears. It set up a parallel structure with civilian and military leadership to coordinate the pandemic response and introduced measures to protect the vulnerable and support businesses. The centralized civilian-military leadership model has been demonstrably effective in enhancing capacity, collecting and collating data, and improving facilities and communication. However, these developments are also a cause for concern in a country with a history of military intervention and where civilian supremacy is fragile. The bypassing of existing constitutional bodies designed for coordination between the provinces and the federation and encroachments on provincial autonomy by the courts and by the federal executive are problematic and raise questions about the sustainability of Pakistan's progress in this crisis (Table 18.1).

Table 18.1 Key Statistics on COVID-19 in Pakistan as of 10 January 2021

Cumulative Cases	Cumulative Cases per 100,000 Population	Cumulative Deaths	Cumulative Deaths per 100,000 Population	Case Fatality Percentage
499,517	226.1	10,598	4.8	2.1

Source: *World Health Organization Weekly epidemiological update* – 12 January 2021. Geneva: WHO, 2021. Available from https://www.who.int/publications/m/item/weekly-epidemiological-update

DOI: 10.4324/9781003251217-18

18.2 The impact of COVID-19

Pakistan's first case was officially reported on 26 February 2020. At the federal level, the country spends just 2 percent of its GDP on healthcare, lagging well behind its neighbors, Iran and India, on per capita health expenditure (Shaikh 2020). Access to health care in Pakistan is very uneven with just six hospital beds, nine doctors, and five nurses per 10,000 population (WHO 2018). These gaps in health service provision and outbreaks in the neighboring countries of Iran and China meant that Pakistan was ranked a high-risk country during the initial days of the pandemic.

Pakistan was slow to mobilize its pandemic response, preferring to monitor the situation and then scrambling to test samples and develop a response plan (Javed et al. 2020). Cases increased steadily during March and April and peaked in June (Our World in Data). Since data collection is poor, developing a policy response was difficult (Syed and Malkani 2020). Official records of deaths are not maintained, making it impossible to accurately calculate excess mortality due to the virus (Kermani 2020). However, even though cases and deaths are most likely higher than government figures, Pakistan's case fatality rate remained around 2 percent even at the peak of the first wave in June, considerably lower than countries like Italy and the UK (Our World in Data; Rehman 2020). Most at risk are frontline healthcare workers, especially during shortages of protective equipment in the initial stages of the pandemic (Siddiqui 2020a). In a country with a chronic shortage of health workforce (Farooq 2020), 24 lives had been lost to COVID-19 by June 2020 and over 2,000 had been infected (Bhatti 2020).

18.2.1 Economic impact

In addition to the human cost, the pandemic is expected to have a serious impact on Pakistan's already fragile economic situation (Mandviwalla 2020). In 2019, the IMF approved a $6 billion Extended Fund Facility for Pakistan, with the federal government agreeing to increase revenues, particularly tax collection, to shrink the fiscal deficit (IMF 2019). Current expenditures have risen at both federal and provincial levels, but revenues have not, leading to cuts in development spending at both levels of government (Table 18.2).

Table 18.2 Revenues and Expenditures as Percentage of GDP in Pakistan

	2016	2017	2018	2019	2020 (Provisional)
Total revenue	**15.3**	**15.5**	**15.1**	**12.9**	**15.0**
Federal tax revenue	11.6	11.4	11.7	10.7	10.4
Provincial tax revenue	1.0	1.0	1.2	1.1	1.0
Federal non-tax revenue (excluding interest from the provinces)	2.4	2.8	1.8	0.9	3.4[a]
Provincial non-tax revenue	0.3	0.2	0.4	0.2	0.2
Total expenditure	**19.9**	**21.3**	**21.6**	**22.0**	**23.1**
Federal current expenditure	10.8	10.9	10.9	12.6	14.4
Provincial current expenditure	5.3	5.4	6.0	6.1	6.0
Federal development expenditure	2.5	2.3	1.7	1.3	1.1
Provincial development expenditure	2.0	2.7	2.5	1.3	1.5

Source: State Bank of Pakistan Annual Report-Statistical Supplement 2019–2020, Chapter 4
a 2.2 percent of this revenue was profits for the State Bank of Pakistan, mainly from lending to the government

The IMF program was paused at the start of the pandemic and remains suspended as negotiations continue between the parties over monetary tightening and systemic reform (Ansari 2020). Meanwhile, the UNDP (2020) projected that nearly 40 percent of Pakistan's population will be living below the poverty line after the pandemic. GDP growth is estimated to be ‒0.4 percent in 2020 (IMF 2020), and the unemployment rate is projected to rise to 28 percent by 2021 (Saleem 2020), especially since Pakistan's extensive informal sector, which employs 72 percent of the labor force (Syed and Malkani 2020), was hit particularly hard by lockdown disruptions. The Federal Budget 2020–2021 projects Pakistan Rupee (PKR) 900 billion in revenue loss due to the pandemic and the government faced considerable criticism for allocating PKR 1,289 billion for defense, a 12 percent increase on the previous budget, and PKR 25 billion for health (Budget in Brief 2020). With provincial health budgets added to this amount, health spending in Pakistan stands at a third of defense spending (Siddiqui 2020b). With declining revenues, Pakistan's economy is susceptible to shocks and will remain reliant on bilateral and multilateral aid flows.

18.3 Pakistan's constitutional structure

The Constitution of 1973 defines Pakistan as a 'federal republic.' The Islamic Republic of Pakistan is composed of the Islamabad Capital Territory (ICT), four provinces – Punjab, Sindh, Khyber Pakhtunkhwa (including the former Federally Administered Tribal Areas or FATA), and Baluchistan and the territories of Azad Kashmir and Gilgit Baltistan. The four provinces and ICT have full constitutional, legal, and political status. However, the Gilgit Baltistan and Azad Kashmir have not been fully integrated into the federation as provinces.

Pakistan follows the parliamentary system with the President as the Head of the State and the Prime Minister as the Head of the Government.[1] The legislature is bi-cameral with the National Assembly (*Majlis-e-Shoora*) as the lower house and the Senate as the upper house. The provinces are equally represented in the Senate with additional seats for FATA and ICT.[2] Membership of the National Assembly is divided amongst the four provinces and the ICT on the basis of population.[3] The four provinces each have their own legislative assemblies headed by a Chief Minister and a Governor. Under Article 140A of the 1973 Constitution, each of the four provinces is required to establish their own local government systems. However, provinces have struggled to devolve meaningful power to local government representatives (S.M. Ali 2018). Sindh

Table 18.3 Composition of the National Assembly of Pakistan

Province/Area	General Seats	Women Seats	Non-Muslim	Total Seats
Balochistan	16	4	–	20
Khyber Pakhtunkhwa	45	10	–	55
Punjab	141	32	–	173
Sindh	61	14	–	75
Federal Capital	3	–	–	3
–	–	–	10	10
Total	266	60	10	336

Source: Composition – National Assembly of Pakistan. Available from: http://www.na.gov.pk/en/content.php?id=2

was the only province that had an elected local government in place during the pandemic response; however, their term ended at the end of August (Table 18.3).

18.3.1 Decision-making in the federation

The 1973 Constitution originally divided legislative powers into two lists: federal and concurrent. Most items came under the concurrent list, including education and health, and the federal government retained the power to overrule the provinces on any of the items on it. In 2010, the 18th Amendment to the 1973 Constitution abolished the Concurrent list, shifting most subjects to the provinces and establishing a Federal Legislative List with two parts. The first part contains subjects solely under the federal government's jurisdiction. The second part contains subjects to be overseen by the Council of Common Interests (CCI), a body with the constitutional mandate to ensure inter-provincial and federal–provincial coordination in decision-making. Its members include the PM, the Chief Ministers of each of the provinces, and the Ministers of Planning, Inter-Provincial Coordination, and Power. The CCI must meet once in 90 days, but this rule has frequently been violated by PMs in the past as well as in the present, and the council has remained under-utilized as a coordinating body (PILDAT 2020).

Though the 18th Amendment was a landmark achievement backed by consensus amongst the political elite (Adeney 2012), the implementation of its provisions was slow and subject to reversals. The federal government transfers 57.5 percent of its revenues to the provinces and is locked into these transfers by Article 160-3A which states that the share of funds received by the provinces from the federation cannot be lower than the share for the previous year (Adeney 2012). These funds have allowed the provinces to legislate and develop their own contextualized policies with regard to health programs, service delivery, and expenditure, but they have struggled to enhance their own revenue collection. This leaves the provinces heavily dependent on federal transfers and because the federal government has persistently failed to meet revenue collection targets, provincial governments are unable to accurately forecast transfers and plan expenditures.

There has also been considerable contention over jurisdictional and coordination issues between the center and the provinces with regard to (amongst other matters) drug licensing and regulations, population welfare, and the delivery of donor funded preventative countrywide programs such as the polio program. These concerns led to the creation of the Ministry of National Health Service Coordination and Regulation (MoNHSCR) at the federal level in 2013 headed by a State Minister for Health. Health research is also conducted by the National Institute for Health (NIH). However, coordination between the federation and the provinces on health care in Pakistan has remained consistently poor (Zaidi et al. 2020). At no time has this been more evident than when the first cases of the novel coronavirus were confirmed in Pakistan at the end of February 2020.

18.4 Emergency management in the federation

Initially, the Pakistan government's response to the pandemic was marred by indecision, confusion, and mismanagement. The federal government prevaricated on a countrywide lockdown, citing valid concerns for the poor who would be disproportionately impacted but failing to substantiate concrete steps for handling the situation (Younus 2020a). Educational institutions were closed mid-March, but the government was unable to convince clerics to shut down mosques or religious gatherings (A. Khan 2020). On 10 March, against government advice, thousands of people gathered in Raiwind, just outside Lahore, for the annual Tableeghi Jamaat gathering. This became a super-spreader event as attendees returned to their homes across the country and across the world without being tested or quarantined (ICG 2020). A quarantine facility at Taftan, near the Iran border, was poorly managed (Afzal 2020a), giving rise to fears regarding government quarantines which prevented people from getting diagnosed.

The PM's opposition to the lockdown motivated the federal government to expedite social protection for vulnerable populations. On 24 March, the federal government announced a COVID-19 relief package of PKR 1.3 trillion, funded in part by the World Bank and Asian Development Bank. Perhaps, the most significant part of the package was the Ehsaas Emergency Cash Program, which incorporates the Benazir Income Support Program. As of July 2020, the federal government had deployed PKR 203 billion to 16.9 million families (Nishtar 2020). In addition, the Pakistan government introduced a range of measures to try and mitigate the economic impact of the pandemic, including cutting interest rates, tax refunds, and deferring interest payments for businesses (IMF 2020; Saleem 2020).

18.4.1 Provincial pandemic response

While the Prime Minister continued to publicly play down the threat of the virus, telling citizens "not to worry" (Malik 2020), the provincial governments were more proactive in their response to the pandemic. They developed their own relief packages, with Punjab allocating PKR 10 billion for cash grants and PKR 18 billion in tax relief, and Sindh PKR 1.5 billion for a cash and ration distribution campaign (IMF 2020). Acting on the National Action Plan issued by the National Institute of Health on 13 March and with the support of the MoNHSCR, the provincial governments set up task forces, designated hospitals for testing and treatment, expanded testing capacity, set up field hospitals and quarantine centers, closed restaurants, cinemas, and marriage halls, and launched helplines and information campaigns to reach citizens. Khyber Pakhtunkhwa declared an emergency in February, began putting in social distancing measures from 18 March, and made data on cases openly available. Sindh ensured that travelers from Taftan were adequately quarantined. However, local governments had little to do with the response. The National Action Plan, for instance, refers to local governments just once, with regard to community awareness. Since the other provinces delayed elections, Sindh was the only province that had elected representatives in place when the pandemic started, but the province's local government law falls well short of devolving meaningful administrative or fiscal powers to those representatives (S.M. Ali 2018). Therefore, their involvement in relief activities was minimal and became a site of political clashes (I. Ali 2020). Overall, the absence of effective local governments led to what Syed and Malkani (2020) refer to as a "misalignment of strategies across government tiers."

Sindh was the first to announce a full lockdown on 23 March. The other provinces soon followed by announcing partial lockdowns (later expanded to complete lockdowns) and calling in the military in aid of civil power (Shehzad 2020). Reports claim that this is where the military leadership intervened, sidelining the vacillating federal executive and working with the provincial governments to enforce lockdowns (Siddiqui 2020b; ur-Rehman, Abi-Habib and Mehsud 2020). However, the government claims that it opted to work closely with the military leadership as they are "on the same page" (Afzal 2020b).

18.4.2 *Centralizing the pandemic response*

The PTI government's 'hybrid governance' (Husain 2020) model is evidenced by their decision to bypass the CCI and the legislature and set up an alternate infrastructure including both civilian (federal and provincial) and military leadership to coordinate the pandemic response. On 13 March, the Prime Minister authorized the formation of a National Coordination Committee (NCC) to curb the spread of the virus (The Nation 2020). In making decisions with regard to the pandemic, the NCC is supported by the National Command and Operations Centre (NCOC), set up by the Prime Minister on 31 March. Led by the Planning Minister, its members include the Health and Interior ministries and representatives from the provincial and regional governments and Inter-Services Intelligence (ISI).

The NCOC became the "nerve center to synergize and articulate [the] unified national effort against COVID-19" (Prime Minister's Office Press Release 2020b). It took charge of data gathering, coordinating messaging, and track, trace, and quarantine protocols using the ISI's surveillance systems. Policy recommendations based on the data are then forwarded to the NCC. Pakistan's National Disaster Management Authority (NDMA), set up in the wake of the devastating earthquake of 2005, is designated as the "lead operational agency" for coordinating the pandemic response between the provinces through provincial Disaster Management Authorities (Prime Minister's Office Press Release 2020a). By 1 April, the civilian and military leadership was committed to a lockdown strategy despite the misgivings of the Prime Minister who used a public address to urge the provincial governments to "discuss and reassess" their lockdowns (*Dawn* 2020a). In a briefing held at the NCOC in the presence of the Chief of Army Staff and various federal ministers and advisers, but with the Prime Minister notably absent, the Chief of Army Staff is quoted as saying, in contradiction to the Prime Minister's stated position, that, "The planned measures, if implemented timely [sic], will contribute to safety and well-being of every Pakistani and society at large" (Syed 2020).

18.5 COVID-19 and provincial autonomy

In April, the Prime Minister announced the easing of the lockdown despite opposition by medical professionals and provincial governments (ICG 2020). On 9 May, two weeks before the religious festival of Eid ul Fitr and with cases on an upward trend, the lockdown was lifted entirely. Though the provincial governments each developed their own plans for phased lifting of lockdown restrictions (*Dawn* 2020b), they struggled to manage the spike in cases during May and early June. Throughout these months, the federal and Sindh governments took a combative approach toward each other, with each side criticizing the other in a series of press statements (Raza 2020).[4] The Supreme Court of Pakistan further cut into provincial autonomy by ordering provincial governments, particularly Sindh, to lift any remaining lockdown restrictions (Shahzad 2020). In a suo moto case, the Court ordered the lifting of any remaining lockdown restrictions as it questioned why significant funds were being spent on the response when it was "not a pandemic in Pakistan" (Bhatti 2020; Shahzad 2020). The bench questioned Sindh's decision to keep certain lockdown restrictions in place by comparing it to the other provinces' decision to reopen fully and ordered the Sindh government to reopen fully immediately (Supreme Court of Pakistan, S.M.C. 01/2020), effectively overruling the provincial government's autonomous decision. The bench's rulings also impacted decision-making in Punjab. A report by the Primary and Secondary Healthcare Department to the Chief Minister of Punjab, dated 15 May, summarized the findings of an expert "smart sampling project" conducted in Lahore and recommended a strict lockdown. The study found an average 6 percent positivity rate and estimated that the city had about 0.7 million cases of the virus as "no workplace and residential area of any town is disease-free" (Gabol 2020). However, the Punjab Health Minister, Dr Yasmin Rashid, claimed that the recommendation was ignored due to the Supreme Court's ruling to lift the lockdown (Greenfield and Farooq 2020).

By the first week of June, the test positivity rate was 23 percent, and Pakistan was amongst the ten countries most affected by the pandemic (The Express Tribune 2020). Testing remained low, trace and quarantine measures seemed insufficient, health services in cities like Lahore were under massive strain (Hashim 2020), and the government scrambled to prepare procedures and regulations to ensure the supply of drugs, plasma, Personal Protective Equipment (PPE), and ventilators (Greenfield and Farooq 2020). On 9 June, the WHO issued a recommendation to the provincial governments to impose intermittent lockdowns to contain the spread of the virus (The Express Tribune 2020). The same day, the Supreme Court bench commented that the federal government and the provinces must work together to develop a uniform response to the pandemic, effectively strengthening the center's control over the pandemic response (ICG 2020; Iqbal 2020; S. Khan 2020).

18.5.1 The smart lockdown strategy

By this point, the NCOC had finalized its own "smart lockdown" strategy based on a test, trace, quarantine protocol developed with the help of the army (*Dawn* 2020c; Siddiqui 2020c) and drawing on the infrastructure of the Pakistan Polio Eradication Program (Mirza 2020). On 14 June, the federal government announced that it was identifying "hot spots" of cases and advising the provinces to impose strict lockdowns in these areas (*The News* 2020). This strategy was implemented across the country without any differences being expressed (Ayub 2020a), perhaps a sign that coordination amongst the federation and provinces had improved or perhaps that space for provincial autonomy had shrunk.

Cases in Pakistan dipped around the same time as the smart lockdowns began and started to decline steadily a week later (Our World in Data). Explanations vary, but it is difficult to be conclusive since testing has remained below recommended levels (ICG 2020). Markets reopened, religious gatherings were held, and services that had been disrupted due to the lockdown resumed. Though essential health care services continued operating, Chandir et al. (2020) found a just over 50 percent decrease in routine immunization visits in Karachi, and some critical services such as polio immunization campaigns were suspended during the lockdown. The polio campaign resumed at the end of July (WHO 2020). Though Pakistan seemed to have averted disaster, government officials continue to remind citizens to observe SOPs since the virus has not gone away.

18.6 Conclusion

In dealing with the first wave, Pakistan improved coordination, built capacity, and enhanced social protection for the most vulnerable. The question is whether or not these gains are sustainable and are institutionalized for the second wave, which began in late October 2020, and for other crises in the future.

Pakistan's federal structure allowed its provinces latitude during the initial onset of the pandemic as the federal government struggled to formulate a coherent response. However, by April, the response was being coordinated at the center by the civilian and military leadership. Provincial autonomy in implementing lockdown measures was further eroded by the Supreme Court's directives. The easing of the lockdown and reopening of the economy allowed for cautious optimism (ADB 2020), but inflation remains high, and export growth is likely to be hindered by a range of domestic and international factors (Younus 2020b).

With the second wave, recommendations on pandemic response continue to come from the National Command and Operations Centre. Perhaps, due to the centralized nature of the first wave response, the provincial governments were slower to react to the spike in cases that heralded the second wave (Ayub 2020b; *Dawn* 2020d). Though smart lockdowns are being instituted, fatigue has set in amongst the population with respect to following distancing, hand washing, and masking guidelines (Hassan 2020b), and conspiracy theories continue to undermine government attempts to enforce SOPs (ur-Rehman and Schmall 2020). Furthermore, a resurgent opposition is placing the government under pressure, holding massive rallies in contravention of government restrictions on large gatherings to limit the spread of the coronavirus (Hassan 2020a). The government's response has been a crackdown on opposition leaders and on dissent more generally, leading to greater domestic discord. From an economic standpoint, the consensus is that serious structural reforms are essential for there to be a sustained economic recovery (ADB 2020; World Bank 2020; Younus 2020b). For the provinces, this uneven recovery has meant that, in drawing up their budgets, they were asked by the federal government to cut costs and enhance provincial revenues (Kiani 2020). Though there is significant variation across the provincial budgets, they all reveal increases in health spending and the introduction of relief and stimulus packages (Khawar 2020).

The civilian-military model has proven to be very effective in coordinating and operationalizing the response to the first wave of the pandemic. But the creation of a parallel set of institutions by executive fiat, while quick and efficient, undermines democratic consensus-based processes, particularly in a context with limited parliamentary oversight (Azad 2020), and weakens existing constitutional arrangements such as the CCI, whose potential for enhancing federal–provincial coordination remains untapped. It is important, therefore, to tread carefully so as not to damage civilian supremacy, provincial autonomy, and democratic processes in the long term.

Notes

1 Military interventions and constitutional engineering shifted the country toward a semi-presidential system. These changes to the 1973 Constitution were reversed through the 18th Amendment in 2010.
2 FATA was integrated into Khyber Pakhtunkhwa through the 25th Constitutional Amendment in May 2018. Senators from FATA will finish their terms, and these seats will be removed from the Senate, bringing membership from 104 to 96.
3 Seats from FATA have been added to the tally for Khyber Pakhtunkhwa.

4 The Sindh government is led by an opposition party, the Pakistan People's Party (PPP). The other provinces are held by the Pakistan Tehreek-e-Insaaf (PTI), Punjab, and Balochistan as part of a coalition and KP outright.

Bibliography

Adeney, K., 2012. A Step towards Inclusive Federalism in Pakistan? The Politics of the 18th Amendment. *Publius: The Journal of Federalism*, 42 (4), 539–565. Available from: https://doi.org/10.1093/publius/pjr055 [Accessed 23 March 2021].

Afzal, M., 2020a. Pakistan Teeters on the Edge of Potential Disaster with the Coronavirus. Brookings Institute Order from Chaos blog, March 27. Available from: https://www.brookings.edu/blog/order-from-chaos/2020/03/27/pakistan-teeters-on-the-edge-of-potential-disaster-with-the-coronavirus/ [Accessed 23 March 2021].

Afzal, M., 2020b. The Pandemic Deals a Blow to Pakistan's Democracy. Brookings Institute Order from Chaos blog, August 6. Available from: https://www.brookings.edu/blog/order-from-chaos/2020/08/06/the-pandemic-deals-a-blow-to-pakistans-democracy/ [Accessed 23 March 2021].

Ali, I., 2020. Favouritism, Political Infighting Mar Covid-19 Relief Operations in Sindh. *Dawn*, April 20. Available from: https://www.dawn.com/news/1550601/favouritism-political-infighting-mar-covid-19-relief-operations-in-sindh [Accessed 23 March 2021].

Ali, S.M., 2018. Devolution of Power in Pakistan. Special Report, United States Institute of Peace. Available from: https://www.usip.org/publications/2018/03/devolution-power-pakistan [Accessed 23 March 2021].

Ansari, I., 2020. Talks with IMF on Subsidies Remain Inconclusive. *The Express Tribune*, September 26. Available from: https://tribune.com.pk/story/2265795/talks-with-imf-on-subsidies-remain-inconclusive [Accessed 23 March 2021].

Asian Development Bank (ADB), 2020. Pakistan Could See 2021 Economic Recovery if COVID-19 Subsides, Structural Reforms Resume — ADB Report. News Release, September 15. Available from: https://www.adb.org/news/pakistan-could-see-2021-economic-recovery-if-covid-19-subsides-structural-reforms-resume-adb#:~:text=ISLAMABAD%2C%20PAKISTAN%20(15%20September%202020,structural%20reforms%2C%20says%20an%20Asian [Accessed 23 March 2021].

Ayub, I., 2020a. Sindh Govt Imposes 'Smart Lockdown' in Province's Select Areas. *Dawn*, June 17. Available from: https://www.dawn.com/news/1563955 [Accessed 23 March 2021].

Ayub, I., 2020b. Sindh Govt in Sate of Indecision on Tough SOPs to Contain Second Covid-19 Wave. *Dawn*, November 23. Available from: https://www.dawn.com/news/1591860 [Accessed 23 March 2021].

Azad, A., 2020. Parliament and the Health Response to Second Wave of COVID-19 in Pakistan. Democracy Reporting International's COVID-19 Policy Brief Series, December. Available from: https://democracy-reporting.org/wp-content/uploads/2021/01/DRI-Brief_Health_small.pdf [Accessed 23 March 2021].

Bhatti, H., 2020. SC Finds 'No Valid Reason' for Keeping Malls Closed, Says No Need to Keep Markets Closed on Weekends. *Dawn*, May 19. Available from: https://www.dawn.com/news/1558005 [Accessed 23 March 2021].

Bhatti, M.W., 2020. Facing Covid-19 and Violence Simultaneously, Healthcare Community in Pakistan Has Lost 24 Colleagues So Far. *The News*, June 2. Available from: https://www.thenews.com.pk/print/666539-facing-covid-19-and-violence-simultaneously-healthcare-community-in-pakistan-has-lost-24-colleagues-so-far [Accessed 23 March 2021].

Chandir, S., Siddiqi, D.A., Setayesh, H. and Khan, A.J., 2020. Impact of COVID-19 Lockdown on Routine Immunisation in Karachi, Pakistan. *The Lancet*, 8, e1119. Available from: https://doi.org/10.1016/S2214-109X(20)30290-4 [Accessed 23 March 2021].

Dawn, 2020a. PM Imran Urges Provinces to 'Reassess' Complete Lockdowns as Strategy against Virus. March 25. Available from: https://www.dawn.com/news/1543642/pm-imran-urges-provinces-to-reassess-complete-lockdowns-as-strategy-against-virus [Accessed 23 March 2021].

Dawn, 2020b. Provinces Announce Easing Lockdown Even as Pakistan Witnesses Record Rise in Coronavirus Cases. May 9. Available from: https://www.dawn.com/news/1555575 [Accessed 23 March 2021].

Dawn, 2020c. Army to Help Govt Adopt 'Test, Trace and Quarantine' Strategy. April 23. Available from: https://www.dawn.com/news/1551531 [Accessed 23 March 2021].

Dawn, 2020d. Lethal Second Wave. Editorial. December 27. Available from: https://www.dawn.com/news/1598082 [Accessed 23 March 2021].

Farooq, M., 2020. Covid-19 to Increase Urgency of Healthcare Sector Reforms in Pakistan: Fitch Solutions. *Pakistan Today*: Profit, August 13. Available from: https://profit.pakistantoday.com.pk/2020/08/13/covid-19-to-increase-urgency-of-healthcare-sector-reforms-in-pakistan-fitch-solutions/ [Accessed 23 March 2021].

Gabol, I., 2020. 'No Disease-Free Area': Summary to Punjab CM Estimates 670,800 Cases in Lahore Alone. *Dawn*, June 2. Available from: https://www.dawn.com/news/1560616 [Accessed 23 March 2021].

Government of Pakistan, 2020a. Federal Budget 2020–21 – Budget in Brief. Finance Division, Islamabad. Available from: http://www.finance.gov.pk/budget/Budget_in_Brief_2020_21_English.pdf [Accessed 23 March 2021].

Government of Pakistan, 2020b. National Action Plan for Corona Virus Disease (COVID-19) Pakistan. Ministry of National Health Services, Regulations & Coordination. Available from: https://www.nih.org.pk/wp-content/uploads/2020/03/COVID-19-NAP-V2-13-March-2020.pdf [Accessed 23 March 2021].

Greenfield, C. and Farooq, U., 2020. After Pakistan's Lockdown Gamble, COVID-19 Cases Surge. *Reuters*, June 5. Available from: https://www.reuters.com/article/us-health-coronavirus-pakistan-lockdown/after-pakistans-lockdown-gamble-covid-19-cases-surge-idUSKBN23C0NW [Accessed 23 March 2021].

Hashim, A., 2020. 'Smart Lockdown' in Pakistan to Target 500 Coronavirus Hotspots. *Al Jazeera*, June 23. Available from: https://www.aljazeera.com/news/2020/06/lockdown-pakistan-target-500-coronavirus-hotspots-200623072202544.html [Accessed 23 March 2021].

Hassan, S.R., 2020a. Pakistan Opposition Holds Mass Rally Calling for PM Khan to Go. *Reuters*, October 18. Available from: https://www.reuters.com/article/us-pakistan-politics-protests-idUSKBN2730S5 [Accessed 23 March 2021].

Hassan, S.R., 2020b. Pakistan's Second Wave of Coronavirus Infections Gathers Momentum. *Reuters*, November 16. Available from: https://www.reuters.com/article/uk-health-coronavirus-pakistan-idUKKBN27W10F [Accessed 23 March 2021].

Husain, F., 2020. Command & Control Governance. *Dawn*, July 11. Available from: https://www.dawn.com/news/1568272 [Accessed 23 March 2021].

Hussain, K., 2020. How Did Pakistan Avert Disaster? *Dawn*, August 31. Available from: https://www.dawn.com/news/1577135/how-did-pakistan-avert-disaster [Accessed 23 March 2021].

International Crisis Group (ICG), 2020. Pakistan's COVID-19 Crisis. Crisis Group Asia Briefing No 162, 7 August. Available from: https://www.crisisgroup.org/asia/south-asia/pakistan/b162-pakistans-covid-19-crisis [Accessed 23 March 2021].

International Monetary Fund (IMF), 2019. IMF Executive Board Approves US$6 billion 39-Month EFF Arrangement for Pakistan. Press Release 19/264, July 3. Available from: https://www.imf.org/en/News/Articles/2019/07/03/pr19264-pakistan-imf-executive-board-approves-39-month-eff-arrangement [Accessed 23 March 2021].

International Monetary Fund (IMF), 2020. Policy Responses to COVID-19- Policy Tracker: Pakistan. Available from: https://www.imf.org/en/Topics/imf-and-covid19/Policy-Responses-to-COVID-19#top [Accessed 23 March 2021].

Iqbal, N., 2020. SC Tells Govt to Take Covid-19 Seriously. *Dawn*, June 9. Available from: https://www.dawn.com/news/1562326 [Accessed 23 March 2021].

Javed, B., Sarwar, A., Soto, E.B. and Mashwani, Z.R., 2020. Is Pakistan's Response to Coronavirus (SARS-CoV-2) Adequate to Prevent an Outbreak? *Frontiers in Medicine* 7, 158. doi: 10.3389/fmed.2020.00158 [Accessed 23 March 2021].

Kermani, S., 2020. Coronavirus: Youthful Pakistan Appears to Avoid Worst of Pandemic. *BBC News*-Asia, August 21. Available from: https://www.bbc.com/news/world-asia-53742214 [Accessed 23 March 2021].

Khan, A., 2020. Why Pakistan Isn't Closing Mosques Despite the Coronavirus Threat. *TRT World*, March 27. Available from: https://www.trtworld.com/opinion/why-pakistan-isn-t-closing-mosques-despite-the-coronavirus-threat-34913 [Accessed 23 March 2021].

Khan, S., 2020. Centre Has Introduced Uniform National Policy for Covid-19, Supreme Court Told. *The News*, May 17. Available from: https://www.thenews.com.pk/print/660064-centre-has-introduced-uniform-national-policy-for-covid-19-sc-told [Accessed 23 March 2021].

Khawar, H., 2020. Provincial Budgets: Exceeding Expectations. *The Express Tribune*, June 23. Available from: https://tribune.com.pk/story/2248246/provincial-budgets-exceeding-expectations [Accessed 23 March 2021].

Kiani, K., 2020. Provinces Free to Act on Own Budget Projections. *Dawn*, June 14. Available from: https://www.dawn.com/news/1563383 [Accessed 23 March 2021].

Mahmood, S., 2020. The Curious Case of Reduced Testing in Pakistan. *Business Recorder*, July 18. Available from: https://beta.brecorder.com/news/40005839 [Accessed 23 March 2021].

Malik, M., 2020. No Curfew Like Lockdown, PM Imran Khan Insists. *The Nation*, March 23. Available from: https://nation.com.pk/23-Mar-2020/no-curfew-like-lockdown-pm-imran-khan-insists [Accessed 23 March 2021].

Mandviwalla, S., 2020. Federalism and the COVID-19 Crisis: A Pakistani Perspective. Forum of Federations. Available from: http://www.forumfed.org/wp-content/uploads/2020/04/PakistanCOVID.pdf [Accessed 23 March 2021].

Mirza, Z., 2020. Rise and Fall of Covid-19. *The News*, August 28. Available from: https://www.thenews.com.pk/print/706671-rise-and-fall-of-covid-19 [Accessed 23 March 2021].

Nishtar, S., 2020. Ehsaas Emergency Cash: A Digital Solution to Protect the Vulnerable in Pakistan during the COVID-19 Crisis. Ehsaas Program, Government of Pakistan. Available from: https://www.pass.gov.pk/Document/Downloads/EECreportAugust10.pdf [Accessed 23 March 2021].

Our World in Data. Pakistan: Coronavirus Pandemic Country Profile. Available from: https://ourworldindata.org/coronavirus/country/pakistan?country=~PAK [Accessed 23 March 2021].

PILDAT, 2020. Infographic: CCI Meetings under Various Prime Ministers 1973–2020. Pakistan Institute of Legislative Development and Transparency (PILDAT), July 16. Available from: https://web.facebook.com/PILDAT/posts/the-council-of-common-interests-cci-is-an-important-constitutional-forum-to-form/4647759241917080/?_rdc=1&_rdr [Accessed 23 March 2021].

Prime Minister's Office, 2020a. Press Release: PM Chaired the National Security Committee Meeting, Especially Called to Review the Current Status of and Pakistan's Response to the Coronavirus. Prime Minister's Office, March 13. Available from: https://pmo.gov.pk/news_details.php?news_id=1066 [Accessed 23 March 2021].

Prime Minister's Office, 2020b. Press Release: Prime Minister Imran Khan Visited National Command and Operation Centre (NCOC) for COVID-19 in Islamabad. Prime Minister's Office, April 03. Available from: https://pmo.gov.pk/news_details.php?news_id=1068 [Accessed 23 March 2021].

Raza, S.I., 2020. Centre Assails Sindh Govt over 'Stricter' Lockdown Measures. *Dawn*, April 16. Available from: https://www.dawn.com/news/1549621 [Accessed 23 March 2021].

Rehman, M., 2020. Covid-19 and Pakistan's Data Narrative. *Dawn* Prism, blog, May 27. Available from: https://www.dawn.com/news/1552905 [Accessed 23 March 2021].

Saleem, A., 2020. How the COVID-19 Crisis Is Affecting Pakistan's Economy. *DW*, July 23. Available from: https://www.dw.com/en/how-the-covid-19-crisis-is-affecting-pakistans-economy/a-54292705 [Accessed 23 March 2021].

Shahzad, A., 2020. Coronavirus 'Not a Pandemic in Pakistan' Says Top Court, Ordering Curbs Lifted. *Reuters*, May 18. Available from: https://www.reuters.com/article/us-health-coronavirus-pakistan-lockdown/coronavirus-not-a-pandemic-in-pakistan-says-top-court-ordering-curbs-lifted-idUSKBN22U2NV [Accessed 23 March 2021].

Shehzad, R., 2020. PM Imran Approves Provinces' Request for Army Deployment Amid COVID-19 Outbreak. *The Express Tribune*, March 23. Available from: https://tribune.com.pk/story/2182335/pm-imran-approves-provinces-request-army-deployment-amid-covid-19-outbreak [Accessed 23 March 2021].

Shaikh, H., 2020. COVID-19: Pakistan's Preparations and Response. International Growth Centre (IGC), blog, 6 April. Available from: https://www.theigc.org/blog/covid-19-pakistans-preparations-and-response/ [Accessed 23 March 2021].

Siddiqa, A., 2020. Why Is Pakistan Spending So Much Money on Defence Amid COVID-19? *Al Jazeera*, July 1. Available from: https://www.aljazeera.com/indepth/opinion/pakistan-spending-money-defence-covid-19-200625115702999.html [Accessed 23 March 2021].

Siddiqui, Z., 2020a. Doctors without Armour. *Himal South Asian*, March 30. Available from: https://www.himalmag.com/doctors-without-armour-pakistan-2020/ [Accessed 23 March 2021].

Siddiqui, Z. 2020b. In Pakistan, the Army Tightens Its Grip. *Foreign Policy*, July 8. Available from: https://foreignpolicy.com/2020/07/08/in-pakistan-the-army-tightens-its-grip/ [Accessed 23 March 2021].

Siddiqui, Z., 2020c. Pakistan Is Using a Terrorism Surveillance System to Monitor the Pandemic. *Slate*: Future Tense Series – Privacy in the Pandemic, July 15. Available from: https://slate.com/technology/2020/07/pakistan-isi-terrorism-surveillance-coronavirus.html [Accessed 23 March 2021].

Supreme Court of Pakistan, 2020. Suo Moto Action Regarding Combating the Pandemic of Corona Virus (COVID-19). S.M.C. 01/2020. Available from: https://www.supremecourt.gov.pk/downloads_judgements/s.m.c._01_2020_18052020.pdf [Accessed 23 March 2021].

Syed, B.S., 2020. Bajwa Calls for National Unity to Fight Covid-19. *Dawn*, April 02. Available from: https://www.dawn.com/news/1545740 [Accessed 23 March 2021].

Syed, M.A. and Malkani, A., 2020. The Analytical Angle: How Smart Containment, Along with Active Learning, Can Help Mitigate the Covid-19 Crisis. *Dawn* Prism, April 19. Available from: https://www.dawn.com/news/1550037 [Accessed 23 March 2021].

The Express Tribune, 2020. WHO Recommends 'Intermittent, Targeted' Lockdowns in Pakistan. June 9. Available from: https://tribune.com.pk/story/2239223/recommends-intermittent-lockdown-punjab [Accessed 23 March 2021].

The Nation, 2020. High-level NCC Constituted to Help Curb Coronavirus. March 14. Available from: https://nation.com.pk/14-Mar-2020/high-level-ncc-constitutes-to-help-curb-coronavirus [Accessed 23 March 2021].

The News, 2020. Strict Lockdown on Hot Spots: PM Imran Khan. June 14. Available from: https://www.thenews.com.pk/print/672214-strict-lockdown-on-hot-spots-pm [Accessed 23 March 2021].

UNDP, 2020. COVID-19 – Pakistan Socio-Economic Impact Assessment and Response Plan. May 1. Available from: https://reliefweb.int/sites/reliefweb.int/files/resources/PAKISTAN-Preparedness-and-Response-Plan-PPRP-COVID-19_0.pdf [Accessed 23 March 2021].

ur-Rehman, Z., Abi-Habib, M. and Mehsud, I.T., 2020. 'God Will Protect Us': Coronavirus Spreads through an Already Struggling Pakistan. *The New York Times*, March 26. Available from: https://www.nytimes.com/2020/03/26/world/asia/pakistan-coronavirus-tablighi-jamaat.html [Accessed 23 March 2021].

ur-Rehman, Z. and Schmall, E., 2020. A Covid-19 Surge and Conspiracy Theories Roil Pakistan. *The New York Times*, December 19. Available from: https://www.nytimes.com/2020/12/19/world/asia/pakistan-coronavirus.html [Accessed 23 March 2021].

WHO, 2018. Eastern Mediterranean Region (EMRO) – Framework for Health Information Systems and Core Indicators for Monitoring Health Situation and Health System Performance. WHO-EM/HST/244/E. Available from: https://applications.emro.who.int/docs/EMROPUB_2018_EN_20620.pdf?ua=1 [Accessed 23 March 2021].

WHO, 2020. Pakistan: Essential Polio Vaccination Campaigns Resume under Strict COVID-19 Prevention Measures. EMRO, July 20. Available from: http://www.emro.who.int/pak/pakistan-news/essential-polio-vaccination-campaigns-resume-under-strict-covid-19-prevention-measures.html [Accessed 23 March 2021].

World Bank, 2020. The World Bank in Pakistan: Overview. October 8. Available from: https://www.worldbank.org/en/country/pakistan/overview [Accessed 23 March 2021].

Younus, U., 2020a. Coronavirus Hits Pakistan's Already-Strained Economy, and Its Most Vulnerable. New Atlanticist, Atlantic Council. Available from: https://www.atlanticcouncil.org/blogs/new-atlanticist/coronavirus-hits-pakistans-already-strained-economy-and-its-most-vulnerable/ [Accessed 23 March 2021].

Younus, U., 2020b. Pakistan Faces a Long Road to Sustainable Growth. United States Institute of Peace. October 7. Available from: https://www.usip.org/publications/2020/10/pakistan-faces-long-road-sustainable-growth [Accessed 23 March 2021].

Zaidi, S.A., Bigdeli, M., Langlois, E.V., Riaz, A., Orr, D.W., Idrees, N. and Bump, J.B., 2020. Health Systems Changes after Decentralisation: Progress, Challenges and Dynamics in Pakistan. *BMJ Global Health*, 4 (1), e001013. Available from: https://doi.org/10.1136/bmjgh-2018-001013 [Accessed 23 March 2021].

19 Federalism and the Russian response to the first waves of COVID-19

Nataliya Golovanova

19.1 Introduction

The COVID-19 pandemic has changed much of the traditional world. At the individual level, personal habits and interactions have changed vastly. At the governmental level in policies around economics, education, and health care, much is different. Federalism has also changed as a result of the pandemic. The emergency management responses to COVID-19 by some governments have involved centralization in decision-making. Many governments have justified such centralized policy choices as the urgent national response of "emergency federalism" (Kurlyandskaya 2020). However, in Russia, powers were already centralized, so there was not much need to change the distribution and balance of powers.

The new revision of the Constitution of the Russian Federation (RF), adopted in the summer of 2020, formally expanded the list of powers of the President. However, centralization occurred much earlier, and the amendments only fixed on paper the already established practices. Over the past decade in Russia, the federal government has strengthened political control over the regions, but the financial levers have always been in the hands of the center.

On the one hand, the central government in Russia issues a large number of regulatory documents: decrees, recommendations, resolutions, bylaws, and orders that subnational governments must follow. On the other hand, regional governments had the right to choose their own instruments for fighting the pandemic. The federal budget generously provided additional transfer payments to the regions, though at the same time, higher rates of cases or high mortality from COVID-19 have been the reasons to blame regional governments directly. COVID-19 has created a new reality in all spheres of our life (Table 19.1).

Table 19.1 Key Statistics on COVID-19 in Russia as of 31 December 2021

Cumulative Cases	Cumulative Cases per 100,000 Population	Cumulative Deaths	Cumulative Deaths per 100,000 Population	Case Fatality Percentage
3,159,297	2,156.6	57,019	38.9	1.8

Source: Data source: Yandex DataLens, 2021. All Known Cases in Russia [dataset]. Available from: https://datalens.yandex/covid19 [Accessed 1 February 2021].

DOI: 10.4324/9781003251217-19

19.2 The impact of COVID-19 on Russia

COVID-19 was first transmitted to Russia by tourists returning from abroad. The lack of the quarantine measures in the first weeks of the outbreak allowed the virus to spread, especially in large cities. Russia faced the consequences of COVID-19 in the second half of March 2020.

Travel agencies, the hospitality industry, and retail trade in Russia were affected by the pandemic from February 2020 on. Lockdowns added to the list of the economic areas significantly affected by the spread of COVID-19. The sectors affected were transportation, leisure and entertainment, sports, public catering, domestic services (repair, laundry, dry cleaning, hairdressing, and beauty salons), non-food retail trade, stomatology, private education, and mass media.[1] The decline in economic activity resulted in an unemployment increase from 4.7 percent in March to 5.8 percent in April with a smooth growth to 6.4 percent in August and a slow decline to 5.9 percent in December (see Figure 19.1).

Small business suffered dramatically from the quarantine, and the support measures resulted in a budget revenue decrease. These declines showed up in consolidated (regional plus local) budget revenues in Q2–Q3 of 2020. On the other hand, online retail and delivery increased in volume, while advertising then shifted from city streets to the internet. According to the research agency Data Insight, the number of orders in online stores in 2020 increased by 78 percent and reached 830 million. In monetary terms, these orders increased by 47 percent to 2.5 trillion rubles. In 2020, the share of online trade reached 9 percent of all Russian retail.[2]

The ripple effect of COVID-19 has had a number of economic and social impacts on the RF. The decline in oil prices also led to a decrease in federal budget revenues. As a response, the additional federal expenses and transfer payments to the regions from the federal budget were covered by the Reserve Fund of the government of the RF.

The World Bank has predicted a 6 percent drop in GDP in Russia as a result of the pandemic (World Bank 2020). The Rosstat – Russia's statistics bureau – was more

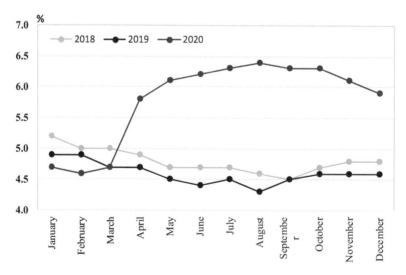

Figure 19.1 Monthly Unemployment Rate in Russia from 2018 to 2020 (According to the Methodology of the WTO) (Operational Data) (Percentage).

optimistic: it listed a 3.1 percent decline in 2020.[3] The decrease in GDP in 2020 was a result of the restrictive measures introduced to combat COVID-19 infection and the decrease in global energy demand. The value-added component has significantly reduced in service industries: hotels and restaurants (−24.1 percent), cultural and sports institutions (−11.4 percent), transport enterprises (−10.3 percent), organizations that provide other services to the public (−6.8 percent). Unfavorable export conditions and lower energy prices contributed to the decline in the value-added physical volume index (−10.2 percent). Increased demand for financial services led to a value-added increase in finance and insurance sphere (+7.9 percent). The increase in Housing and Utilities tariffs affected the value-added deflator indices of enterprises providing electricity, gas and steam (+3.9 percent), water supply, sanitation, and waste disposal (+6.2 percent). The growth of the value-added deflator index compared to last year in health care (+11.9 percent) and other sectors of the public administration are associated with an increase in the average salary in these industries.

The population of the RF has decreased by 510,400 people (0.3 percent of the total population) by the end of the year.[4] In addition to the increase in mortality, many families postponed their childbirth decisions that will have negative effect in the future. Furthermore, it is unknown how the necessary shift to online education during shutdown will affect the future workforce.

The labor market has also changed. According to Ministry of Labor[5] data, about 3.7 million Russians work remotely in 2020, which is about 7 percent of all employed citizens of the country. That number increased 110 times from previous year.

Despite the all measures taken by the all levels of government, this was not sufficient to stop the epidemic although in the summer the number of cases reduced. However, in the fall, the number of cases grew again (see Figure 19.2).

As of 31 December 2020, the number of total COVID-19 cases from the beginning of the year was 3,159,297 people (2 percent of the total population of the RF).

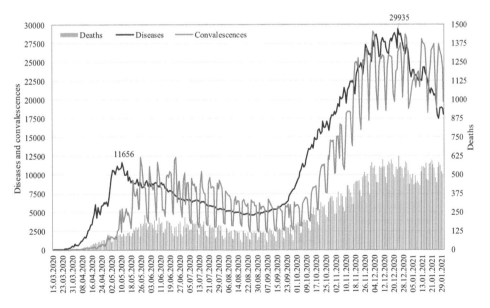

Figure 19.2 Daily Dynamics of Diseases (Cases), Recoveries (Convalescences), and Deaths from COVID-19 in Russia.

The number of deaths reached 57,019 (0.04 percent of the total population). The daily numbers of new cases have grown dramatically from September. The disease's peak (29,935 people per day) was passed on 24 December 2020, and the number of cases has started to decrease.

The numbers of cases and deaths per 100,000 people varies considerably between regions (see Figure 19.5 in the Annex). The highest death rates to the number of people infected by COVID-19 on 31 December 2020 are in the Republic of Dagestan (4.8 percent of all infected), Rostov Oblast (4.0 percent), and Perm Krai and Krasnoyarsk Krai (3.7 percent).[6]

19.3 COVID-19 and federalism in Russia

19.3.1 *Administrative and territorial divisions*

According to the RF Constitution, Russia is a federal state.[7] The Federation consists of 85 regions (*subjects of the federation*). Local self-government system is represented

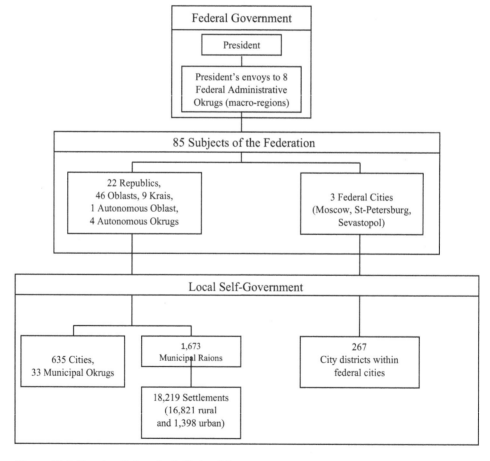

Figure 19.3 Russian Federation's Federal Structure.
Source: Updated from de Silva et al. (2009) based on Rosstat data on 1 January 2020.

by 635 city municipalities (*gorodskoi okrugs*) and 33 *municipal okrugs*[8] (both types are one-level local governments), plus 1,673 *municipal raions*[9] with over 18,000 associated rural and urban settlements inside (two-tier local governments).[10] Administratively, Russia is also divided into eight *federal okrugs* that are deconcentrated branches of the federal government (see Figure 19.3).

According to the new revision of the 2020 RF Constitution, federal territories (like territories in Canada) may be established in the RF. Russian legislation assigns powers and revenue sources across all levels of government. However, reassignment of revenues and expenditures during the last 15 years has made Russia a more and more centralized country. Besides, there is one phenomenon not typical in federal countries, namely "vertical of power." This vertical is exerted when regional governments have to account for their performance to the federal government, and local governments report to the regional ones. So, Russian intergovernmental relations usually are "top-down": thus, when the central government makes a decision, subnational governments have to agree and must try to perform according to those decisions.

This leads to the problem of accountability. The heads of the regions must look to the federal government for money and political survival. Thus, they are accountable upward and not downward, meaning that sometimes the federal orders are more important for regional governments than local needs.

Federal regulations often became unfunded mandates because of the lack of adequate resources transferred from the central level. In recent years, the heaviest mandates, such as raising wages in the public sector, were initially funded from the federal budget through grants to ensure a balance. After some time, funding for these items was stopped. In addition, the principles of distribution of these grants are not set up in legislation, unlike equalization grants.

19.3.2 *The Russian federation government's response to COVID-19*

In the middle of March 2020, a Coordination Council under the Government of the Russian Federation was formed to fight the spread of COVID-19 in the country. The Council's goal was to provide cooperation between the central government, governments of the subjects of the Russian Federation, local governments, and different organizations. Members of the Council discuss the effectiveness of the measures already taken to combat COVID-19 and the introduction of new ones.

The Government of Russia developed a "Priority plan."[11] This document contained a number of measures including provision of essential goods and services to the population, support for the sectors of economy at risk, support for small and medium business and other measures including extension of support to regional budgets faced with a decline in tax revenues.

The list of priority measures to ensure sustainable development of the economy included:

- Deferred payment of taxes and social contributions for certain categories of taxpayers;
- Suspension of audits and checks;
- Zeroing of customs duties for some socially important goods;
- Employment support; and
- Other targeted measures for certain sectors of the economy.

For all small and medium enterprises (SMEs), a twofold reduction in the social contributions rate and loan restructuring was proposed.

Following the federal authorities, regional governments have also adopted measures to support economic activities. The most frequently used measures were:

- Reducing the property tax rate for taxpayers from the sectors of economy affected by COVID-19;
- Providing property tax benefits for landlords in exchange for rent reduction and/or rent deferral for tenants;
- Reducing regional property rent;
- Reducing the rates of the SME taxes for certain sectors; and
- Canceling the transportation tax for certain sectors.

Local (municipal) governments took part in disinfection of public spaces, courtyards, public transport,[12] and in some cases with the help of the reserve funds of local administrations (e.g., Podolsk, Smolensk, and Yakutsk) and control over the application of markings at retail outlets.

Besides, local governments allowed to defer payments for the lease of municipal property and local taxes.

Federal government social support measures included:

- Increasing the minimum sick leave payment for 2020;
- Increasing the unemployment benefit;
- Introducing additional benefit for an unemployed parent with children under 18;
- Additional one-time payments for families with children.

The Ministry of Healthcare[13] and Federal Service for Surveillance on Consumer Rights Protection and Human Wellbeing (*Rospotrebnadzor*)[14] plays a pivotal role in anti-epidemic response. The latter has regional offices, which include scientific research institutes, hygienic, and epidemiological centers and laboratories. The Ministry of Healthcare has adopted the "Interim methodical recommendations prevention, diagnosis and treatment of new coronavirus infections (COVID-19)" that have become the guideline for the regional health care authorities in their response to the pandemic.

The existing federal legislation gives the regional governments the power to establish restrictive measures in emergency situations.[15] The Presidential Decree issued on 2 April 2020[16] declared that regional governors have the power to implement any additional anti-COVID-19 restrictive measures to expand the federal ones. However, some regional governors (e.g., the head of Moscow) introduced restrictive measures even before the Presidential Decree was issued. Experts say that the Presidential Decree "transformed the opportunity into a duty." Presidential Decree also implies a personal responsibility of governors for the epidemic situation in regions. As a result, regional governors started to impose strict restrictions, often excessive ones (such as the prohibition against walking outdoors in Moscow that negatively affected the health of older people), so that the federal center could not accuse them for the insufficient measures.

All regional authorities eventually introduced a state of high alert. The first to do so were the regions in the Far East: Amur Oblast (27 January 2020), Jewish

Autonomous Oblast (5 February 2020), the Republic of Buryatia (10 February 2020), and Yaroslavl Oblast (7 February 2020). In March, all other regions joined the list. The City of Moscow proclaimed a state of high alert on 5 March 2020. In St. Petersburg, Moscow, and Leningrad Oblasts, it was proclaimed on 13 March 2020. The last to do so was Voronezh Oblast (20 March 2020).[17] In all, 43 regions out of 85 (including the City of Moscow, Moscow, and Leningrad Oblasts) declared a *force majeure* situation – the pronouncement of the existence of a crisis or disaster often called "an act of God."

The first self-quarantine order was introduced in the City of Moscow on 26 March 2020 and Moscow Oblast on 29 March 2020. By the end of March, 26 regions had adopted self-isolation measures. In the summer, most of the restrictions were canceled. However, in October, some isolation measures were reimposed. In spite of all the measures taken by all levels of government, this was not sufficient to stop the epidemic (see Figure 19.2).

As a result of the economic support measures (mostly tax deferrals), during the first half of the year, the main sources of regional budget revenues declined predictably.[18] Profit tax revenues dropped 15.2 percent from the corresponding period of the previous year, personal income tax revenues decreased by 2.7 percent, small business taxes declined by 12.8 percent, and property taxes by 7.7 percent. The only increase was 3.2 percent in excise taxes. The steep drop in consolidated regional budgets revenue was made up for by a 57.4 percent growth in transfer payments from the federal budget. The federal government increased in grants by 64.1 percent, subsidies by 82.6 percent, and other intergovernmental transfer payments by 52.1 percent.

But, by the end of 2020, the deferrals were over, the economy began to recover, and the volume of tax and non-tax revenues of consolidated regional budgets almost returned to the level of 2019 (see Figure 19.6 in the Annex for monthly dynamics). Tax revenues from consolidated regional budgets shrank to 98.2 percent of those in 2019.[19] Personal income tax rose by 7.5 percent from the corresponding period of the previous year, excise taxes by 5.6 percent, property taxes by 0.5 percent. Small business taxes declined by 0.7 percent. A 12.8 percent drop was seen in the profit tax. The largest profit tax revenue decline was in the regions with a high share of the oil and gas sector as well as the extraction and processing of metals in the industry. In the regions with a diversified economy, however, there was an increase in total tax revenues (this took place in 22 regions, including Tambov, Voronezh, Amur, Leningrad, and Tver Oblasts).

Transfer payments from the federal budget grew by 53.9 percent in 2020: grants were enlarged by 41.1 percent, subsidies by 81.6 percent, and other intergovernmental transfer payments by 48.5 percent.

Other tools for supporting subnational budgets were the loans from the federal budget. In December, the Ministry of Finance provided 224 billion rubles of budget loans maturing no later than 1 July 2021. These loans were available to 75 regions (Russian Ministry of Finance 2021).

Federal tax and non-tax revenues have fallen by 12.5 percent in 2020 compared to 2019. For that reason, all additional federal budget expenses (including intergovernmental transfer payments, see Table 19.2 in the Annex) were covered from the Reserve fund of the Government of the Russian Federation.

Federal transfer payments for supporting the implementation of anti-COVID-19 measures in 2020 account for 15 percent of consolidated regional budget expenditures on health care and 6 percent of consolidated budgetary and extra-budgetary health care expenses (Consolidated Budgets of the Russian Federation 2021).

19.3.3 Assignment of powers in health care

In 2001, the federal government launched intergovernmental relations reforms based on the fiscal federalism development strategy.[20] The main objectives of these reforms were the following:

- To clarify and optimize the assignment of expenditure responsibilities across tiers of government;
- To eliminate unfunded federal and regional mandates;
- To reassign revenue sources to levels of government in accordance with their newly reassigned expenditure responsibilities;
- To establish transparent and fair rules for allocating federal and regional intergovernmental transfer payments.[21]

The new rules have been in effect since 2005. However, a transparent system of intergovernmental relations did not last long.

Soon numerous amendments were made to the laws that contradicted the original strategy of federalism. New federal unfunded mandates have appeared in the legislation, the change in the assignment of revenue sources did not fully correspond to the change in the allocation of expenditures and part of intergovernmental transfer payments became untransparent.

After the intergovernmental relations reforms, health care was funded by the level of government according to the type of services (2005–2011). Primary health care and ambulances were the responsibilities of the local governments, regional governments were in charge of the specialized health care in hospitals, and R&D and specialized expensive treatment were assigned to the federal level.

Since 2012, the legislation has changed: provision of medical (including emergency) and palliative care have been assigned according to the ownership of the medical organization. Now, the federal government is responsible for the health care provided in federal hospitals while regional governments are responsible for all types of health care provided in regional hospitals and policlinics (Figure 19.4).[22] Some regions delegate primary health care to the local level if local governments have their own health care institutions.[23] According to the federal legislation, local self-government bodies just have to ensure the *availability* of medical care without an obligation to provide services.

Most health care services are funded by extra-budgetary Mandatory Medical Insurance Funds.[24]

Federal Mandatory Medical Insurance Fund (FMMIF) revenues include the following:

- Employer's insurance payments (5.1 percent of payroll) for the working population;
- The contribution from regional budgets for the non-working population (children, elderly people, and unemployed citizens);
- Specific purpose intergovernmental transfer payments from the federal budget.

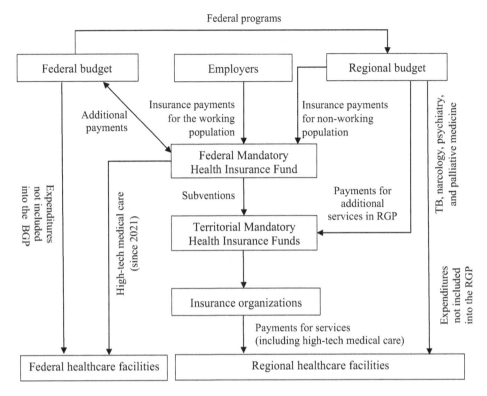

Figure 19.4 Public Financing of Healthcare Services in Russia.
Source: Author's sources, based on RF legislation and budget execution reports.

A total of 95 percent of the FMMIF budget is spent on transfer payments to the Territorial Mandatory Medical Insurance Funds (TMMIF). The allocation of these targeted subsidies to the TMMIF is based on a *per capita* amount and adjusted to account for the regional cost of living.

FMMIF also issues regulations on the management of public health care sector in regions. FMMIF and TMMIF pay for services included into the Basic Guarantee Program (BGP) on providing medical assistance to the residents of particular region. Regional governments may also include additional services into the Regional Guarantee Program (RGP) and finance it through the transfer from the regional budget to the TMMIF. Regions also finance tuberculosis, narcology, psychiatry, and palliative medicine.

In 2019, 60 percent of health care expenditures have been contributed by the Medical Insurance Funds, about 30 percent from the consolidated regional budgets and only 10 percent from the federal level (final expenditures without intergovernmental transfer payments) (Russia Federal Treasury 2021). In 2020, the figures were 50 percent, 37 percent, and 13 percent, respectively.

Total health care expenditures (budgetary and extra-budgetary) grew from 3.5 percent of GDP in 2019 to 4.6 percent of GDP[25] in 2020 (at the same time GDP decreased by 3.1 percent). Most of the additional expenses associated with COVID-19 were carried out through regional budgets. Consolidated regional health care budgetary expenditures grew by 71 percent in 2020 while TMMIF expenditures increased by only 10 percent.

19.3.4 COVID-19 impact on the RF health care system

The Russian health care system was not prepared for the pandemic. The recent financial crisis and the growth of regional debts impacted the subnational governments' capacity to combat COVID-19. The effect of the previous economic shocks meant that the RF had to enact austerity measures across the regions that were called cost optimization programs. These programs involved stringent planning and approval processes for regional government from the federal Ministry of Finance. All regions receiving equalization grants had to prepare and approve such programs. One of the outcomes of the program was the optimization of the network of health care institutions and the reduction of the number of hospital beds.

Donor regions were also forced to optimize health care spending because of changes in the system of financing expenditures through the FMMIF. The health care financing became more even due to changes in the allocation formula. The new distribution formula was based on a *per capita* sum, adjusted for regional cost of living coefficients. Equalization resulted in the redistribution of FMMIF resources from "rich" to "poor" regions. Therefore, "rich" regions like "poor" ones had to optimize their medical institutions to make the health care sector more economically efficient.

Therefore, when faced with the first wave of COVID-19, the health care system began to adjust the number of hospitals and hospital beds to the new requirements. The federal structure of the state provides some leeway, allowing the regions to choose the way of adjusting, whether it is building new temporary or permanent hospitals or changing an existing hospital's profile or capacity.

For example, a new infectious disease hospital was built in the Republic of Tatarstan (a donor region), a hospital from prefabricated modules was constructed in only 55 days in Bashkortostan. In the City of Moscow, temporary hospitals were opened in the Trade Center "Moscow" and at the VDNKh exhibition center. The federal government helps to increase the number of beds with special grants (see Table 19.2 in the Annex).

Besides the insufficient number of beds, previous health care reforms resulted in the lack of doctors and nursing staff in the public sector. Some regions (e.g., Nizhny Novgorod Oblast and Republic of Tatarstan) successfully used the help of volunteers in organizing information about patients.[26] District doctors received statistics from ambulance, call centers, and social workers – statistics that were processed by these volunteers. This information helped in making decisions about the urgency of assistance and the need for hospitalization.

With a lack of professionals, telemedicine began to play a significant role. Regional hospitals had online consultations with the specialists from the federal medicine centers.

Unfortunately, another impact on the health care system during the pandemic was a reduction in providing health services in other areas. One of the orders from the Ministry of Health[27] recommended postponing planned medical care and suspending regular medical examinations.

19.4 Case study of innovation/transformations in COVID-19 and federalism in Russia

19.4.1 Fiscal policy

According to Russian laws, regional governments have to follow the federal government's orders. However, the pandemic dramatically changed the fiscal policy goals.

Before 2020, subsidized regions had to adopt expenditure optimization and revenue increasing programs to receive equalization grants. Now, due to an increase in the number of disease cases, regional governments had to change policy guidelines. Regions had to increase health care expenses to open new inpatient or mobile hospitals, redesign existing ones, and attract additional personnel.

Following the federal recommendations, regional governments started to provide tax benefits for the small business and hard-hit economic sectors. So, budgetary policy has turned from saving costs and generating the highest possible revenues to increasing health care expenses and reducing budgetary income in the short term in order to save the tax base for the future.

Russia experienced a re-assignment of powers in the middle of 2000s and a gradual move to a less transparent governance system. Surprisingly, in the aftermath of this less than clear health care expenditure allocation, public health care is still able to provide services and still works normally in practice. The existing health care system *de facto* assigns the responsibility for providing most of the services to the subnational levels of government.

The federal government supports regions in their fight against COVID-19 in three ways:

1   Through in-kind purchasing and distributing equipment and supplies among the regions – including ambulances, medical personal protective equipment, medical ventilators, ECMO equipment, and medicines (see Kurlyandskaya 2020);
2   Through intergovernmental transfer payments; and
3   Through short-term loans from the federal budget.

However, regional governments do not know how long this support will last. For example, how long will the federal budget fund additional payments to doctors and nurses working in hospital with COVID-19? The regions already had a negative experience when the central government stopped providing transfer payments for financing the obligations established by the federal legislation after a couple of years. This practice turned an obligation into an unfunded mandate.[28] This uncertainty provides for a murky and potentially inconsistent policy environment for providing these essential services and is a concern for regions and significantly, for citizens. Besides, as often happens with emergency grants, new intergovernmental fiscal transfer payments are non-transparent. The results of the allocation of transfer payments are set by legislation but not the formulas. For example, three regions (Ivanovo Oblast, Murmansk Oblast, and Kabardino-Balkar Republic) received special *ad hoc* transfer payments (see Table 19.2 in the Annex).

A high degree of centralization in emergency management looks like an effective measure. However, Russia is a very centralized country, so further centralization is not necessary. On the contrary, it would be positive to see the regions freer in decision-making as it were in mid-2000th and not overloaded with federal mandates. Nevertheless, the world pandemic is not a good moment for the re-distribution of powers. Many are of the opinion that, if the system 'isn't broke, don't fix it.'

19.4.2 New practices

Several new features have appeared in the practice of Russian health care after the COVID-19 pandemic began.

First of all, temporary and mobile hospitals were built. It became clear that having permanent beds reserve for the case of emergency in stationary hospitals was too expensive. So light and mobile constructions helped to decide this problem for the required period.

One of the problems with COVID-19 is the lack of specialists (doctors and nurses) who could work with infected people. Life has shown that public health care needs more general practitioners because not all specialists can change their profile. This problem was partly solved with the help of volunteers and by hiring personnel from the private sector.

Besides, the pandemic gave a push to the use of telemedicine. Online conferences with professors from federal medicine centers also helped to develop the course of treatment in difficult cases.

The common threat also pushed interregional horizontal cooperation. Groups of doctors from hospitals in regions most successful in treatment (like Tatarstan[29]) visited neighboring regions and the former CIS countries to share their experience.

Different initial conditions and different strategies for fighting COVID-19 led to different results. The numbers of infections and deaths per 100,000 people vary considerably (see Figure 19.5 in the Annex). This is especially noticeable when comparing the two regions with the highest death rates per 100,000 people, Moscow and St. Petersburg. Both cities faced a high number of cases due to population density and intensive tourist traffic through the airport at the beginning of the epidemic. But St. Petersburg's death rate for the number of people infected by COVID-19 is more than twice as high as that in Moscow.

The COVID-19 infection has a seasonal spread, so in the fall, the number of cases and deaths began to grow. But now, both federal and regional governments can consider the previous experience and change policies so the next wave will be less damaging. The Ministry of Health also hopes that vaccinations, which began in December 2020, could help to reduce the spread of the disease.

Annex

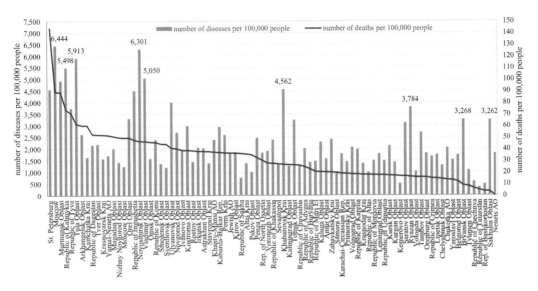

Figure 19.5 Number of COVID-19 Cases (Diseases) and Deaths by Regions as of 31 December 2020. Data source: Yandex DataLens, 2021. All Known Cases in Russia [dataset]. Available from: https://datalens.yandex/covid19 [Accessed 1 February 2021].

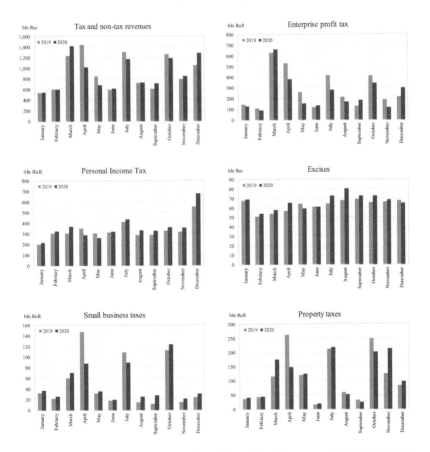

Figure 19.6 Consolidated Regional Budgets: Tax Revenues in 2019–2020. Data source: consolidated budgets of Russian Federation reports https://roskazna.gov.ru.

Table 19.2 Additional Intergovernmental Transfer Payments Financed through the Reserve Fund of the Government of the Russian Federation in 2020

No	Intergovernmental Transfer Payments	Budgeted, Million Rubles
1	Grants to support balanced budgets for equipping (re-equipping) additionally created or re-profiled beds in medical organizations to provide medical care for patients with the COVID-19 infection	68,180
2	Grants to support measures to ensure balanced budgets that offer additional payments to medical and other workers of medical and other organizations providing medical care for the diagnosis and treatment of a new COVID-19 infection in contact with patients who have the COVID-19 infection	10,000
3	Grants to support measures to ensure the balance of budgets for the financial support of measures to combat the COVID-19 infection	10,000
4	Grants to support the balance of budgets for the provision of subsidies to legal entities and individual entrepreneurs to partially compensate for the costs associated with their activities in the context of a worsening situation as a result of the spread of the COVID-19 infection, including for maintaining employment and remuneration of their employees	4,900
5	Intergovernmental transfers for the purchase of drugs for the treatment of patients with the COVID-19 infection receiving medical care on an outpatient basis	7,833
6	Intergovernmental transfers for the implementation of incentive payments for the performance of especially important work to medical and other workers directly involved in the provision of medical care to citizens who have the COVID-19 infection	109,898
7	Intergovernmental transfers for the implementation of incentive payments for special working conditions and additional workload for medical workers providing medical care to citizens who have the COVID-19 infection and people at risk of contracting the COVID-19 infection	66,379
8	Intergovernmental transfers for the implementation of incentive payments for special working conditions and additional workload for employees of stationary social service organizations, stationary departments created in non-stationary social service organizations, providing social services to citizens who have the COVID-19 infection, and people at risk of the COVID-19 infection	17,856
9	Intergovernmental transfers to equip laboratories of medical organizations with medical devices that carry out etiological diagnostics of the COVID-19 infection with nucleic acid amplification methods	1,000
10	Intergovernmental transfers to the budget of the Kabardino-Balkar Republic for co-financing the expenditure obligations arising from the implementation of measures to counter the spread of the COVID-19 infection	704
11	Subsidy to the budget of the Murmansk Oblast to co-finance the expenditure obligations for the deployment in the village Murmashi of the Kola District of the Murmansk Region of a pre-fabricated field hospital to provide medical care to patients with the COVID-19 infection	969
12	Subsidy to the budget of the Ivanovo Oblast to co-finance expenditure obligations for the deployment in the territory of the Ivanovo region of a pre-fabricated infectious diseases hospital with a bed capacity of 360 beds to provide medical care to patients with the COVID-19 infections	2,580
	Total	300,299

Source: http://budget.gov.ru accessed on 1 February 2020.

Notes

1 RF Government resolution N 434 on 3 April 2020.
2 The research agency Data Insight, 2021. [website]. Available from:_https://datainsight.ru/ [Accessed 8 April 2021].
3 Rosstat presents the first GDP estimate for 2020. Available from: https://rosstat.gov.ru/ storage/mediabank/Ytm0lG1M/GDP-2020-1.pdf [Accessed 8 April 2021].
4 Federal State Statistics Service, 2021. Estimate of the resident population as of 1 January 2021. Available from: https://rosstat.gov.ru [Accessed 8 April 2021].
5 Ministry of Labor and Social Protection, 2021 [website]. Available from: https://mintrud. gov.ru/ [Accessed 8 April 2021].
6 Yandex DataLens, 2021. All Known Cases in the World [dataset]. Available from: https:// datalens.yandex/covid19 [Accessed 8 April 2021].
7 Nevertheless, the old Federal Constitutional Law of December 17, 1997 N 2-FKZ "On the Government of the Russian Federation" stated that the Government of the RF was guided by the principles of federalism and separation of powers. The new Federal Constitutional Law of November 6, 2020 N 4-FKZ "On the Government of the Russian Federation" doesn't mention federalism at all.
8 A municipal okrug – a newly established – in 2019 – type of local government that includes several localities with common borders (usually city or town and its surrounding *raion*).
9 A *raion* (also rayon) is an administrative unit in rural areas typical for several post-Soviet countries.
10 For more on administrative divisions, such as regions and local self-government in Russia see: de Silva, Migara, Galina Kurlyandskaya, Elena Andreeva, Natalia Golovanova. *Intergovernmental Reforms in the Russian Federation: One step forward, two steps back?* Washington: The World Bank Press, 2009.
11 Russian Federation Government, 2020. COVID-19 Response in the Russian Federation. *In*: *Russian Federation 2020*. 17 March 17. Translated in United Nations, New York City. See also report prepared by Deloitte Consulting LLC: "Support measures for those affected by COVID-19". Available from: https://www2.deloitte.com/ru/en/pages/tax/ articles/podderzhka-economiki.html [Accessed 8 April 2021].
12 Monitoring and atlas, 2020. Regions, municipalities and local communities against COVID-19. *All-Russian Congress of Municipalities*. Available from: http://okmo.news/ event.php?42 [Accessed 7 May 2021].
13 Russian Ministry of Healthcare, 2021 [website]. Available from: https://minzdrav.gov.ru/ [Accessed 8 April 2021].
14 Federal Service for Surveillance on Consumer Rights Protection and Human Wellbeing. Available from: https://www.rospotrebnadzor.ru [Accessed 8 April 2021].
15 *Federal law No. 68-FZ of 21 December 1994*. Protection of the Population and Territories in Case of Natural and Man-made Disasters. Duma, Moscow. Translated in International Labour Organization, Geneva, Switzerland. Available from: https://www.ilo.org/ dyn/natlex/natlex4.detail?p_lang=en&p_isn=93583 [Accessed 8 April 2021].
16 *Decree of the President of the Russian Federation of 2 April 2020 N 239*. Moscow. Translated in Washington, DC: Food and Agriculture Organization. Available from: http:// www.fao.org/faolex/results/details/en/c/LEX-FAOC194256/ [Accessed 8 April 2021].
17 All data on alert mode from Consultant Plus legislation database. Available from: http:// www.consultant.ru/online/
18 Monitoring of Russia's Economic Outlook No.13 (115) August 2020. Available from: https://www.iep.ru/en/publications/publication/monitoring-of-russia-s-economic-outlook-no-13-115-august-2020.html [Accessed 8 April 2021].
19 Data on consolidated budgets of RF reports. Available from: https://roskazna.gov.ru and http://budget.gov.ru [Accessed 8 April 2021].
20 Decree of the Government of the Russian Federation N 584 of August 8, 2001 "On the Program for the development of fiscal federalism in the Russian Federation for the period up to 2005."
21 For more on fiscal federalism reform in Russia, *see*: De Silva et al. (2009).

22 Federal law No. 323-FZ of 21 November 2011. "On the basics of public health protection in the Russian Federation."
23 This is the remainder of the system that was in effect in 2005–2011. In most regions, since 2012, local health care institutions have been transferred to the regional level.
24 See more on financing health care in Russia and Medical Insurance Funds: Popovich, L., Potapchik, E., Shishkin, S., Richardson. E., Vacroux, A. and Mathivet, B., 2011. Russian Federation: Health System Review. *Health Systems in Transition*, 13 (7), 1–190. Available from: https://www.euro.who.int/en/countries/russian-federation/publications/russian-federation-hit-2011 [Accessed 8 April 2021].
25 Preliminary estimates.
26 The conference, "Pandemic 2020: Challenges, Solutions, Consequences." Available from: https://confpandemic.com/ [Accessed 8 April 2021].
27 Order of the Ministry of Health of Russia No. 198N, 19 March 2020. Translated in Commonwealth of Independent States, Moscow. Available from: https://cis-legislation.com/document.fwx?rgn=123310 [Accessed 8 April 2021].
28 For example, financial support for families with children has been assigned to the regions since 2005 and for the first two years was financed through subsidies from the federal budget. However, since 2007, this intergovernmental transfer has been canceled although responsibility for the provision of appropriate benefits is still assigned to the regional authorities by federal legislation.
29 The Republic of Tatarstan was one of the regions that first faced COVID-19 infections. But thanks to good governance, Tatarstan had the lowest infection rate per 100,000 people on 31 December 2020.

Bibliography

Consolidated Budgets of the Russian Federation, 2021. Federal Budget Execution in 2021. Portal for the Russian Federal Budgetary System. Available from: http://budget.gov.ru [Accessed 8 April 2021].

De Silva, M., Kurlyandskaya, G., Andreeva, E. and Golovanova, N., 2009. *Intergovernmental Reforms in the Russian Federation. One Step Forward, Two Steps Back?* Washington: The World Bank Press.

Federal Constitutional Law No. 2-FKZ of 17 December 1997, "On the Government of the Russian Federation" (with Amendments and Addenda of December 31, 1997). Duma, Moscow. Translated in World Trade Organization. Geneva, Switzerland. Available from: https://www.wto.org/english/thewto_e/acc_e/rus_e/WTACCRUS48_LEG_79.pdf [Accessed 8 April 2021].

Federal State Statistic Service, 2020. Estimate of Russia's GDP for 2020. *The Russian Government*. Available from: https://rosstat.gov.ru/storage/mediabank/Ytm0lG1M/GDP-2020-1.pdf [Accessed 8 April 2021].

Federal State Statistic Service, 2021. Estimate of the Resident Population of the Russian Federation. *The Russian Government*, 1 January. Available from: https://rosstat.gov.ru [Accessed 8 April 2021].

Kurlyandskaya, G., 2020. Federalism and the COVID-19 Crisis: 'Emergency Federalism' Russian Style. *Forum of Federations*. Available from: http://www.forumfed.org/2020/05/federalism-and-the-covid-19-crisis-federalism-and-the-covid-19-crisis-emergency-federalism-russian-style/ [Accessed 8 April 2021].

Monitoring of Russia's Economic Outlook No.13(115), August 2020. Gadar Institute for Economic Policy, Moscow. Available from: https://www.iep.ru/en/publications/publication/monitoring-of-russia-s-economic-outlook-no-13-115-august-2020.html [Accessed 8 April 2021].

Russia Federal Treasury, 2021. Consolidated Budgets of the Russian Federation. *The Russian Government*. Available from: https://roskazna.gov.ru [Accessed 8 April 2021].

Popovich, L., Potapchik, E., Shishkin, S., Richardson. E., Vacroux, A. and Mathivet, B., 2011. Russian Federation: Health System Review. *Health Systems in Transition*, 13 (7), 1–190. Available from: https://www.euro.who.int/en/countries/russian-federation/publications/russian-federation-hit-2011 [Accessed 8 April 2021].

Russian Federation Government Resolution N 434 on 3 April 2020. Commonwealth of Independent States, Moscow. Available from: https://cis-legislation.com/document.fwx?rgn=125277 [Accessed 8 April 2021].

Support measures for those affected by COVID-19. Deloitte Consulting LLC. 2021. Available from: https://www2.deloitte.com/ru/en/pages/tax/articles/podderzhka-economiki.html [Accessed 8 April 2021].

World Bank, June 2020. *Global Economic* Prospects. Washington. doi: 10.1596/978-1-4648-1553-9. Available from: https://www.vsemirnyjbank.org/ru/publication/global-economic-prospects [Accessed 8 April 2021].

20 South Africa's response to COVID-19

The multilevel government dynamic

Nico Steytler and Jaap De Visser

20.1 Introduction

When the COVID-19 pandemic reached South Africa in March 2020, the country already faced severe social, economic, and political difficulties. Socially, half of the population was poor, many in the urban areas living in informal settlements, and with an unemployment rate of 30 percent. The country's economy was not growing and was in recession. Politically, the divisions in the country, between black and white, poor and rich, rural and urban, were stark. South Africa's multilevel system of government – the national government, provinces, and municipalities – was struggling to meet these difficulties. The COVID-19 pandemic made these difficulties more intense, resulting, among other things, in a more centralized system of multilevel government (Table 20.1).

20.2 COVID-19 in South Africa

South Africa recorded its first Coronavirus infection on 5 March 2020. Since then, the number of infections has increased steadily, reaching a peak by June/July, before declining significantly over the next three months, but by the end of October, the infection rate spiked dramatically in some parts of the country as a second wave seemingly gathered moment.

By 31 July, South Africa placed among the top five in the world in terms of confirmed COVID-19 infections with a total of 493,183 infections (Department of Health 31 July 2020). However, the number of COVID-19-related deaths remained significantly low (8,005) compared to other countries in the top five. Gauteng and the Western Cape, the two most urbanized provinces, took turns in being the epicenter of the virus. Other provinces such as North West and Northern Cape, which are generally sparsely populated, experienced low levels of infections and deaths.

Table 20.1 Key Statistics on COVID-19 in South Africa as of 10 January 2021

Cumulative Cases	Cumulative Cases per 100,000 Population	Cumulative Deaths	Cumulative Deaths per 100,000 Population	Case-Fatality Percentage
1,214,176	2,047.2	32,824	55.3	2.7

Source: *World Health Organization Weekly epidemiological update* – 12 January 2021. Geneva: WHO, 2021. Available from https://www.who.int/publications/m/item/weekly-epidemiological-update

DOI: 10.4324/9781003251217-20

As of 30 September 2020, South Africa was at the lowest level of its five-level scale of restrictions (Level 1), with a total of 674,339 COVID-19 confirmed cases and 16,734 COVID-19-related deaths. By the end of December 2020, on the back of a second wave, the cumulative total of COVID-19 cases identified stood at 1,057,161, a recovery rate of 83 percent and 28,469 fatalities (Department of Health 31 December 2020). These official fatality figures are, however, an undercount. The South African Medical Research Council reported 110,000 excess deaths in South Africa since May 2020 to mid-January 2021, measuring the total number of fatalities from natural causes compared with the expected death rate in a "normal" year. The vast majority of these deaths, it suspects, are linked to COVID-19. And the end of the second wave is still far off, so too, is the economic and social recovery. Both the international and domestic economies have shrunk. The forecast for South Africa is that the Gross Domestic Product (GDP) for 2020 will shrink by more than 8 percent, causing unemployment to reach 40 percent. A fiscal crunch is already experienced; due to the recession, less revenue will be collected to meet increased expenditure in health, social, and economic assistance.

20.3 COVID-19 pandemic and South Africa's federal arrangements

20.3.1 General features

South Africa has a national government, 9 provinces, and 257 municipalities. The provincial and local spheres are constitutionally entrenched, with their powers listed in the Constitution. Provinces and municipalities have their own, locally elected, provincial legislatures, and municipal councils are headed by indirectly elected Premiers and Mayors, respectively.

Provinces are responsible for big social functions such as public health, housing, primary, and secondary education, and, importantly, disaster management. They share these functions with the national government, which is also responsible for all residual functions, such as international relations, policing, and the judiciary. The national government collects the vast majority of taxes, such as income, corporate, and value-added tax and distributes this annually across the three levels of government. Municipalities are responsible for the delivery of basic services, such as water, sanitation, waste management, roads, and electricity.

Provinces largely confine themselves to implementing national legislation and are almost entirely reliant on transfers from the national government (Khumalo, Mahabir and Dawood 2015). Together with a number of other design features, this makes South Africa a hybrid federal state, encompassing a strong national government, relatively 'weak' provinces, and a mix of strong cities and weak rural municipalities (Steytler 2013).

20.3.2 National government's response

The national government declared a national state of disaster on 15 March 2020 and on 27 March 2020 imposed one of the harshest lockdown regimes globally. It is important to note that a declaration of a 'national state of disaster' in terms of the Disaster Management Act of 2002 did not require Parliamentary approval, which a declaration of a state of emergency would have. The declaration of a national state of disaster was informed by concerns about high levels of co-morbidity, poverty, and inequality, South Africa's many informal and densely populated settlements and its fragile public health system. The lockdown regime included a strict stay-at-home order, a ban on all gatherings, closure of all external borders and ports, a ban on travel across provincial and municipal boundaries, a closure of the entire economy barring the trade in essential goods and services and even a ban on the sale of alcohol and tobacco. The South African Police Services, municipal law enforcement officers, and even the South African National Defense Force were deployed to enforce the lockdown rules. This was accompanied by a raft of national regulations, determining detailed regimes per sector such as health, education, transport, trade, and home affairs.

The national government also issued a specific set of directions to provincial and local governments. Both municipalities and provinces were instructed to develop COVID-19 Response Plans and establish special disaster management structures (see also below). Municipalities were also instructed to provide emergency water services, identify infection hotspots, and quarantine sites, sanitize public places, monitor social gatherings, and funerals and ensure community awareness.

After five weeks of the 'hard lockdown,' the national government announced a 'risk adjusted strategy' to be implemented from 1 May 2020. This strategy introduced differentiation in two important ways: first different 'alert levels,' ranging from the most severe 'level five' to the most relaxed 'level one,' and second, a place-based approach with possible variations in the severity of the restrictions between provinces and districts. This enabled the national government to determine a different alert level for each province and each district but was not used initially. As the overriding concern was solidarity and manageability, the government shied back from differentiating between provinces and districts. However, in early December 2020, when the second wave manifested itself in certain 'hotspots' – in municipalities along the Western Cape's south coast (the Garden Route) and the Nelson Mandela Bay Metropolitan municipality, stricter rules were imposed on those municipalities only. On 28 December 2020, the government imposed a ban on all gatherings, a curfew (9 PM to 4 AM), a ban on alcohol sales, and closed all beaches, fearing super-spreader events on old year's eve.

South Africa's response to the outbreak was quick, robust, and comprehensive. At first, the restrictions enjoyed broad-based support, in large part due to the re-assuring but realistic and science-based communication of the President and the national Minister of Health. However, the lockdown had a devastating impact on food security, the livelihoods of the marginalized and excluded as well as, essentially, the economy as a whole.

Three weeks into the national lockdown, a social relief and economic stimulus package of R500 billion was announced, totaling 7 percent of the GDP, which is the largest percentage on the continent. It included credit guarantees, support for small businesses, income support (mainly tax measures), and wage protection (through the unemployment insurance fund). Support was also provided to vulnerable households in the form of top-ups to existing grants (such as the Child Support Grant) and emergency food relief. This provided much-needed relief for those hit hardest by the crisis. All of these measures were implemented by the national government.

The package also included an additional R20 billion for health, which was channeled to provinces to augment provincial health budgets for treatment, testing, contact tracing, and the procurement of personal protective equipment (PPE). A further

R20 billion were set aside for local government to assist them with the additional services as well as their loss of revenue. This was important relief for municipalities and a result of successful lobbying by organized local government.

The social relief and economic stimulus package tells the story of South Africa's centralized response to the crisis. All in all, only R40 billion of the R500 billion were channeled through subnational governments with the remainder administered by national government.

20.3.3 Provinces' role

South Africa' nine provincial governments played a key role in fighting the pandemic, although it was limited to assisting national government with the implementation of the national strategy. Provincial governments did not announce, let alone legislate, COVID-19 strategies and/or rules that deviated from the essence of the national approach. This was true to the centralized nature of South Africa's hybrid federal system.

The division of responsibilities with regard to the competency 'disaster management,' at the heart of the management of the pandemic, is a case in point. The Constitution in schedule 4 provides that it is a concurrent power, which means that both national and provincial governments may legislate on it. Conflicts are ultimately resolved by the Constitutional Court. So far, only the national government has adopted a national Disaster Management Act in 2002 (the basis for the current state of disaster and the lockdown regime). Provinces implement this Act as none of them have adopted their own. A key factor is that eight of the nine provinces are controlled by the same African National Congress that controls the national government. Furthermore, as mentioned earlier, provinces rely on national funding. All in all, the legal, political, and financial reality is that the national government managed the disaster, assisted by provinces.

This did not mean that provinces were insignificant. The greatest provincial effort to combat COVID-19 was in the provincial health system. Provincial health departments provided primary and secondary health care. They monitored infection rates, rolled out testing, and screening, conducted contact tracing, raised awareness, equipped provincial hospitals, and treated those who are hospitalized. Second, provincial governments were instrumental in overseeing the implementation of the national strategy to close and re-open public schools. Provinces were also critical in monitoring and supporting municipalities, mainly by working through provincial and district disaster management structures (see below).

When the crisis hit, the national and provincial governments were in their first month of the financial year, which commenced on 1 April. These budget cycles have largely remained intact. The first additional cash injection of R20 billion for increased provincial health spending was appropriated in a special adjustment budget in June, but it came with a slight reduction in the provincial equitable share.

An important question was whether the multilevel nature of South Africa's system of government aided the fight against the pandemic or whether it hampered it. The answer is neither an unequivocal yes nor a definitive no. The relevance of provinces (and local governments) came to the fore in government's 'risk adjusted strategy,' which enabled differentiation across provinces, depending on the infection rate. Indeed, the infection rates differed vastly between provinces. Rural provinces such as the Northern Cape and Limpopo had low infection rates in comparison with the more urbanized provinces, namely the Western Cape, Gauteng, and KwaZulu-Natal. However, this differentiated strategy to combat the virus was never implemented, thus not taking advantage of the multilevel government system and differentiation between provinces and districts. Provinces were able to innovate and distinguish themselves within the national framework. The Western Cape government, for example, adopted a strategy to actively 'chase' infections by aggressively testing in hotspots, a strategy that yielded higher statistics but assisted in managing the pandemic. On the other hand, some of the national government's efforts to contain the spread of the virus were stumbling over weaknesses in provincial administration. For example, the Eastern Cape government is notorious for its weak provincial administration and debilitating political infighting. Its infection rate was high for a rural province, and there was palpable tension between the national government and the Eastern Cape provincial government over the provincial government's inability to contain the virus.

Provinces have generally been loyal partners of the national government in managing the national state disaster. Certainly, during the first five weeks, provincial governments – even the opposition-controlled Western Cape, cooperated, did their lobbying behind the scenes and avoided overt intergovernmental disputes. However, as the economic contraction spiraled and the devastating impact of the lockdown on livelihoods became more and more evident, cracks appeared in the united national–provincial front. As usual, the opposition-controlled Western Cape government was where most of the pushback came from. For example, the Western Cape re-introduced school feeding schemes, a critical lifeline for vulnerable children that the national government had cancelled. It was also openly criticizing lockdown rules and is 'petitioning' the national government for a relaxation to protect its key industries.

20.3.4 Local government's role

Municipalities, already facing tremendous financial and governance challenges, suddenly saw their responsibilities increase and their funding eroded with the onset of COVID-19 (De Visser and Chigwata 2020). Some of their existing mandates suddenly intensified. For example, municipal law enforcement officers, ordinarily focused on traffic control, by-laws, and crime prevention, were enlisted to help enforce the national lockdown. Municipalities had to work on water relief measures to ensure hygiene and sanitize public places such as public transport facilities. When the national government gave approximately 19,000 water tanks to provide underserviced areas with (free) water, municipalities had to now ensure that the tanks remained filled. When national government devised a scheme to exempt informal food traders from the general prohibition on street trading, municipalities were enlisted to issue temporary permits. While these functions generally fell within the remit of municipalities, new responsibilities were also loaded on local government. For example, many municipalities had to organize basic shelter and food for the homeless in order to ensure their social distancing. When the lockdown prevented millions from earning an income food relief became necessary. The national government manages the social welfare system, including emergency food relief. However, municipalities had to assist with the identification of beneficiaries and sometimes by establishing their own food relief schemes.

As national revenue declined, the transfers to local government were consequently also reduced. Because municipalities, on average, are responsible for raising 70 percent of their revenue, the financial impact of the lockdown was immediate. They rely on households and businesses paying property taxes and fees for municipal services. An immediate reduction in payments inevitably followed and is likely to endure as the continuing economic crisis reduces households' and businesses' ability to pay. Municipalities were also reluctant to use their main credit control mechanism (disconnecting electricity) during these times. A few municipalities even responded to the economic hardship by announcing 'payment holidays,' permitting those hardest-hit by the crisis to defer the payment of municipal bills. Municipalities in any event already provided free basic services to the indigent, the numbers of whom have grown substantially during 2020; they had to budget more for free basic services as the lockdown has forced many more people into poverty.

The financial year for municipalities starts annually on 1 July, so budget preparations had already started in earnest when the pandemic struck. The disaster management regulations instructed municipalities to prioritize COVID-19 related spending in their upcoming budgets. They were also given a once-off power to pass an additional adjustments budget, thereby changing the priorities of the 2019/2020 financial year. Not many municipalities have made use of this, given the fact that the lockdown period coincided with preparations for their regular budget anyway.

20.4 Inter-governmental structures

The crisis intensified the need for collaboration between national, provincial, and local governments. At a national level, the President established a National Coronavirus Command Council (NCCC), comprising a selection of national Ministers. A few weeks into the national state of disaster, it became clear that, in effect, the NCCC was the key decision-maker. All executive measures (including the regulations to govern the lockdown) passed through the NCCC before they were officially passed by the full Cabinet and the relevant Ministries. The role of the NCCC was challenged in court, but the latter found that it was a legitimate cabinet committee.

The NCCC was not used for national–provincial cooperation, but the President's Coordinating Council (PCC), South Africa's apex intergovernmental coordination body, was. This body is provided for in law and brings together the President, key Ministers, nine Premiers, and a representative of organized local government. Ordinarily, it meets a few times each year. However, at the early phases of the crisis, it met weekly and coordinated the national–provincial response at a political level. Sector IGR forums (so-called MinMECS) also operated in the fields of health, education, and local government. A hands-on sectoral IGR forum was the Council of Education Ministers, which brings together the national minister and his or her provincial counterparts in a statutory body. It was very active and cooperative during 2020 seeking to save the school year from the ravages of the pandemic.

Intergovernmental coordinating platforms also existed at provincial and local levels. Provincial governments convened provincial command councils, largely mirroring the national structure. Local government was sometimes invited to their meetings. At an administrative level, there was close interaction between local and provincial governments, mainly through Joint Operating Centres (JOCs), established in terms of the Disaster Management Act at both provincial and district level. At the height of the crisis, they met almost daily, and the general sentiment was that they are functioning reasonably well.

During the early phase of the state of disaster, there was close collaboration between the national government and the nine provincial Premiers. However, six weeks into the lockdown, some provinces were starting to resent the highly centralized management of the disaster. In developing lockdown regulations, the national government gave provinces the same rights as citizens, namely, to send in their comments on drafts. Concerns in respect of the power of the NCCC were mounting. There was no provincial or local government representation on the NCCC with government rather relying on the PCC for high-level consultation with provinces. This is despite the fact that the Disaster Management Act actually calls for a dedicated intergovernmental committee of national, provincial, and local representatives to coordinate disaster management among the spheres of government.

20.5 Conclusion

Although the key policy areas concerning combating the Covid-19 pandemic were concurrent responsibilities – health, disaster management, education, and social welfare – calling for cooperation and coordination, during the first wave of the pandemic, the response was decidedly centralized. Instead of using existing intergovernmental relations structures as the main coordinating vehicles, the national government concentrated power in an informal cabinet committee, the National Coronavirus Command Centre, with no provincial or local government presence on them. In its shadow operated the existing IGR forums – the President's Coordinated Councils and sector IGR forums dealing with health and education.

Although provided for in the Disaster Regulations, there was no provincial differentiation on key issues such as the lockdown rules and the key tenets of the public health response. Provinces played a crucial role in implementing, but not in designing, the response to the disaster. Given that national government collects all major revenue, the fiscal response was also designed and paid for by the national government, with little input from provinces. However, the performance of provinces has been highly uneven, some did well while others struggled to provide the necessary services. Local government has been confronted with additional mandates and the prospect of drastically reduced revenue with national government promising some relief. Some municipalities managed well in delivering these services, while others were hamstrung in their performance by maladministration and corruption.

Intergovernmental relations have worked reasonably well to address implementation challenges, but not as a mechanism to co-design policy or regulation. Contestation over policy was limited as the ruling party controlled most provinces and municipalities. It was only the Western Cape and the City of Cape Town, in the hands of the main opposition party, where some contestation emerged. As attempts at divergence stemmed from the opposition party, it was not readily tolerated by the national government in control of the legal levers of power. All in all, South Africa's response to COVID-19 underscores that it is a hybrid federal state or, if you like, a unitary state with federal features. Its constitutional, financial, and political reality makes it prone to centralizing reflexes, even more so in times of crisis. The severe social, economic, and political difficulties the countries faced before the pandemic have been exacerbated by that pandemic. Whether the government will opt for a more differentiated approach to decentralization – where the capable do more, and the capacity-challenged subnational governments do less – to confront these challenges, is not likely. However, it may become possible when the government runs out of options for a way out of the crisis that the COVID-19 pandemic has deepened.

Bibliography

Department of Health, 2020. Update on Covid-19. July 31. Available from: https://sacoronavirus.co.za/2020/07/31/update-on-Covid-19-31st-july-2020/ [Accessed 2 October 2020].

Department of Health, 2020. Update on Covid-19. December 31. Available from: https://sacoronavirus.co.za/2020/12/31/update-on-covid-19-31st-december-2020/ [Accessed 20 January 2021].

De Visser, J. and Tinashe C., 2020. Municipalities and COVID-19: What the National Disaster Management Directions Mean for Municipal Governance. *Local Government Bulletin*, 15 (1). Available from: https://dullahomarinstitute.org.za/multilevel-govt/local-government-bulletin/volume-15-issue-1-march-2020/municipalities-and-covid-19-what-the-national-disaster-management-directions-mean-for-municipal-governance [Accessed 10 January 2020].

Khumalo, B, Mahabir, J. and Dawood, G., 2015. South Africa's Intergovernmental Fiscal Relations System. *In*: Steytler, N. and Yash, P.G., eds. *Kenya-South Africa Dialogue on Devolution*. Cape Town: Juta, 201–226.

Medical Research Council (MRC), 2020. *Report on Weekly Deaths in South Africa*. December 31. Available from: https://www.samrc.ac.za/reports/report-weekly-deaths-south-africa [Accessed 20 January 2021].

Steytler, N., 2013. South Africa: The Reluctant Hybrid Federal State. *In*: Loughlin, J., Swenden, W. and Kincaid J., eds. *The Routledge Handbook of Regionalism and Federalism*. London and New York: Routledge, 442–454.

21 COVID-19 and federalism in Spain

Mario Kölling

21.1 Introduction

In 2018, Spain was ranked as healthiest in the world by the Bloomberg Healthiest Country Index. The Index also ranked its highly decentralized health system as third in terms of efficiency. However, the country's aging population and the accompanying increase in the incidence of chronic diseases are potential risks to the system's sustainability. Funding cuts to healthcare following the 2008 financial crisis have led to increasing variability in the quality of healthcare services in Spain. This variability can be seen across the 17 Autonomous Communities (ACs) and 2 autonomous cities – the constituent units in Spain – which assume the responsibility for the delivery of these services.

Taken together with earlier funding constraints, the COVID-19 pandemic remains an unprecedented challenge. COVID-19 is severely testing both the Spanish federal territorial model and the National Health System (NHS). During 2020, Spain was one of the worst-hit countries in the world both in terms of infections and deaths (Table 21.1). The first nationwide "state of alarm" based on Article 116 of the Spanish Constitution (SC) lasted from 14 March to 21 June 2020. During this state of alarm, in which the central government took over the decision-making in the NHS, Spain entered a "new normalcy" in late June, during which social distancing measures remained in place. Since late June, the ACs governments gradually re-assumed powers to deal with the pandemic and took the main decisions in health care. However, in September 2020, a second wave outbreak once again pushed Spain to the bottom of the European Union's rankings, although the impact throughout the country was very different. Following requests from most of the ACs – including Catalonia and the Basque Country – the central government adopted a second "state of alarm" at the national level on 25 October.

Several Spanish scientists explained the high number of infections and deaths in Spain as due to the low capacity for PCR tests, scarcity of personal protective equipment, and critical care equipment but also due to delayed reactions by central and ACs governments, and the poor coordination among central and ACs authorities were all contributing factors (Garcia-Basteiro et al. 2020). In fact, I argue in this paper that the COVID-19 crisis has above all revealed the structural weaknesses of the Spanish territorial model. In particular, it has become clear that vertical and horizontal intergovernmental coordination instruments and joint decision-making bodies were insufficient to respond to the crisis appropriately. Nevertheless, during the crisis, the coordination and common decision-making among the levels of government improved and later reached unprecedented levels across the board.

DOI: 10.4324/9781003251217-21

Table 21.1 Key Statistics on COVID-19 in Spain as of 10 January 2021

Cumulative Cases	Cumulative Cases per 100,000 Population	Cumulative Deaths	Cumulative Deaths per 100,000 Population	Case-Fatality Percentage
2,025,560	4,332.3	51,690	110.6	2.6

Source: *World Health Organization Weekly epidemiological update* – 12 January 2021. Geneva: WHO, 2021. Available from https://www.who.int/publications/m/item/weekly-epidemiological-update

21.2 COVID-19 in Spain

Spain has been hit hard by COVID-19, with more than 1,000,000 cases and more than 50,000 confirmed deaths, as of the end of December 2020 (Ministerio de Sanidad 2020). More than 50,000 health workers had been infected, and nearly 25,000 deaths were in nursing homes. With a population of 47 million, these data place Spain among the worst-affected countries.

The situation from March to June 2020 and from July to December 2020 created two very different maps across Spain, with varied effects between ACs. At the top of the list was the AC Madrid, with 13,236 cases per 100,000 inhabitants. It was followed by the AC Navarre with 12,594 cases for every 100,000. There are several reasons for the asymmetry and for the different map.

Most of the Spain's COVID-19 cases occurred in large urban areas during the first wave for these reasons:

- High population density;
- High mobility;
- A tendency toward physical proximity and greetings; and
- More than 20 percent of the population over the age of 65.

At the beginning of the second wave, the role of seasonal workers in the agriculture sector and their poor living conditions led to higher numbers of cases in rural areas. But the numbers soon increased in the urban centers as well reaching new maximum levels at the beginning of November.

The confinement measures taken in response since mid-March 2020 have resulted in an unprecedented contraction of economic activity in the first half of the year, with the service sector – especially tourism – being the most affected. The economic indicators improved in May, when restrictions started to be lifted in a gradual and differentiated way across sectors and ACs. However, changes in consumer behavior, reduced flight connectivity, disruptions in global value chains, and weak demand impeded a normalization of economic activities during 2020 and for the foreseeable future. According to the European Commission autumn forecast, the annual GDP growth in 2020 is forecast at almost –12.5 percent. Activity may continue recovering during the second half of 2021 and then moderate gradually in 2022. This would bring annual GDP growth to about 5.1 percent in 2021 (European Commission 2020). The public budget balance (% of GDP) will rise to 12.2 and the Gross public debt (% of GDP) to 120.3 at the end of 2020. The impact of the crisis on labor-intensive sectors will result in a significant rise in the unemployment rate, while the pandemic is having a disproportionate impact on the poorest and most vulnerable.

21.3 COVID-19 and federalism in Spain

Since the 1980s, Spain has developed from a unitary state with a longstanding central-ist tradition to a strongly decentralized state. The territorial division is based on three levels of territorial organization: 19 ACs (*Comunidades Autonomas*) among them 2 Autonomous Cities, 50 provinces (*Provincias*); and 8,124 municipalities (*Municipios*). According to the constitution, the ACs can adopt their own statutes which define their institutions and powers (Article 148 SC). The statutes must be approved by the re-gional assembly and the national Parliament. In the constitutional division of powers, some competences are expressly attributed to the central state (Article 149), whereas the AC competences can extend to all matters not allocated to the central state. The exclusive powers of the Spanish state include, among other, the regulation of the basic conditions guaranteeing the equality of all Spaniards. Articles 148, 149, and 150 SC specify the competences which the ACs may assume. These include competences re-lated to social assistance, health, among other matters. Today, the ACs have assumed most competences they possibly could (Tudela and Kölling 2020).

The NHS is highly decentralized and based on the principles of universality, free access, and equity. Although the NHS is financed from general tax revenue, the ACs assume the responsibility for the delivery of healthcare services. The central gov-ernment retains the responsibility for certain strategic areas as well as for the over-all coordination and national monitoring of the health system. Since 2001, the ACs have developed strong administrative capacity to implement national regulations and develop region-specific policies. Coordination on health matters between the cen-tral government and ACs is routed through the Interterritorial Council for the NHS (OECD 2019).

The General Public Health Law of 30/2011 establishes the model for the manage-ment of any epidemiological or pandemic crisis. In 2013, the National Early Warn-ing and Rapid Response System (SIAPR) was created, which assumes the functions of coordination, notification, and evaluation of epidemiological or pandemic crisis. The system received a positive assessment by the Global Health Security Index 2019. The assessment approved both the healthcare capacity of the NHS and the warning capacity of SIAPR. Nevertheless, the model was criticized for its ability to prevent and react to pandemic challenges. The Interterritorial Council merely takes care of coordinating technical measures between health officials among the ACs and the cen-tral government within the SIAPR. However, the Council cannot guarantee the coor-dination of political measures among the central government and the ACs (Arteaga 2020). Several research projects have produced similar results for other policy areas in the past. While the coordination works at the level of technicians, this coordination does not exist at the political level (Arbos et al. 2009). In normal times, the meetings of the Council are held at technical level, and everything goes well. However, during the COVID-19 crisis, it was mainly the health ministers of the ACs and the Spanish health minister who attended the meetings.

Compared to other countries, Spain was a laggard in raising the level of response to the surge of reported cases. The first restrictive measures became effective on 9 March 2020, when the number of confirmed cases already exceeded 1,500. This contrasts with the responsiveness of other countries, most of which adopted measures when they reached 1,000 confirmed cases. Prime Minister Sánchez declared a nationwide state of alarm on 13 March, following a videoconference with Presidents of all ACs when the number confirmed cases already exceeded 7,500 (Timoner 2020). The state of alarm is based on Article 116 SC and on the Organic Law 4/1981. The Royal Decree 463/2020, which came in force on 14 March), conferred full responsibility to the Spanish government to implement measures to deal with the COVID-19 crisis. The Royal Decree contained measures related to the limitation of the free movement of persons or vehicles, the suspension of procedural and administrative time periods, and necessary action to ensure the supply of property and services needed for health, food, power, and other essential services. The declaration of the state of alarm allowed the central government to suspend the powers devolved to the ACs for a period of 15 days. The Prime Minister delegated authority to the Ministers for Defence, Internal Affairs, Transport, Mobility, and Urban Matters as well as to the Minister for Health in their respective areas of responsibility, with any residual responsibility being assumed by the Minister for Health. With the creation of the *mando único* (single command), the Minister for Health formally assumed the responsibility for decision-making and coordination of health policy decisions in the 17 ACs. Although the declaration suspended the ACs powers, it did not suspend the State of Autonomies or reduce the power of the ACs, the central government assumed their power for a very detailed period of time and in response to a very specific situation.

The first state of alarm has been extended six times by parliament at the request of the government and ended on 21 June 2020. The measures undertaken were supported by all ACs at the political and technical level. Nevertheless, considering that decision-making and management have been in the hands of the ACs for almost two decades, the central government's coordination competence has been shown to be very weak. It was very difficult for the Ministry of Health to obtain and provide even basic operational data as well as to coordinate joint actions with the ACs, such as organization of joint trade in the procurement of protective clothing and masks and data management. Besides the *mando único*, the first reactions consisted of 17 different reactions by the ACs. Because of shortages of equipment and medical supplies, ACs started to compete for these scarce resources and to purchase this material by their own at the international markets.

Some ACs demanded stronger measures to tackle the crisis, like Murcia, or decided to start with COVID-19 tests on their own, like Andalucía. Moreover, the decision of the central government to limit activities which were not considered essential has disproportionately hit industrialized regions such as the Basque Country or tourist regions in Valencia. Although party politics were not very noticeable during the first weeks of the first state of alarm, the Basque nationalist party (PNV) had been very critical about the lockdown measures. It did, however, continue to support the central government in maintaining its majority in the Spanish Parliament. Partisan considerations increased during April and triggered the criticism, especially by the Madrid, ruled by the Partido Popular (PP), a conservative party. The criticism was also based on existing conflicts, as in Catalonia, where the government refused to sign a joint declaration with the central government and the rest of the ACs on coordinating the lockdown. The government there was also reluctant to accept the presence of armed forces for the construction of field hospitals in its territory. However, there was also criticism from the socialist presidents of some ACs due to a lack of information about decision-making processes. The criticism from the head of government in Valencia, the leader of the *Partido Socialista Obrero Español* (PSOE) in May was particularly clear: "Loyalty does not mean submission!"

On 28 April, the central government presented a four-phase plan for a gradual transition to a "new normality." With each phase, the social and economic situation has been further normalized. The transition of the provinces (the administrative unit below the ACs) from one phase to the next one was decided by the central government. In this way, the restrictions in the social sector were gradually and asymmetrically lifted without the participation of ACs. Although the method of asymmetric transition to a "new normality" was criticized by the ACs, they came to an arrangement with the central government, which was also increasingly flexible. With the transition to a "new normality," the ACs took over again the competences in the health sector and other areas affected by the state of alert.

After several coronavirus outbreaks in July, ACs started to adapt their own measures, for example, to make the wearing of face masks mandatory in public spaces. Following a legal wrangle due to unclear responsibilities, courts greenlighted most of the restrictions. However, ACs did not get clear legal coverage to adapt several full measures, such as selective confinements or restrictions on mobility. Since coronavirus infections continued to rise, similar strategies were progressively adopted by all ACs. But mainly Partido-Popular-governed ACs – such as Madrid – also demanded that the central government should again take over the control. The Spanish government announced new legal mechanisms in May that would allow to implement measures in "co-governance" with the ACs without having to impose another state of alarm. However, no legislative proposals were submitted by the government to Parliament for nearly four months. Then, at the end of September, the central government and the majority of ACs governments reached an agreement. They would impose restrictions in areas with more than 100,000 residents only if they reached three benchmarks: 500 cases of COVID-19 per 100,000 inhabitants, 35 percent COVID-19 patient occupancy in intensive care units, and positive test results of 10 percent or greater. Nevertheless, the ACs demanded a new nationwide state of alarm in order to impose more severe social restrictions. The second state of alarm was declared by the central government on 25 October and extended until 9 May 2021. This new state of alarm was implemented in a decentralized manner, primarily managed by the Autonomous Community governments.

21.3.1 Management of fiscal impact and response

On 17 March, the central government announced a package of €200 billion to fight the economic fallout of the coronavirus crisis, made up of public and private funds. On July 15, the parliament approved a €16 billion aid package to help ACs cover the health, social, and educational expenses of the pandemic. A total of €9 billion of this was provided as transfers for healthcare, plus €2 billion to cover the needs of the education system, and €5 billion to compensate ACs for the decline in their tax revenues. The criteria to distribute these funds among the ACs included population weighted by age, population density and insularity, the number of admissions to intensive care units, total hospitalizations, and total numbers of PCR tests for COVID-19 performed. For education funds, the main criteria included the size of the population under 16 years of age. Finally, the compensation for the decrease in economic activity was allocated according to local taxation revenues, population size, and mobility requirements.

However, this was clearly not enough. A report published at the beginning of 2020 already had warned of the "fragility" of the ACs finances in the face of a possible slowdown of the economy (de la Fuente 2020). The COVID-19 crisis was more than a slowdown, and the ACs were facing it with the financing system that was adopted in 2009 and which had been waiting for a reform for years. On 8 May, a new EU regulation allowed ACs to use up to €3.2 billion of the European Regional Development Fund to cover healthcare extraordinary expenditures such as spending for healthcare equipment, tests, personal protective equipment, and additional workforce or surveillance apps development. In general terms, the relief packages have been smaller in Spain than in other advanced economies, and direct aid has been low. The crisis arrived in Spain when the government had a very small spending margin both in terms of debt and deficit. These restrictions prevented the government from adopting more aggressive measures. For this reason, the government placed all its faith in the European recovery funds.

21.3.2 *Intergovernmental relations*

One of the mayor weaknesses of the Spanish "State of Autonomies" is intergovernmental relations (IGR). The Constitution did not establish an institutional framework that would guarantee continuous political dialog and IGR. Thus, there is neither a permanent institutionalized representation of regional interests at the national level nor a framework for intergovernmental relations. IGR are mainly developed informally or at the bilateral level between the ACs and the central government and are strongly influenced by party politics and parliamentary arithmetic. However, the institutional framework for cooperation and coordination has expanded over the past 30 years and has been extensively used during the COVID-19 crisis. Today, sectoral conferences form the most commonly used IGR mechanism. The legal nature of the conferences is that of a consultative and deliberative body that does not have executive powers; therefore, its resolutions are merely recommendations. Whether sectoral conferences will be convened and which topics will be discussed both depend on the central government. Although sectoral conferences have a political composition, their functioning has shown that they are bodies in which the more technical dimension predominates. While in 2019, 49 sectoral conferences had been held (the average of previous years was 60), in 2020, 166 conferences were celebrated.

The sectoral conference on public health (Interterritorial Council for the NHS – *Consejo Interterritorial del Sistema Nacional de Salud*) has in the past been quite effective and less affected by partisan divisions and considerations when dealing with crises. In early January 2020, the Ministry of Health activated the COVID-19 protocol in coordination with the Departments of Health in the ACs. On February 4, the conference adopted an emergency protocol reinforcing the coordination and surveillance mechanisms among the central and AC health authorities. During the state of alarm, the conference met online twice a week for information interchange at the highest political level. Even Catalonia, which had not attended these meetings since 2018, participated in the search for common agreements. Since the beginning of the new normality at the end of June 2020, the conference continued to meet very frequently reaching agreements, for example, regarding common standards for PCR tests, closure of bars, the benchmarks to impose social restrictions, and measures in seniors residences. In total, 82 sectoral conferences on public health were held in 2020 – as opposed to 5 in 2019. All ACs implemented most of these agreements, within which they developed their own legislation. Central and ACs authorities also reached asymmetrical agreements involving different sectorial conferences, such as health and agriculture, or at the bilateral level.

The Conference of Presidents is also an example of the increasing dynamic of intergovernmental cooperation and also of the lack of constitutionally guaranteed joint decision-making. This conference has been held since 2004 on a *de facto* basis and represents the highest political level for multilateral cooperation between the Prime Minister and the presidents of the 17 ACs and the Autonomous Cities of Ceuta and Melilla. The Conference was convened only seven times between 2004 and 2020 but met in weekly online meetings during the first state of alarm. All presidents participated in these meetings. At the end of the state of alarm, after 14 meetings, most of the presidents of the ACs stressed the usefulness of the Conference during the management of the COVID-19 crisis. In fact, according to Carolina Darias, Minister for Territorial Policy of the Spanish government, the plan to move from the state of alarm to the "new normality" in late June was elaborated in close collaboration with the ACs. Once the ACs assumed again their competences during the new normality, the meetings have been convoked with less intensity. However, during the three conferences held between June and October, several common agreements were reached, including one on the redistribution of the EU recovery fund. In this sense, the vertical IGR improved on a quantitative and qualitative level, but the horizontal IGR continue to show traditional patterns of IGR in Spain and therefore do not exist.

21.4 Transformations in COVID-19 and federalism in Spain

The COVID-19 crisis has above all revealed the structural weaknesses and cyclical problems of the Spanish territorial model. From the central government to the municipalities, vertical intergovernmental coordination instruments and joint decision-making bodies were insufficient to respond to the crisis appropriately. From Catalonia to the Canary Islands, horizontal intergovernmental coordination is non-existent. During the pandemic, the tension between the constitutionally determined framework legislation of the central government and the reality of heterogeneous regional health systems was also revealed.

Furthermore, decisions were taken very late and slowly due to the institutional weakness, the unclear division of competences and lack of legal endorsements as well as party politics and territorial cleavages. This assessment is not new. "The limits and vitiated dynamics of the Spanish decentralization that, long before we knew about this virus, was already an ill-equipped territorial model to cope with any serious challenge in a federal way" (Grau, Sanjaume-Calvet 2020). Many initiatives to reform the system, especially after the economic and financial crisis, have not been successful. These failures were due to many reasons, including party politics and the conflict in Catalonia which hindered reforms of the territorial model for a decade.

The pandemic has not served to build "trust and loyalty" (Munarriz 2020), but there are also positive lessons that could be learned. During the past months, there has been an unprecedented level of interaction and common decision-making between the different levels of government. This activity may be the ground for an institutionalization of the Conference of Presidents, including rules of procedure for joint decision-making and a permanent secretariat.

A further strong point was the flexibility of the model. During the first state of alarm, the central government imposed comprehensive restrictions throughout Spain, with severe impact on the economy and social life. Then, since the end of June, the ACs took decisions by their own depending on the health situation in their territory. Finally, the second state of alarm was adopted with fewer restrictions, allowing ACs to specify measures within a certain common range. This policy divergence reduced the limitations to specific hot spots and contributed to learning effects among ACs. The most important effect was the move toward coordinated actions, such as the framework agreement for centralized purchase for healthcare products signed at the beginning of August by all ACs – with the exception of Valencia – and the central government (Ministerio de Sanidad 2021). The expected savings with this aggregate purchase will exceed €300 million.

Another positive effect was the role of the Spanish government within the EU. Since the beginning of the pandemic, the government demanded a strong European mechanism to face the consequences of the crisis and presented several initiatives. Accordingly, the EU Council decision issued in July commits the EU to support Spain during the coming years in economic terms but may also connect this support with certain conditions such as reforms of the labor market and the pension system. Spain will receive close to €140 billion over the next six years from a €750 billion coronavirus recovery fund. Resources will be mobilized to support recovery and to reorient the economy toward a more inclusive and sustainable kind of growth. Spain also will receive €21.3 billion from the EU SURE program to assist the country in addressing the increases in public expenditure to preserve employment.

Drawing from the experience of the crisis management so far, the Health ministry and the ACs have already drafted their reflections on the challenges that the NHS must address. This document, now an Action Plan, includes initiatives aimed at strengthening the NHS to prepare it to tackle and even anticipate future challenges. The Plan will also strengthen the essential capacities which the NHS needs in times of normality. Moreover, some specific proposals have already been announced to improve the co-governance between the central government and ACs.

Bibliography

Arbós, M.X., Colino, C.C., García, M.M.J. and Parrado, D.S., 2009. *Las relaciones intergubernamentales en el Estado autonómico. La posición de los actores.* Barcelona: Institut d'Estudis Autonómics. Barcelona: Generalitat de Catalunya. Available from: http://www.gencat.cat/drep/iea/pdfs/IEA_64.pdf [Accessed 3 February 2021].

Arteaga, F., 2020. *La gestión de pandemias como el COVID-19 en España: ¿enfoque de salud o de seguridad?* Madrid: Real Instituto Elcano, ARI 42/2020-13/4/2020. Available from: http://www.realinstitutoelcano.org/wps/portal/rielcano_es/contenido?WCM_GLOBAL_CONTEXT=/elcano/elcano_es/zonas_es/ari42-2020-arteaga-gestion-de-pandemias-covid-19-en-espana-enfoque-de-salud-o-de-seguridad [Accessed 2 February 2021].

de la Fuente, Á. 2020. *Una mini-reforma de urgencia de la financiación autonómica para una mejor respuesta a la crisis,* Fedea Policy Papers – 2020/05 Available from: https://www.fedea.net/una-mini-reforma-de-urgencia-de-la-financiacion-autonomica-para-una-mejor-respuesta-a-la-crisis/ [Accessed 11 March 2021].

Garcia-Basteiro, A., Alvarez-Dardet, C., Arenas, A., Bengoa, R., Borrell, C., Del Val, M. Franco, M., Gea-Sánchez, M., Gestal Otero, J., González López Valcárcel, B., Hernández, I., Carles March, J., Martin-Moreno, J., Menéndez, C., Minué, S., Muntaner, C., Porta, M., Prieto-Alhambra, D., Vives-Cases, C. and Legido-Quigley, H. 2020. The Need for an

Independent Evaluation of the COVID-19 Response in Spain. *The Lancet*, 396 (10250), 529–530. doi: 10.1016/S0140-6736(20)31713-X [Accessed 11 March 2021].

Grau-Creus, M., Sanjaume-Calvet, M. «Loyalty does not mean submission!»: On the Covid19 measures and the apparently surprising features of the Spanish territorial model. UACES Territorial Politics Available from: https://uacesterrpol.wordpress.com/2020/05/26/loyalty-does-not-mean-submission-on-the-covid19-measures-and-the-apparently-surprising-features-of-the-spanish-territorial-model/ [Accessed 11 March 2021].

Ministerio de Sanidad, 8 April 2020. *Actualización n° 177: Enfermedad por el coronavirus (COVID-19).* Available from: https://www.mscbs.gob.es/en/profesionales/salud Publica/ccayes/alertasActual/nCov-China/documentos/Actualizacion_177_COVID-19.pdf [Accessed 11 March 2021].

Ministerio de Sanidad, 2021. Notas de Prensa: El Ministerio de Sanisterio de Sanidad licita un acuerdo marco para adquirir material sanitario y equipos de protección individual para el SNS por un valor de mas de 2.500 millones de euros [*The Framework Agreement for Buying Personal Protective Equipment by the Central Government for the ACs*]. Available from: https://www.mscbs.gob.es/gabinete/notasPrensa.do?id=5023 [Accessed 11 March 2021].

Munarriz, A., 2020. El "test de estrés" del virus destapa los fallos y lagunas del Estado autonómico [online]. *infoLibre*, 6 July. Available from: https://www.infolibre.es/noticias/politica/2020/06/29/la_pandemia_pone_prueba_estado_autonomico_test_estres_muestra_fatiga_materiales_107485_1012.html [Accessed 11 March 2021].

OECD and European Observatory on Health Systems and Policies. 2019. *Spain: Country Health Profile 2019, State of Health in the EU*. Paris: OECD Publishing.

Tudela, J. and Kölling, M. 2020. The Kingdom of Spain. *In*: Griffiths, A., Chattopadhyay, R., Light, J. and Stieren, C. eds. *Handbook of Federal Countries*. London: Palgrave – Forum of Federations.

Timoner, A. 2020. Policy Responsiveness to Coronavirus: An Autopsy. *Agenda Pública – El País*, 8 June.

22 Switzerland

Overnight centralization in one of the world's most federal countries

Rahel Freiburghaus, Sean Mueller and Adrian Vatter

22.1 Introduction

This chapter examines Switzerland's response to the first wave of the COVID-19 pandemic from the perspective of federalism. The analysis covers the period from 28 February to 19 June 2020. Noteworthy aspects addressed in this chapter are the almost overnight centralization of political power not just at the federal level but also within the seven-member executive following the adjournment of the federal parliament; the rapid enactment of a nationwide shutdown in mid-March 2020, just two weeks after the first case had been diagnosed; and the simultaneous dialogs, coordination efforts, and learning processes among the 26 cantons as well as between the cantons and the national and local levels of government.

Two main lessons can be distilled. First, *experimental policy innovation has contributed to leveling inter-regional asymmetries* in administrative and fiscal capacity. The 26 Swiss cantons are both highly autonomous and deeply interconnected. This encourages not only innovation but also communication and mutual learning. Hence, experimentation and willingness to share emerge as key conditions for effective policy responses. Second, a *"deliberative layering" of intergovernmental cooperation has enhanced the crisis management capacity* of existing institutions. Even though the Swiss intergovernmental relations landscape was already crowded when the pandemic erupted, and the legal framework allowed for almost overnight centralization, the cantons remained assertive in demanding differentiated policy responses. Moreover, at the peak of intergovernmental conflict over how best to deal with rising infections, a "crisis summit" with all 26 presidents of cantonal governments was convened by the central government. Designed on the premise of deliberation among equals rather than minimal majorities, a compromise could thus be found. Rather than simple centralization or outright decentralization, the key to successfully tackle the first wave thus rested in finding new ways of intergovernmental coordination—and quickly so.

Ironically, when later in 2020, the second wave hit Switzerland, much of the failure to adequately deal with that stage of the pandemic was also due to the relative success experienced during the first wave. More specifically, it was felt that the federal level had infringed too much on regional autonomy and that the cantons could very well coordinate with each other only. The result of this was that, as most cantonal governments, afraid of electoral sanctions if imposing strict containment measures, were waiting for their neighbors to enact restrictions, few did so in time. Most cantons had also underestimated the complexity of "track and trace," which, in principle, all had agreed was preferable to a second nationwide shutdown. Nevertheless, a second

DOI: 10.4324/9781003251217-22

Table 22.1 Key Statistics on COVID-19 in Switzerland as of 10 January 2021

Cumulative Cases	Cumulative Cases per 100,000 Population	Cumulative Deaths	Cumulative Deaths per 100,000 Population	Case-Fatality Percentage
475,604	5,495.4	7,545	87.2	1.6

Source: *World Health Organization Weekly epidemiological update* – 12 January 2021. Geneva: WHO, 2021. Available from https://www.who.int/publications/m/item/weekly-epidemiological-update

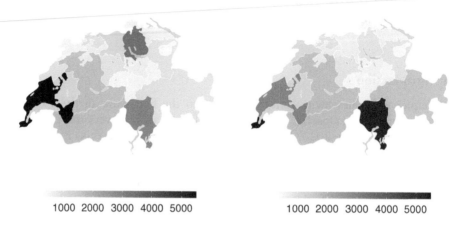

1000 2000 3000 4000 5000   1000 2000 3000 4000 5000

Figure 22.1 Cumulative Number of COVID-19 Cases (left) and Number of COVID-19 Cases Per Capita (right) in Switzerland by Canton as of 19 June 2020.

shutdown was decreed by the federal government in January 2021, albeit with slightly fewer restrictions and more room for cantonal exceptions (e.g., on ski resorts) than a year before (Table 22.1).

22.2 COVID-19 in Switzerland: first wave human and economic damage

In mid-February 2020, the Swiss authorities and citizenry were confident that they would survive the COVID-19 outbreak in distant China without any significant damage (Duttweiler 2020)—just as the country had come through two world wars largely unscathed.[1] But as hospital beds in the Italian region of Lombardy began to fill increasingly quickly, even optimists had to acknowledge that Switzerland too would slip into an unprecedented public health crisis. The proximity to northern Italy, one of the epicenters of the first wave of the pandemic in Europe, presented a particular challenge: some 68,000 cross-border workers (*"frontalieri"*) commute from Italy into mainly canton Ticino on a daily basis (FSO 2020). Inevitably, the coronavirus would thus simply travel northward, and indeed, on 25 February 2020, the first ever Swiss citizen, a traveler returning from Milan (the capital of Lombardy), was confirmed as the first-recorded Swiss case of COVID-19 (FOPH 2020a) (Figure 22.1).

As elsewhere, the disease spread rapidly throughout Switzerland. On 5 March, the country recorded its first deaths from COVID-19 (NCS-TF 2020). Given the exponential increase in the number of daily-confirmed cases (R_e: 2.61–2.1), at this time, Switzerland was "among the countries with the highest number of [...] COVID-19 cases per capita in the world" (Salathé et al. 2020, p. 1; cf. Mueller et al. 2021). Since the capacity to conduct testing in the country was initially relatively low, there were likely many people with an undetected infection (*ibid.*). At the same time, however, the first wave hit Switzerland very unevenly, as shown in Figure 22.1: While the rate of confirmed COVID-19 cases per capita was highest in Geneva, Ticino, Vaud, Valais, and Basel-City, that is, along Switzerland's border with France and Italy, the small and sparsely populated cantons in Central Switzerland were only marginally affected (NCS-TF 2020, p. 4; cf. FOPH 2020b). To contain the spread of the virus, the federal government imposed a nationwide shutdown in mid-March 2020, stopping short of an all-out lockdown—that is, it was still possible to go outside for walks and see friends, provided official hygiene and distancing guidelines were followed (see below).

The COVID-19 pandemic and the subsequent government measures caused a sharp drop in Swiss economic activity between March and June 2020, when social and economic life in Switzerland virtually ground to a halt (Rathke et al. 2020). According to the scenarios modeled by the *KOF Swiss Economic Institute* at ETH Zurich, the Swiss economy lost between 22 and 35 billion CHF between March and June 2020, corresponding to some 10–17 percent of GDP. The bulk of these high losses can be attributed to the decline of the global economy (44–71 percent). The shutdown measures implemented in Switzerland caused 19–45 percent of the economic losses, while illness-related absence from work and quarantine requirements was estimated to account for the remaining 8–14 percent (*ibid.*).

22.3 COVID-19 and Swiss federalism: centralization versus cantonal voice

Switzerland is widely known to be one of the most decentralized federal countries worldwide. Not only do all of its 26 cantons possess their own constitution, elected authorities, and wide-ranging legislative and fiscal powers but they are also responsible for implementing the majority of federal law.[2] This affords cantons an exceptionally strong political position, particularly since the electoral districts for all federal elections overlap perfectly with cantonal borders and political parties too are organized in a bottom-up fashion. At the same time, there is a wide variation among the cantons in terms of their size, wealth, official language, majority religion, and the political preferences of their citizens. For instance, the largest canton has 1.5 million inhabitants, the smallest 15,000. The wealthiest canton receives no annual fiscal equalization payments, while these payments comprise some 20 percent of the total income of the poorest canton. What is more, the six westernmost, exclusively or predominantly French-speaking cantons often feel overruled by the German-speaking majority—not least during the pandemic, when they demanded even stricter measures.

In terms of the competences relevant to fight a pandemic, the cantons are mainly responsible for health and also operate their own hospitals. Furthermore, they exclusively run the police, justice, and prison systems and regulate most economic activities (e.g., licensing and opening hours). They also administer unemployment and other social services and grant health care insurance subsidies. Fragmentation into 26 completely different policy spaces is avoided by extensive bilateral and multilateral coordination and cooperation processes across the cantons. The main instruments of such horizontal federalism are some 800 treaties (Arens 2020) and around 50 conferences, that is, regular meetings of cantonal ministers or entire governments (cf. Mueller et al. 2021; Schnabel 2020; Vatter 2018).

By the time the pandemic hit Switzerland, the country had just fully revised its legal framework to deal with public health crises: the "Epidemics Act" (henceforth EpidA) has been in force since early 2016. It regulates the timely detection, monitoring, prevention, and control of communicable human diseases. The cantons themselves had pushed for the fundamental revision of the earlier framework as the risk of pandemics rose as a consequence of global mobility (e.g., the 2002–2004 SARS outbreak; cf. FOPH 2013; Rüefli and Zenger 2018, pp. 90–92). The EpidA distinguishes between "normal," "particular," and "extraordinary situations" (Art. 6–7). Each one divides tasks differently between the federal government and the 26 cantons (Table 22.2).

The *"normal" operating mode (stage 1)* corresponds to customary levels of rather high decentralization in the health sector (Dardanelli and Mueller 2019; Gerritzen and Kirchgässner 2013, p. 250). The cantons not only have the majority of powers but also pay more than 80 percent of all of the public money invested in the system (*ibid.*; cf. Vatter 2018). Costs add up quickly, as Switzerland has an extensive network of doctors, well-equipped hospitals (both private and public), and clinics. Patients are free to choose their own doctor just as they enjoy unlimited access to specialists. By law, comprehensive medical treatment is guaranteed to all 8.6 million residents; in exchange, there is mandatory contracting with one of the officially licensed private health care insurers. With regard to the detection, monitoring, and control of the spread of communicable human diseases, under "normal" circumstances, the federal government is not permitted to instruct the cantons to implement any kind of (preventive) measures. Its prerogatives are limited to information campaigns, vaccination evaluations, and border controls (Rüefli and Zenger 2018, p. 125; cf. FOPH 2020c).

Once a crisis kicks in, the seven-person Federal Council—that is, "the supreme governing and executive authority of the Confederation" (Art. 174 Cst)—alone decides whether a "particular" or even an "extraordinary" situation exists. How a given public health crisis may be classified as either the one or the other is, legally speaking, "yet unclear; just as it is still to be seen how the cantons should be involved politically" (Rüefli and Zenger 2018, p. III).

Prerequisites for the proclamation of the *"particular situation" (stage 2)* are excessive demands on the cantons *and* an increased risk of infection or an increased risk to health or serious consequences for the economy or other areas of life (lit. a). Alternatively, stage 2 may be called if occurrences constitute a public health emergency of international concern according to the WHO (lit. b). In either case, the Federal Council can order various measures, including very far-reaching controls. In doing so, it must first consult the cantons—just as in normal times when the federal level must inform them of its intentions "fully and in good time" (Art. 45 Cst).

The *"extraordinary situation" (stage 3)*, in turn, is not precisely defined. Nor are the measures that the Federal Council can take described in detail. The law merely states that it is empowered to take the all the "necessary measures" which may apply to either the whole or parts of the country. As such, Art. 7 EpidA hardly differs from the general emergency law under Art. 185 Cst (*"polizeiliche Generalklausel"*), that is, government-sponsored ordinances that must be limited in duration ("sunset clause;" cf. Rüefli and Zenger 2018, p. 9; Uhlmann and Scheifele 2020, pp. 116–117).

Table 22.2 The "Three-Part Model" of the Swiss Epidemics Act (EpidA)

| | Stage 1: "Normal situation" | | Stage 2: "Particular situation" (Art. 6 EpidA) | | Stage 3: "Extraordinary situation" (Art. 7 EpidA) | |
| | Until 28 February 2020 | | 28 February to 16 March 2020; 20 June 2020 (ongoing) | | 16 March to 19 June 2020 | |
	Confederation	*Cantons*	*Confederation*	*Cantons*	*Confederation*	*Cantons*
Legislation	Limited competencies (e.g., information programs, vaccination evaluation, border controls, admission of foreign nationals)	Full range of competencies to (preventively) detect, monitor, and control the spread of communicable human diseases	Stipulating the use of certain measures comprehensively outlined in the EpidA—provided that the cantons are consulted beforehand	Limited range of competencies to detect, monitor, and control the spread of communicable human diseases (e.g., bans on public events and early closing time for bars)	Instructing the use of any "necessary measures" to combat the spread of communicable human diseases (i.e., general emergency law)	None (de jure)
Implementation	Supervision of the cantonal implementation of the EpidA	Implementation of the EpidA and the EpV	Supervision of cantonal implementation of federal regulations	Implementation of federal regulations; some leverage	Supervision of cantonal implementation	Mere implementation; no leverage (de jure)

Source: Own collection based on FOPH (2020c), Rüefli and Zenger (2018).
Note: EpidA = "Epidemics Act" (as of 28 September 2012); EpV = Ordinance on the control of communicable human diseases (as of 29 April 2015).

Although "the equilibrium of powers of was modified toward a predominance of the executive" (Sager and Mavrot 2020, p. 301), during the entire first wave of the COVID-19 pandemic, the cantons retained important implementation powers. Even in stage 3, that is, from 16 March 2020 to 19 June 2020, the constituent units had to execute federal policy responses. In theory, implementation should have been a matter of sheer administrative routine (*"Vollzugsauftrag"*). In practice, however, cantonal governments were able to gain leverage by "monitor[ing] compliance with the measures on their territory" (Art. 1*b* COVID-19 Ordinance 2) in several ways.

First, even the most clearly defined *"Vollzugsauftrag"* brings about context-specific implementation challenges that require cantonal and/or local authorities to take further action. An example is the outright closure of popular public spaces (such as parks or terraces) ordered by the local governments in large cities such as Zurich (Stadt Zürich 2020) or Bern (Stadt Bern 2020), where the nationwide ban of gatherings of more than five people[3] and/or social distancing just could not be enforced. Second, subnational implementation of nationwide COVID-19 measures was contingent upon the administrative resources of a given canton or indeed municipality (Loser and Lenz 2020). This resulted in highly divergent "implementation styles" (Howlett 2000)— a defining feature also of normal "Swiss executive federalism" (e.g., Vatter 2018). Hence, even if the coronavirus pandemic temporarily deprived the cantons of their wide-ranging legislative powers in health policy, it could not entirely stop the Swiss federation's characteristically diverse implementation arrangements from producing divergent outputs either.

As the subnational level(s) succeeded in gaining (limited) *de facto* leverage in the implementation of certain COVID-19 policy responses and the cantons were—even in stage 3—still perceived as recognized partners of the national government, intergovernmental relations (IGR) became crucially important. Already, in normal times, they are the indispensable "oil in the federal machinery" (Poirier and Saunders 2015, p. 2). We can distinguish existing, more or less formalized IGR institutions from *ad hoc* fora created during the pandemic. There are also mechanisms that give voice to many cantons at the same time as well as bilateral fora (cf. Mueller 2019). That IGR, in general, would achieve such prominence is hardly surprising. Indeed, Switzerland is known for its long-established, highly institutionalized, and dense web of IGR institutions especially in the horizontal dimension (Schnabel and Mueller 2017, p. 553), where generalist and policy-specific councils or "conferences" support each other (cf. Arens 2020; Bolleyer 2009). The pandemic further accentuated this.

In the early days of the pandemic, the Federal Council primarily consulted the *Conference of Cantonal Directors for Health* (GDK; established in 1919). Before strict nationwide regulations were deemed necessary (e.g., the ban on major public events issued on 28 February 2020), the 26 cantonal governments submitted their opinions to an internal GDK consultation procedure. The content of their submissions was subsequently aggregated into a representation of the general "will of *the cantons*" (Marjanović 2020). Once such a common front is forged, the presidents of intercantonal conferences then speak on behalf of *the cantons*, for example, during joint, televised press conferences with members of the Federal Council. The GDK also enjoys legally guaranteed permanent representation in the *"Koordinationsorgan Epidemiengesetz,"* the "coordinating body" of the EpidA (Art. 82 lit. g EpV). The same is true for the generalist *Conference of Cantonal Governments* (KdK; founded in 1993), which had a delegate in the Federal Council's main "crisis unit" (*"Krisenstab des Bundesrats Corona*") to tackle the coronavirus pandemic side-by-side with top-level federal officials (cf. Federal Chancellery 2020). The different levels of government thus coordinated extensively with each other both vertically and horizontally through *collective* IGR (Hegele and Schnabel 2021).

But individual linkages mattered too. If the long-established, highly institutionalized, and dense network of intercantonal conferences ensured rapid, efficient consultation, minority stances of single (groups of) cantons could—for the sake of an unambiguous crisis response—not be considered accordingly. Just as in "normal times," formalized IGR councils only "protect[ed] the autonomy of the constituent units *as a whole*" (Schnabel 2020, p. 267; emphasis added). As every region was equally affected by COVID-19, individual cantonal governments' specific interests diverged. Alongside the collective approach to talking with the center, they continued to pressure the Federal Council at their own discretion, asking either for stricter measures (e.g., the canton of Ticino which demanded the closure of the border with Italy (St. Galler Tagblatt 2020) or more permissive "waivers" (e.g. special permits for the operation of ski businesses in cantons heavily dependent on tourism (Berner Oberländer 2020). Subnational lobbying was so intense and diverse that, at some point, federal officials could not tell anymore "who '*the cantons*' actually were: the KdK, the GDK, or individual cantonal governments?" (Mr. Walter Thurnherr, Federal Chancellor (Aargauer Zeitung 2020). In order to accommodate the constituent units' collective and individual voice, the coronavirus pandemic thus required additional, *ad hoc* IGR venues to be created—a crucial innovation of Swiss federalism's first wave response.

Overall, the strong collaborative element that existed pre-COVID-19 helped Swiss federalism to tackle the first wave rather well. Although political decision-making was basically centralized overnight, the cantons continued to be in charge of implementing federal rules and remained in touch both with each other and with "the principal." A similarly collaborative and decentralized approach was taken in the government's economic response: to help affected businesses, the federal government coordinated with the Swiss National Bank and commercial banks to provide interest-free loans.

As best illustrated by the government-guaranteed interest-free bridging loans, the fiscal and economic response displayed strong features of the traditional "liberal-corporatist" Swiss model (cf. Katzenstein 1985, pp. 104–105, 129). In "record time" (Economiesuisse 2020), the national government, the Swiss National Bank, and commercial banks rolled out a jointly elaborated emergency relief scheme to provide bridging loans to support SMEs encountering liquidity problems due to the lockdown measures. This "simple, fast, and efficient" (*ibid.*) policy response is typical for Swiss corporatist problem-solving: a "pragmatic approach" was applied, established state-private networks were used, and the action was implemented in a decentralized way.

22.4 Lessons learned

The way Switzerland, in general, and Swiss federalism, in particular, has reacted to the first wave of the pandemic leads us to distil two main lessons learned.

Lesson 1: Leveling asymmetries through experimental policy innovation. Asymmetry has become the "backbone of contemporary federalism" (Palermo 2020) as many federal systems are faced with expanding heterogeneity in terms of economic, social, and fiscal differences among the constituent units. To ensure stability, such differences require at least some leveling, for example, through fiscal equalization. In a crisis situation, in particular, federal asymmetries tend to increase further: natural disasters (such as Hurricane Katrina) primarily affect a certain region (and, therewith, certain subnational entities), but their effects spill over, often requiring national-level measures (cf. Birkland and Waterland 2008).

In Switzerland, however, such asymmetries also became *a key supporting condition for experimental policy innovation.* Put differently, "policy diffusion" (Gilardi and Wasserfallen 2019) played out the most fruitfully *because* of asymmetries, fueled, in turn, by crises: Not only did case numbers vary substantially across the cantons (Figure 22.1) but also the unequal distribution of COVID-19 infections also paired with highly divergent administrative capacities. In the early days of the pandemic, asymmetric administrative resources were especially visible in public health campaigns. While nationwide leaflets targeted the entire population, children struggled to make sense of abstract guidelines regarding hand hygiene or social distancing. The canton Basel-City therefore decided to design its own public health campaign tailored to kids. As a financially powerful canton with a highly professionalized, well-equipped administration, it had all the necessary resources to mandate an external advertising agency with CHF 400,000 to launch a catchy, iconic public "sermon" entitled "#SoapBoss" (Kanton Basel-Stadt 2020). Once the information campaign distributed through social media "went viral" (persoenlich.ch 2020), cantons with lower administrative capacity such as Solothurn—one of the nineteen recipients in the national fiscal equalization scheme—asked to adopt the *"SoapBoss"* (Solothurner Zeitung 2020). Basel-City was happy to unconditionally share its pioneering "soft" crisis response to level out administrative asymmetries by letting experimental policy innovation diffuse.

Lesson 2: Enhancing the crisis management capacity of existing IGR institutions by "deliberative layering." Due to the multifaceted nature of crises, disaster management is usually a "shared responsibility" (Birkland and Waterman 2008, p. 692). IGR become crucially important to ensure a certain coherence between the measures taken by the different levels. Yet, crises can also threaten existing IGR institutions because of "federal dominance" (Schnabel 2020, pp. 61–62), inefficiency due to unanimity requirements (Vatter 2018), or growing polarization (Bowman 2017). The dilemma, then, is this: existing IGR might be ill-suited for the quick policy responses that are so desperately needed, but urgent situations simply do not allow for time-consuming institutional reforms either since such structures are essentially path-dependent and, thus, difficult to change (cf. Broschek et al. 2018). So, disaster management must evolve within existing IGR settings. This is particularly true for federal systems with highly institutionalized IGR institutions such as Switzerland (cf. Bolleyer 2009). Hence, "disruptive unilateralism" (Schnabel 2020, p. 39) is incentivized: Because existing IGR institutions are too slow to react, heavily affected subnational units may rush ahead alone and thereby further obstruct a coordinated response.

Yet, as illustrated by Swiss federalism's first wave response to the COVID-19 pandemic, the crisis management capacity of existing IGR institutions can be enhanced by *"deliberative layering."* Layering is a familiar notion in the policy science assuming that new goals and means are gradually added to—or, more precisely "layered on" existing ones (Béland 2007). Such onion-like *ad hoc* amendments might offer a "third way" out of the dilemma just described *if new deliberative fora are layered on existing IGR institutions*. The Swiss experience is intriguing: Given the stalemate in intercantonal conferences, individual cantons with particularly high COVID-19 infection rates ordered further measures unilaterally. For example, the canton of Uri imposed an over-65 curfew without consulting the Federal Council (19 March 2020), while the canton of Ticino ordered non-essential industry to temporarily cease production (22 March 2020) (Studer 2020). Both policy responses went further than a previous federal order, bringing them into conflict with the Federal Council. The issue was finally resolved at a "crisis summit" of all 26 presidents of the cantonal governments and the Federal Council. As this forum was designed on the premise of deliberation among equals rather than minimal majorities in collective IGR (i.e., the GDK or KdK), a joint compromise could be achieved (i.e., *ex post* authorization of Ticino's closure of businesses and construction sites that did not meet rules on social distancing and hygiene; cf. The Federal Council 2020).

Notes

1 Cf. Sager and Mavrot (2020) for a detailed account of early policy responses (e.g., toll-free hotline and leaflets at airports).
2 Below the level of the cantons, there are some 2,000 local governments, each with their own elected authorities, administrations, and fiscal powers. The extent and nature of local government autonomy varies from canton to canton (e.g., Mueller 2015).
3 From 21 March 2020 to 30 May 2020, gatherings of more than five persons in public places were forbidden. Anyone found to be infringing this rule could be fined up to CHF 100 (Sager and Mavrot 2020, p. 296).

Bibliography

Aargauer Zeitung, 2020. Die Schweizer begannen sich selbst zu führen. *Aargauer Zeitung*, 14 September, p. 2–3.

Arens, A., 2020. Federal Reform and Intergovernmental Relations in Switzerland. An Analysis of Intercantonal Agreements and Parliamentary Scrutiny in the Wake of the NFA (PhD Thesis). Berne: University of Berne, Switzerland.

Béland, D., 2007. Ideas and Institutional Change in Social Security: Conversion, Layering, and Policy Drift. *Social Security Quarterly*, 88 (1), 20–38.

Berner Oberländer, 2020. Sonderregelung war kein "Buebetrickli". *Berner Oberländer*, 16 March, p. 2.

Birkland, T., and Waterman, S., 2008. Is Federalism the Reason for Policy Failure in Hurricane Katrina? *Publius: The Journal of Federalism*, 38 (4), 692–714.

Bolleyer, N., 2009. *Intergovernmental Cooperation. Rational Choices in Federal Systems and Beyond*. Oxford: Oxford University Press.

Bowman, A.O'M, 2017. Intergovernmental Councils in the United States. *Regional & Federal Studies*, 27 (5), 623–643.

Broschek, J., Petersohn, B. and Toubeau, S., 2018. Territorial Politics and Institutional Change: A Comparative-Historical Analysis. *Publius: The Journal of Federalism*, 48 (1), 1–25.

COVID-19 Ordinance 2 – Ordinance on Measures to Combat the Coronavirus (COVID-19), 13 March 2020. Available from: https://www.admin.ch/opc/en/classified-compilation/20200744/index.html [Accessed 17 October 2020].

Cst – Federal Constitution of the Swiss Confederation, 1999. April 18. Available from: https://www.admin.ch/opc/en/classified-compilation/19995395/index.html [Accessed 17 October 2020].

Dardanelli, P. and Mueller, S., 2019. Dynamic De/Centralization in Switzerland, 1848–2010. *Publius – The Journal of Federalism*, 49 (1), 138–165.

Duttweiler, C., 2020. Die Armee war besser: Corona war ein extremer Stresstest für Bundesrat, BAG und Militär. Wer hat ihn bestanden, was waren die grössten Fehler? Eine erste Bilanz. *Das Magazin*, May 30, p. 10.

Economiesuisse, 2020. Simple, Fast and Efficient: Swiss COVID-19 Bridging Credits for Companies in Need. *Economiesuisse*, June 26. Available from: https://www.economiesuisse.ch/en/articles/simple-fast-and-efficient-swiss-covid-19-bridging-credits-companies-need [Accessed 30 October 2020].

EpidA – Federal Act on the Control of Communicable Human Diseases ("Epidemics Act"), 28 September 2012. Available from: https://www.admin.ch/opc/de/classified-compilation/20071012/index.html [Accessed 10 October 2020].

EpV – Verordnung über die Bekämpfung übertragbarer Krankheiten des Menschen, 29 April 2015. Available from: https://www.admin.ch/opc/de/classified-compilation/20133212/index.html [Accessed 10 October 2020].

Federal Chancellery, 2020. *Krisenstab des Bundesrats Corona (KSBC)*. Available from: https://cdn.repub.ch/s3/republik-assets/assets/article-wer-sitzt-im-krisenstab/ksbc.pdf [Accessed 17 October 2020].

FOPH, 2013 – Federal Office of Public Health, 2013. *Das neue Epidemiengesetz: Informationen*. Fact sheet, July 2013.

FOPH, 2020a – Federal Office of Public Health, 2020a. *Neues Coronavirus COVID-19: Erster bestätigter Fall in der Schweiz*. 25 February 2020. Available from: https://www.bag.admin.ch/bag/de/home/das-bag/aktuell/medienmitteilungen.msg-id-78233.html [Accessed 17 October 2020].

FOPH, 2020b – Federal Office of Public Health, 2020b. *Geografische Verteilung im Zeitverlauf: Laborbestätigte Fälle, Normalisierte 14-Tages-Inzidenz*. Available from: https://www.covid19.admin.ch/de/epidemiologic/case/d/geo-regions?geoDate=2020-02-24 [Accessed 10 October 2020].

FOPH, 2020c – Federal Office of Public Health, 2020c. *Normale, besondere und ausserordentliche Lage*. Fact sheet, 28 February 2020. Available from: https://www.newsd.admin.ch/newsd/message/attachments/60477.pdf [Accessed 17 October 2020].

FSO, 2020 – Federal Statistical Office, 2020. *Cross-Border Commuters*. Available from: https://www.bfs.admin.ch/bfs/en/home/statistics/work-income/employment-working-hours/employed-persons/swiss-foreign-nationals/cross-border-commuters.html [Accessed 10 October 2020].

Gerritzen, B.C. and Kirchgässner, G., 2013. Federalism in Health and Social Care in Switzerland. *In*: Costa-Font, J. and Greer, S.L., eds. *Federalism and Decentralization in European Health and Social Care*. Basingstoke: Palgrave Macmillan, 250–271.

Gilardi, F. and Wasserfallen, F., 2019. The Politics of Policy Diffusion. *European Journal of Political Research*, 58 (4), 1245–1256.

Hegele, Y. and Schnabel, J., 2021. Federalism and the Management of the COVID-19 Crisis: Centralisation, Decentralisation and (Non-)coordination. *West European Politics*, 44 (5/6), 1052–1076.

Howlett, M., 2000. Beyond Legalism? Policy Ideas, Implementation Styles and Emulation-Based Convergence in Canadian and U.S. Environmental Policy. *Journal of Public Policy*, 20 (3), 305–329.

Kanton Basel Stadt. 2020. *#SeifenBoss*. Available from: https://www.coronavirus.bs.ch/Aktuelle-Situation/so-schuetzen-wir-uns/seifenboss.html [Accessed 17 October 2020].

Katzenstein, P.J. 1985. *Small States in World Markets*. Ithaca: Cornell University Press.

Loser, P. and Lenz, C., 2020. Krampf der Kantone: Die Corona-Krise ist auch eine Krise des Föderalismus. Hält unser System das aus? *Tages-Anzeiger*, March 27, p. 6.

Marjanović, P., 2020. Interne Dokumente zeigen, welche Kantone Berset und Koch bremsen wollten. *Watson*, 28 March. Available from: https://www.watson.ch/schweiz/

coronavirus/631137094-dokumente-zeigen-welche-kantone-den-schweizer-bundesrat-bremsen-wollten [Accessed 16 October 2020].

Mueller, S., 2015. *Theorising Decentralisation: Comparative Evidence from Subnational Switzerland*. Colchester: ECPR Press.

Mueller, S., 2019. Federalism and the Politics of Shared Rule. *In*: Kincaid, J., ed. *Research Agenda for Federalism Studies*. Cheltenham: Edward Elgar Publishing, 162–174.

Mueller, S., Freiburghaus, R. and Vatter, A. (2021). La pandemia, una vaccinazione per il federalismo svizzero? *In*: Mazzoleni, O. and Rossi, S., eds. *In movimento, nonostante il lockdown. L'esperienza Svizzera del Covid-19*. Locarno: Armando Dadò editore, 173–189.

NCS-TF, 2020 – Swiss National COVID-19 Science Taskforce, 2020. *Situation Report: Effective Reproductive Number*. Available from: https://ncs-tf.ch/en/situation-report [Accessed 10 October 2020].

Palermo, F., 2020. Asymmetry as the Backbone of Contemporary Federalism. *Paper presented at the ECPR Virtual General Conference*, 24–28 August 2020.

persoenlich.ch, 2020. #SeifenBoss: Basler Aufklärungskampagne geht viral. March 11. Available from: https://www.persoenlich.com/kategorie-werbung/basler-aufklarungskampagne-geht-viral [Accessed 30 October 2020].

Poirier, J. and Saunders, C., 2015. Comparing Intergovernmental Relations in Federal Systems: An Introduction. *In*: Poirier, J., Saunders, C. and Kincaid, J., eds. *Intergovernmental Relations in Federal Systems*. Oxford: Oxford University Press, 1–13.

Rathke, A., Samand, S., Sina, S. and Sturm, J.E., 2020. KOF Konjunkturforschungsstelle: Szenario-Analysen zu den kurzfristigen wirtschaftlichen Auswirkungen der COVID-19-Pandemie (April 2020). Available from: https://ethz.ch/content/dam/ethz/special-interest/dual/kof-dam/documents/Medienmitteilungen/Prognosen/2020/Corona_Krise.pdf [Accessed 10 October 2020].

Rüefli, C. and Zenger, C., 2018. Analyse besondere Lage gemäss EpG: Aufgaben, Zuständigkeiten und Kompetenzen des Bundes (Schlussbericht Büro Vatter Politikforschung und-beratung & Zenger Advokatur und Beratung in Zusammenarbeit Büro Elser). 31 August 2018. Available from: https://www.bag.admin.ch/bag/de/home/krankheiten/ausbrueche-epidemien-pandemien/pandemievorbereitung/fachinfo.html [Accessed 17 October 2020].

Sager, F. and Mavrot, C., 2020. Switzerland's COVID-19 Policy Response: Consociational Crisis Management and Neo-Corporatist Reopening. *European Policy Analysis*, 6 (2), 293–304.

Salathé, M., Althaus, C.L., Neher, R., Stringhini, S., Hodcroft, E., Fellay, J., Zwahlen, M., Senti, G., Battegay, M., Wilder-Smith, A., Eckerle, I., Egger, M. and Low, N., 2020. COVID-19 Epidemic in Switzerland: On the Importance of Testing, Contact Tracing and Isolation. *Swiss Medical Weekly*, 150 (1), 1–3.

Schnabel, J., 2020. *Managing Interdependencies in Federal Systems. Intergovernmental Councils and the Making of Public Policy*. Basingstoke: Palgrave Macmillan.

Schnabel, J. and Mueller, S., 2017. Vertical Influence or Horizontal Coordination? The Purpose of Intergovernmental Councils in Switzerland. *Regional & Federal Studies* 27 (5), 549–572.

Solothurner Zeitung, 2020. Kampf gegen Corona-Virus: Neue Kampagne macht Schüler zum "Seifenboss". *Solothurner Zeitung*, 9 March. Available from: https://www.solothurnerzeitung.ch/solothurn/kanton-solothurn/kampf-gegen-corona-virus-neue-kampagne-macht-schueler-zum-seifenboss-136780480 [Accessed 30 October 2020].

Stadt Bern, 2020. *Gemeinderat schliesst vier weitere städtische Parkanlagen*. March 20. Available from: https://www.bern.ch/mediencenter/medienmitteilungen/aktuell_ptk/gemeinderat-schliesst-vier-weitere-staedtische-parkanlagen [Accessed 16 October 2020].

Stadt Zürich, 2020. *Coronavirus: Zürich definiert Sperrgebiete*. March 20. Available from: https://www.stadt-zuerich.ch/pd/de/index/das_departement/medien/medienmitteilung/2020/maerz/2003201.html [Accessed 16 October 2020].

St. Galler Tagblatt, 2020. Grenze dicht? Tessin streitet mit Bundesrat. *St. Galler Tagblatt*, 11 March, p. 2.

Studer, R., 2020. Bundesrat prüft "Krisenfenster" für Kantone: Tessin hält am Shutdown fest. *Blick*, 24 March, p. 2.

The Federal Council, 2020. *Coronavirus: Kantone können in Ausnahmefällen kurzfristig zusätzliche Massnahmen beantragen.* 27 March 2020. Available from: https://www.admin.ch/gov/de/start/dokumentation/medienmitteilungen.msg-id-78606.html [Accessed 31 October 2020].

Uhlmann, F. and Scheifele, E., 2020. Legislative Response to Coronavirus (Switzerland). *The Theory and Practice of Legislation* 8 (1/2), 115–130.

Vatter, A., 2018. *Swiss Federalism. The Transformation of a Federal Model.* London and New York: Routledge.

23 Perfect storm

The pandemic, Brexit, and devolved government in the UK

Clive Grace

23.1 Introduction

The context for COVID-19 in the UK has been strongly shaped by the devolved structures of UK Government and the unusual character of intergovernmental relations to which it gives effect. But if we are looking for the echoes of genuinely federal systems, it is not 'cooperative' or 'competitive' federalist themes which stand out. The quality of relationships has instead been more about unilateral action by the center and frustration on the part of the devolved nations. However, like devolution itself, intergovernmental relationships during the pre-vaccine waves have been a 'process rather than an event' and a process of several interwoven threads. On the pandemic itself, the four UK governments began to work somewhat more cooperatively toward the end. But that became increasingly difficult to untangle from the consequences of delayed and last-minute Brexit negotiations with the EU, and with the underlying pressures for Scottish independence and Irish re-unification.

It might all have been quite different, and the UK's devolved 'federalized' arrangements could have been mobilized effectively to tackle COVID-19 Collaboration and coordination could have been uppermost, with regular Heads of Government engagement and strong, positive, and open lines of communication. Information and early sharing of thinking and options, and views on what the 'science' had to say, could have been a significant feature. Marshaling of local government expertise, knowledge, and capacity could have been a natural part of the strategy.

What might have been the outcome of such an approach in governmental terms, notwithstanding the inevitable economic and health consequences of the pandemic, and even if the death rates were not very different from what actually transpired? A probable outcome would have been a strengthening of the centripetal influence of crises, making people across the UK feel that they were all 'in it together' and that they were stronger together than apart. Indeed, this effect was evident early on in support for the UK Government's handling and through deployment of the power of collective institutions and common sentiments and symbols, such as when Her Majesty the Queen addressed the UK as a whole with a message of care, compassion and resolve.

In the event, the UK Government's handling of COVID-19 and its approach to governing turned the crisis into a catastrophe. It was the centrifugal forces which were made ascendant. The UK had the worst performance of the G7 in both health and economic terms. A massive Conservative opinion poll lead and strong majority support for its approach have both been transformed into a neck and neck position with the Labour Opposition and widespread disapproval ratings. These ratings contrast

DOI: 10.4324/9781003251217-23

Table 23.1 Key Statistics on COVID-19 in the United Kingdom as of 10 January 2021

Cumulative Cases	Cumulative Cases per 100,000 Population	Cumulative Deaths	Cumulative Deaths per 100,000 Population	Case-Fatality Percentage
3,017,413	4,444.8	80,868	119.1	2.7

Source: *World Health Organization Weekly epidemiological update* – 12 January 2021. Geneva: WHO, 2021. Available from https://www.who.int/publications/m/item/weekly-epidemiological-update

strongly with those of the leadership of the three devolved Nations despite relatively minor difference in death rates from those in England.

Initially, the devolved Governments in the UK had limited influence on the handling of the pandemic. Centripetal forces were strong, and crisis and economic measures were paramount. Despite their powers in key areas of domestic policy and service delivery, they followed the UK Government lead. But their influence grew into a significant factor in handling matters differentially and especially in when and how to ease lockdown restrictions. Collaboration between the UK Government and those in the devolved Nations and local government was very limited and mainly conducted on UK Government terms except when coordination was absolutely required, such as in relation to quarantine measures associated with international travel. Even that alignment subsequently broke down.

Paradoxically, the UK Government's handling of the pandemic looks likely to have a potentially profound effect on the future course of devolution and federalized arrangements in the UK. It has overlain and reinforced divisions created by Brexit, fueling support for Scottish independence and encouraging independence debate in Wales, whilst proposed Brexit arrangements nudge Northern Ireland toward reunification. Brexit itself threatens to weaken the current devolution settlement, but the combination of COVID-19 and Brexit may even drive the devolved parts of the UK further apart. This could lead either to separation or perhaps to greater devolution as a means to try and hold the Union together.

23.2 COVID-19 in the UK

The Management of COVID-19 in the UK has been a disaster. It would be wrong to temper that overall judgment with weasel words and the mitigation that these are 'unprecedented' times. The UK was judged by WHO as recently as 2019 as the second best prepared country in terms of ability to respond to a pandemic (the country judged as best prepared was the USA), and the UK had plenty of opportunity to learn from the early experiences of Italy, in particular (McCarthy 2019). But it failed to do so. Its vaunted preparations were overwhelmed by disastrous errors of policy and politics. After the first COVID-19 death at the end of January, the UK was slow into lockdown some six weeks later and so suffered huge health consequences. It was correspondingly slow out of lockdown and suffered enormously in economic terms also and then failed to thwart or manage well the emerging second wave.

As of the end of August 2020, the UK had experienced one of the very highest figures for deaths from COVID-19 per 1 m population (610), one of the highest absolute numbers of COVID-19 recorded deaths (over 41,000), and a level of excess deaths that was the highest in Europe (a 6.9 percent increase in the death rate for the period from January to the end of May 2020). From the end of March 2020 until the middle of May, the UK recorded more than 2,500 new cases every day. From early April, death levels climbed rapidly to a peak of more than 1,000 a day, before dropping to an average of under 50 a day by early July and negligible numbers by the end of August. The number of new cases remained at what then seemed to be stubbornly high at 1,000+ a day – rather put into context by the 60,000+ cases a day which the UK experienced during the second wave.

The NHS was nearly, but not quite, overwhelmed, and it has been widely and deeply celebrated for the effort and the sacrifices which its staff made. New hospitals were created in record time, although for the most part, their capacity was only lightly used, principally because of a shortage of qualified staff. However, alongside the heroic efforts of the NHS, the key-associated components of a strategy to combat a pandemic were widely perceived as a shambles. They included a failure to 'test and trace,' a systematic and persistent absence of PPE, and a very poor response to the severity and consequences of the outbreak in care homes exacerbated by years of austerity-driven funding reductions.

There was also a widespread failure of trust in government and in governmental competence – on which the UK generally prides itself. This was partly due to the failures in health policy and approach outlined above and then magnified by the flagrant and highly publicized breach of the lockdown rules by the Prime Minister's principal (and highly controversial) adviser, Dominic Cummings. It was then further amplified by a succession of policy U-turns culminating in the chaos of badly handled summer examination results. One could barely script what a mess it has been, and how it has damaged the UK's reputation for good government and trust amongst its own population and overseas.

The economic costs to the UK have also been amongst the worst of anywhere in the world. The Q2 2020 GDP figure for the UK was 22 percent below the Q4 2019 figure, twice the fall in the US, far worse than Germany, and worst in the G7, ahead even of France. However, notwithstanding such huge economic consequences, the one area of government which has been seen as having a 'good' crisis has been the Chancellor of the Exchequer and the Treasury and Bank of England. The measures introduced have not been especially innovative in international terms, but they were introduced quickly and boldly, notwithstanding that they represented a major departure from fiscal and economic orthodoxy as practiced by Conservative Governments for more than 40 years.

The Chancellor introduced tax and spending measures to support households and families including:

- Additional funding for the NHS, public services, and charities (£48.5 billion);
- Measures to support businesses (£29 billion), including property tax holidays, direct grants for firms and a 'furlough' scheme, and compensation for sick pay leave;
- Strengthening the social safety net to support vulnerable people (by £8 billion);
- Three separate loans schemes to facilitate business' access to credit.

Key monetary measures included:

- Reducing the bank rate;
- A liquidity stimulus of £300 billion;

- Additional incentives for lending to the real economy and especially SMEs;
- A COVID-19 Corporate Financing Facility which makes £330 bn of loans and guarantees available to businesses (15 percent of GDP).

By mid-May, a roadmap to ease lockdown had been put in place to re-open the economy, with continued support via an extended furlough scheme and more targeted help for key sectors. The UK economy began to grow back but remained shrunken and severely weakened. The pandemic has exacerbated some underlying negative trends for UK retailing and High Streets as consumers switch to purchase online as well as disrupting supply chains. Unemployment is expected to be high, and to stay high for some considerable time. The UK economy had barely begun its recovery when the second wave, almost equally badly handled, dealt it a series of further hammer blows, intensified in some sectors by the economic consequences of Brexit.

23.3 COVID-19 and devolved government in the United Kingdom

The relationship between 'federalism' (devolved government) and COVID-19 in the UK, and the role of the three devolved Nations, has been heavily influenced by the underlying demographic and geographical structure of the UK, and the specific histories associated with devolution to all three.

23.3.1 The topography of UK 'federalism'

The UK has a devolved and 'federal-lite' system of government which has been created top down (albeit largely in response to bottom-up pressure) and which could still, in theory, be reversed. The UK central government devolved powers to the three 'Home Nations' of Scotland, Wales, and Northern Ireland, each of which has a specific historical, political, and geographical relationship with the central government, and with England being ruled by the UK central government itself and having no specific devolved government. If it is federalism, it is not as we usually know it.

Whilst England has a population of 53 m, Scotland has 5.3 m, Wales 3.1 m, and Northern Ireland 1.8 m. The size differential is even greater in GDP terms, with London and the South East of England producing a disproportionate share of UK national wealth, and all three devolved Nations having a GDP shortfall as compared to their population ratios. Geographically, Scotland is part of mainland Britain but has a relatively impervious physical barrier to England. Wales has a long and very porous boundary with England, and many trade and transport routes run east–west between Wales and England rather than north–south within Wales itself. Northern Ireland, of course, is physically part of the island of Ireland and separated from Great Britain by the sea.

Scotland achieved devolution in 1998 following a referendum and built upon a network of distinctly 'Scottish' institutions and cultures, many of which traced roots back to when Scotland was still an independent country before 1707. Wales similarly achieved devolution in 1998, but had further to go in creating its own institutional infrastructure having been more strongly integrated into union with England, starting in the 13th century (although Welsh is the most widespread indigenous language of all three devolved nations). Northern Ireland was part of Ireland and in union with Great Britain, formally dating from 1801. It remained as part of the UK on the creation of an independent Irish

State in 1922. The Good Friday Agreement of 1998 triggered a modern, power sharing devolved government for Northern Ireland following the long period of the 'troubles' and inter-community conflict. In the Brexit referendum, a majority in Scotland and in Northern Ireland voted to remain and a majority in Wales to leave.

All three devolved nations have extensive powers in relation to domestic policy, but very constrained fiscal resources. They get a guaranteed share of national expenditure, but the aggregate total (and thus the size of the annual budgets of the devolved nations) is controlled by the UK government. In turn, the devolved national governments control local government spending closely. Healthcare and social care are devolved, along with many of the powers for managing emergencies, such that the devolved nations were able to diverge from the UK government's approach in England. Initially, they did so hardly at all, but more significant differences emerged as lockdown restrictions began to be eased.

All three devolved Nations also have effectively just one other order of government at local level in the form of local authorities with broad powers and responsibilities including housing, transport, leisure and environmental matters, and with Scottish and Welsh local authorities also having extensive powers in the fields of social services and education especially. Compared to almost any other jurisdiction, UK local authorities are, on average, very large, have very wide powers, employ a lot of people, and spend a significant proportion of national public expenditure, notwithstanding the decade of austerity which hit their funding very hard.

Overall, devolution in the UK has been seen as a success (Paun and Mcrory 2019), albeit differentially. As Bronwen Maddox summarizes the position:

> Devolution has had the most surefooted development in Scotland where, from the start, there was strong public support and the Scottish Parliament had extensive powers. In Wales, public support took time to build; so did the powers of the National Assembly. In Northern Ireland, the devolved government's ability to function has been dogged by splits between rival parties which the devolution settlement itself was designed to try to heal.
>
> (Cheung and Valsamidis 2019, p. 2)

And whereas Tony Blair initiated the referenda which led to Scottish and Welsh devolution in order to save the Union, when combined with COVID-19 and Brexit, the forces unleashed may yet have the power to destroy it.

23.3.2 *COVID-19 in the devolved nations*

The course and consequences of COVID-19 across the four Home Nations have often felt quite different, but, in reality, the similarities outweigh the differences in most major respects. When the UK government finally woke up to the need for lockdown, the character and scale of the crisis was so pronounced that the devolved nations followed suit almost to the letter, notwithstanding that the lockdown powers they relied on were substantially matters for self-regulation. The major fiscal and economic measures were in any event largely a matter for the UK government to determine and it did so in a relatively unilateral manner.

The key coordinating mechanism for emergencies which are UK wide or of broad significance is COBRA, the committee for dealing with crisis contingencies (Haddon

2020). The devolved Nations had access to COBRA, and it did play some part. For example, the Welsh Government declared that it was working in collaboration with the other governments in the UK to take an aligned approach where it was beneficial to do so, coordinated by the UK Government through meetings of COBRA. However, power to impose the lockdown in Wales rested with the Welsh Government, which decided how it should be implemented, along with responsibility for health and social care.

The relative lack of coordination has led to unnecessary differences and confusion for citizens. Commentators have called for greater collaboration not as a matter of principle and not in order to impose inappropriate uniformity but to optimize the collective effort. More extensive use of such collaborative intergovernmental machinery as the UK possesses has been strongly encouraged (Sargeant 2020).

The variations in handling between the UK's four 'Home Nations' showed some of the strengths of devolved government as well as its limitations in what remains a highly centralized country in fiscal terms. The devolved Nations increasingly deployed their powers to diverge from the UK Government's approach across the course of the pandemic and especially in relation to the 'when' and 'how' to ease lockdown. But, overall, the response to the pandemic reflected the fundamentally centralist character of UK Government associated with its political culture and history and the sheer weight and dominance of England.

This was reinforced and amplified by a centralizing political impulse of the new Conservative Government. By early July, the First Ministers of Scotland and Wales launched a coordinated attack on the UK Government for being 'shambolic' and failing to provide coherent information from UK Ministers on key issues of international travel and quarantine. They claimed that consultation with the devolved Governments was being treated as an afterthought, even though all three had clear legal duties to make sure that their decisions were lawful and proportionate. But whilst feeling like 'rubber stamps,' in practice, the devolved Nations initially accepted the UK government position on which countries should be exempt from travel restrictions – before then diverging both from the UK Government and from each other. Conversely, on some issues, the devolved Nations moved first, and the UK Government found itself under public pressure to follow suit.

Much of this criticism was reinforced and echoed by the Westminster Scottish Affairs Committee in its interim report on intergovernmental working during the pandemic. It spoke of a vacuum in ministerial-level communication between the UK and Scottish Governments and deterioration in collaboration as lockdown measures started to be eased. It saw the growing divergence of approach as creating public confusion and criticized the UK Government for not being clear when its messaging applied only to England.

The concerns of the devolved Nations about an over-centralized approach were exacerbated by what were seen as further centralizing moves arising from Brexit such as legislation to establish an internal 'single market' for the UK as a whole. *Inter alia*, this would potentially impose uniform regulatory standards on the devolved Nations, including on matters on which they currently have devolved powers. The UK Government's apparent unwillingness to engage with the devolved Governments unless it absolutely had to was also evident in the lack of consultation about post-Brexit trade agreements and migration policy.

Whereas 'strengthening the Union' was one of the Prime Minister Teresa May's five tests for a successful Brexit (Jack et al. 2018, p. 5), in fact, Brexit has imposed severe strains on the Union. It has "highlighted the stark divide between how exist-ing devolution arrangements are interpreted in Westminster and Whitehall, and how they are interpreted in Cardiff and Edinburgh. And it has divided the main parties in Northern Ireland" (Blair 2019). It seems less likely that Brexit will aid the Union than further weakening along the lines predicted by Tony Blair.

The devolved Governments felt shut out of the negotiations with the EU and other countries about future trade deals. They were keen to see key sectors of their econo-mies taken account of and feared that the UK Government would not be sufficiently concerned about these. Scotland argued for a different approach to migration policy to avoid damaging rural communities which need in-migration to sustain birth rates and basic services. The same issue applies to Wales. So, an optimally effective UK-wide post-Brexit policy on migration would have needed more consultation and en-gagement with the devolved Nations than was the case.

The verdict as to whether devolution has helped or hindered the management of the pandemic in the UK is that it certainly has not been a hindrance, although the multi-ple messaging may have added somewhat to the sometimes confused communications of the UK Government. More positively, it has permitted the devolved Nations to tai-lor lockdown-easing plans more closely to their own concerns and judgments on what the 'science' was telling them. It also provided an element of competitive federalism as people were able to compare the various approaches being taken and thus supported greater accountability of all the governments. The more interesting question, how-ever, is not so much what devolution did for the pandemic as to what the pandemic may well do to the future of devolution.

23.4 New directions in devolution: the impact of the pandemic

The pandemic has exacerbated intergovernmental tensions within the UK. It has not stimulated greater enduring collaboration but rather fuelled resentment and exaspera-tion on the part of the devolved Nations. The policy divergences and the experience of the pandemic have been relatively minor, in fact, but have generated disproportionate confusion and irritation, notwithstanding that they were based in genuine differences of view and genuine differences in context between the four Nations.

Most strikingly, the pandemic made devolution visible in a much stronger and starker way. For many people, it brought devolution to life as they realized that things were being done differently in different parts of the UK, and that crossing from one jurisdiction to another meant that different rules and approaches applied.

The political impact of how the virus was handled has been profound. The UK Government is widely perceived as having handled it badly – its approval rating fell from 65+ percent in late March to 36 percent by July (see Savanta 2021). This has not been so in the devolved Nations. Broadly, they were slower than England to ease lock-down measures and have higher approval ratings for their handling of the pandemic. In part, they appear to have been more in tune with risk-averse public sentiment but perhaps did more harm to their economies. But, on many measures, all four Home Nations failed as badly as each other. So, the approval ratings in the devolved Nations seem to be as much about presentation and perception as more effective handling of the crisis as such.

The UK Government's failure was amplified by a series of U-turns on both ma-jor and relatively minor matters of policy. These culminated in the fiasco over the examination results of hundreds of thousands of 16- and 18-year-old pupils which created chaos in the higher education and vocational education sectors. The UK Government has lost a huge lead in opinion polls over the Labour Opposition and a huge positive approval rating for its handling in the early days of the crisis. The Prime Minister's personal approval rating plummeted. In contrast, the leaders in the devolved Nations have been continuously visible and have had continuously solid positive approval from their populations (see Davies-Lewis 2021; YouGov 2021). The policy divergence and the political tensions have been inevitable in the absence of any continuing positive and collaborative intergovernmental machinery. The limitations and lack of resilience of existing intergovernmental relations processes, such as they are, have been cruelly exposed. Collaboration between the UK Government and the devolved Nations, and between central/regional government and local authorities, should have been the hallmark of a nationwide response to the pandemic, but for the most part was missing or under-developed.

Interestingly, what might be thought of as being an 'obvious' place for international collaboration in the UK has been notably absent throughout. The 'Council of the Isles' (also known as the British-Irish Council) was created as part of the Good Friday Agreement and comprises high level and ongoing engagement between all four Home Nations and others on a broad range of matters of intergovernmental concern and with a permanent secretariat. A search of the official website found no results for 'coronavirus,' and 'pandemic' produced just one result – that a planned creative industries meeting had been cancelled because of the pandemic. The 34th summit (they average two a year) scheduled for June was also postponed. So, rather than building on and using existing collaborative machinery, it was actually put to one side.

The character and history of devolution in each of the devolved Nations, and their specific geographies, heavily influenced their relationships with the UK Government during the pandemic. Scotland, with its relatively impervious land border with England, was able to contemplate a 'COVID-19-free' policy approach. The Scottish First Minister even threatened to close the Scotland/England border to help give effect to this policy (but with the UK Prime Minister dismissing the very idea that such a border existed at all). Wales also made its 'border' with England part of its COVID-19 travel restrictions at one stage in a minor way, whilst knowing that its physical connectivity with major English conurbations along and across that border made major policy divergence difficult to justify and maintain.

The realities of the immediate consequences of the pandemic were not, in practice, so very different across the four Nations, although Northern Ireland's figures for deaths stand out as best, and on some other measures the devolved Nations did comparatively better than England. Care homes were a major problem almost everywhere, and especially in Scotland, partly from weak resources and capacity as a result of years of under-funding, and partly from policy errors. But the messaging and leadership was significantly different and perceived as such by the respective populations.

What may also be different in the longer term is that the pandemic has exposed and amplified the impacts of inequality on health and employment. The populations of the devolved nations are, on average, poorer, older, and sicker than the UK as a whole, and their economies are less resilient than England's. So, the ensuing increase in inequality will likely fall hardest on the devolved Nations. There will also be differences in post-pandemic recovery policy, with Wales, for example, already demonstrating difference by attaching high priority to tackling inequality, climate change and fair work, and less emphasis on inward investment, innovation, and economic growth (see Russell 2020 and WCPP 2020). There will (or ought to) be a great deal of learning to harvest and share both about the course of the pandemic and its handling and the various post-pandemic paths that are and will be taken.

The wider consequences of the pandemic for devolved government and even the breakup of the Union will likely be potentially major. The Scottish National Party expects to win an overall majority in the Scottish national elections in 2021 on a platform of another independence referendum, which this time may well be won, if it is allowed to take place. The UK Government has already signaled that it will reject such a proposal, and their consent is required. But it will not be easy for Brexiteers, in particular, to argue that Scotland's people do not have the right to determine their own independence from the 'yoke' of Union within the UK.

The issues for Wales and for Northern Ireland are less stark and immediate, but the combination of the politics of the pandemic and the consequences of Brexit appear to be encouraging separatist sentiment. The push from within Wales for a more federalized UK is relatively longstanding in a devolved context (see Melding 2013) and that seam of opinion has grown through the pandemic (Jones 2021). The federalism/independence sentiment remains at a far lower level than in Scotland, but that example may have big ripple effects for Wales if Scotland does become independent and makes a success of it, or if Brexit departure arrangements impact on Northern Ireland as adversely as some fear. Positive sentiment toward re-unification has shifted visibly, albeit lacking a consistent majority (LucidTalk 2021).

However, the twists and turns of UK politics over the past five years have been so violent and remarkable, even without COVID-19's unique contribution, that such a linear prediction feels inherently unsafe. It may be that events take a more elliptical path. Stronger pressures for independence may lead to thwarted aspirations for immediate separation, but nonetheless trigger grants of greater devolved powers in an effort to assuage independence sentiment. That, in turn, could facilitate a longer-term independence path. Or it may even lead to a willingness to look more fundamentally at the structure of UK Government itself, perhaps even to contemplate a constitutional equivalence between the four Home Nations. We might yet see the eventual emergence of a system much more akin to a federalized government than could possibly have been imagined not so very long ago by anyone other than federalist dreamers.

Bibliography

Blair, T., 2019. *Devolution, Brexit, and the Future of the Union*. London: Institute for Government.

Cheung, A., and Valsamidis, L., 2019. *Devolution at 20*. London: Institute for Government.

Cheung, A., 2021. *The Barnett Formula*. London: Institute for Government.

Davies-Lewis, T., 2021. Wales' Vaccine Problems Mount for Mark Drakeford. *The Spectator*, 18 January. Available from: https://www.spectator.co.uk/article/wales-vaccine-woes-are-becoming-a-problem-for-mark-drakeford [Accessed 31 January 2021].

Haddon, C., 2020. COBRA, Institute for Government, London. Available from: https://www.instituteforgovernment.org.uk/explainers/cobr-cobra [Accessed 31 January 2021].Jack, M.T., Owen, J., Kellam, J., and Pash, Al., 2018. Devolution after Brexit, Institute for Government, London. Available from: https://www.instituteforgovernment.org.uk/explainers/barnett-formula [Accessed 31 January 2021].

Jones, G.C., 2021. *A Sovereign Wales in an Isle-Wide Confederation*. Cardiff: Institute of Welsh Affairs.

LucidTalk Polling, January 2021. *State of the Union Polling*. Available from: https://www.lucidtalk.co.uk/single-post/lt-ni-sunday-times-january-2021-state-of-the-uk-union-poll [Accessed 31 January 2021].

McCarthy, N., 2019. The Countries Best Prepared to Deal with a Pandemic. *Statista* [online]. Available from: https://www.statista.com/chart/19790/index-scores-by-level-of-preparation-to-respond-to-an-epidemic/ [Accessed 31 January 2021].

Melding, D., 2013. *The Reformed Union: The UK as a Federation*. Cardiff: Institute of Welsh Affairs.

Paun, A. and Mcrory, S., eds., 2019. *Has Devolution Worked?* London: Institute for Government.

Russell MSP, M., 2020. *Scotland in a Post Brexit and Post Pandemic World* [online]. Available from: https://policyscotland.gla.ac.uk/scotland-in-a-post-brexit-and-post-pandemic-world/ [Accessed 31 January 2021].

Sargeant, J., 2020. *Co-ordination and Divergence: Devolution and Coronavirus*. London: Institute for Government.

Savanta, 2021. *Coronavirus Data Tracker* [dataset]. Available from: https://savanta.com/coronavirus-data-tracker/ [Accessed 31 January 2021].

Scottish Affairs Committee, October 2020. *Coronavirus and Scotland, Second Report of Session 2019–21*. London: House of Commons.

The National, October 2020. *Record Support for Scottish Independence* [online]. Available from: https://www.thenational.scot/news/18793584.record-public-support-scottish-independence-new-poll-shows/ [Accessed 31 January 2021].

Wales Centre for Public Policy, July 2020. *Planning for a Prosperous, Equal and Green Recovery from the Coronavirus Pandemic*. Cardiff: WCPP.

YouGov, 2021. Nicola Sturgeon is the Most Popular other UK Public Figure and the Most Famous. *Politics & Current Affairs*. Available from: https://yougov.co.uk/topics/politics/explore/public_figure/Nicola_Sturgeon [Accessed 31 January 2021].

24 COVID-19 and American federalism

First-wave responses

John Kincaid and J. Wesley Leckrone

24.1 Introduction

The United States' response to COVID-19 marked an acute failure of cooperative federalism but did not alter the federal system because the federal government under President Donald Trump did not seek centralization; instead, he left the primary response up to the states in the fashion of dual federalism in which the federal and state governments occupy separate spheres of authority. This strategy was not ideal, as evidenced by the country's high numbers of COVID-19 casualties. But given President Trump's unwillingness to forge a cooperatively coherent federal-state-local response, states' constitutional authority to shut down much of the nation's economy limited a contagion that would have been more rampant absent this state authority. Another major factor handicapping the US response was partisan polarization, which pitted the Republican president against Democratic state and local officials, gridlocked Congress, and produced different pandemic policies in Democratic and Republican states and localities (Table 24.1).

24.2 COVID-19 in the United States

The United States experienced three waves of COVID-19 in 2020: spring, summer, and fall/winter. The last wave had, by far, the highest number of infections and deaths. As of 31 December 2020, the United States had recorded 19,943,605 COVID-19 cases (reaching 25,780,144 by 29 January 2021) and 344,497 deaths, which totaled 435,151 by 29 January 2021 (US Centers for Disease Control and Prevention 2021). The highest numbers of cases and deaths occurred from late October 2020 into January 2021.

The first confirmed US case occurred in Washington state on 20 January 2020 in a man who had visited Wuhan, China (although the United States only discovered the first case on 29 February). The first death was in northern California on 6 February.

Table 24.1 Key Statistics on COVID-19 in the United States of America as of 10 January 2021

Cumulative Cases	Cumulative Cases per 100,000 Population	Cumulative Deaths	Cumulative Deaths per 100,000 Population	Case Fatality Percentage
21,761,186	6,574.3	365,886	110.5	1.7

Source: *World Health Organization Weekly epidemiological update* – 12 January 2021. Geneva: WHO, 2021. Available from https://www.who.int/publications/m/item/weekly-epidemiological-update

DOI: 10.4324/9781003251217-24

However, the pandemic's epicenter was the commuter-linked states of Connecticut, New Jersey, and New York that pivot around New York City. On 31 December, these states, with 9.6 percent of the US population, still accounted for 18.2 percent of all US deaths despite the infection's nationwide spread. New York City had the highest death rate (300 per 100,000 population). New York, including New York City, had the highest state death rate (414 per 100,000 population); Vermont had the lowest (21). Among federal and quasi-federal countries on 31 January 2021, only Belgium (184.4 deaths per 100,000) and Bosnia and Herzegovina (140.7) had worse outcomes than the United States (134.3). Other health outcomes are still unknown because many people with non-COVID-19 conditions feared visiting medical facilities during the pandemic, while state governors' stay-at-home orders (SAHOs) probably increased Alzheimer deaths, suicides, domestic violence, depression, and other maladies.

Because most governors began issuing SAHOs in late March, the national unemployment rate leaped from 4.4 percent in March to 14.7 percent in April, then dropping monthly to 6.7 percent in November and December. The absence of a further drop in December was due largely to some governors' reimposition of SAHO's in response to the pandemic's third wave. This slowed the country's economic recovery. Some consumer-goods shortages appeared in late March, but supplies recovered to nearly normal levels by June. International air travel had virtually halted by 11 March, domestic air travel dropped 95 percent by 2 April, and most public interstate surface transportation shut down. However, domestic air travel had increased considerably by the Thanksgiving (26 November) and Christmas (25 December) holidays as millions of Americans disregarded advice against travel issued by the US Centers for Disease Control and Prevention (CDC). Economic recovery will take several years, although long-term economic damages are yet to be determined in terms of more homeless people, damaged careers, interrupted educations, permanent business closures, and perhaps greater income inequality.

24.3 COVID-19 and federalism in the United States

The United States has a dual federal system with three orders of government: national, state, and local, although local governments are the creatures of each state. The federal Constitution of 1788 is one of limited, delegated powers. All other powers are reserved to the states or the people. States retain the most authority to address public health emergencies through their police power, which is the authority to regulate citizens' health, safety, welfare, and morals. All states can enact declarations of emergency or disaster, and 35 states can declare public health emergencies. Such declarations authorize state officials to address pandemics. The federal government can address interstate and international infectious diseases through its commerce power. For example, the federal government lacks authority to require mask-wearing for everyone nationwide but can require mask-wearing on all federal-government land and property and on interstate transportation systems. Trump never issued such a mandate, but President Joseph Biden did so immediately after his 20 January 2021 inauguration. The US Public Health Services Act (1944), in conjunction with presidential executive orders, authorizes other forms of federal responsiveness, with the US Department of Health and Human Services at the forefront.

The states are mainly responsible for health care, but the federal government plays a large role. The United States has no universal health-care program. The national

Medicare program covers all citizens age 65 and over, and Medicaid covers 73.5 million low-income people. Public–private arrangements under the US Affordable Care Act (2010) cover other low-income citizens. Hence, the two populations most vulnerable to COVID-19 mortality have government insurance. About 67.5 percent of citizens are covered by private insurance, which is mostly state-regulated, and about 9 percent lack health coverage. State and local governments own approximately 18.6 percent of all hospitals, while non-profit entities own 56.5 percent, and for-profit companies own 24.9 percent (Kaiser n.d.).

Although the United States ranked first on the 2019 Global Health Security Index, which evaluates capacity to address pandemics, investment in the US public health system languished over the pre-2020 decade. Funding for states' public health departments fell 16 percent per capita and 18 percent for local health departments. At least 38,000 jobs were lost in these fields, with more cutbacks occurring during the pandemic. Some health officials blamed these reductions for problems they faced setting up testing sites, building contact-tracing systems, distributing vaccines, and keeping vaccination records once vaccines become available (Weber et al. 2020).

24.3.1 Management of health impact and response

In mid-January 2020, the US CDC began screening for COVID-19 in travelers passing through the largest US international airports. On 31 January, the US Secretary of Health and Human Services declared a public health emergency, and President Trump barred entry of foreign nationals arriving from China. The president extended this ban to non-Americans travelling from Europe on 11 March. On 13 March, Trump issued 57 simultaneous disaster declarations for all states, Washington, DC, and US territories – the first all-state declaration in US history. The president indicated that the states should lead in combating COVID-19.

Initially, the nation experienced shortages of personal protective equipment for front-line responders, COVID-19 tests, and effective contact tracing. The CDC distributed contaminated test kits in March, requiring more than a month to rectify the problem. Once tests were available, they were in short supply, and processing backlogs delayed results for days. Ventilators were in short supply early in the outbreak, but Trump invoked the US Defense Production Act to require private industry to manufacture them. The president partnered with drug developers and manufacturers to accelerate vaccine development. This successful initiative, called Operation Warp Speed, enabled the US Food and Drug Administration to approve a vaccine developed by Pfizer on 11 December and a Moderna vaccine on 18 December. Trump also relaxed federal regulations to allow Medicare telehealth visits, ease hospital hiring of health workers, and decrease paperwork for federal health-care programs.

SAHOs were the most common tool used by governors, county officials, and mayors. California's Democratic Governor Gavin Newsom issued the first statewide SAHO on 19 March. However, San Francisco and five neighboring counties had issued the country's first SAHO on 16 March. From 19 March to 7 April, 43 governors – 24 Democrats and 19 Republicans – issued SAHOs of varying stringency and geographic scope. Of the first ten governors issuing SAHOs, nine were Democrats. All seven states having no SAHO had Republican governors. However, between 16 March and 1 April, 136 counties (i.e., non-municipal local governments in 48 states) nationwide, accounting for 66.9 million people, imposed SAHOs before their states (Brandtner et al. 2020).

State and local SAHOs varied on prohibited activities and enforcement. Most required people to stay home except for "essential" work and personal activities. SAHOs shut down businesses and public services (e.g., mass transit) deemed "non-essential," though these varied by state and sometimes partisanship. For example, some Republican states tried to close abortion services as "non-essential"; Democratic states deemed them essential. Americans were limiting their activities before SAHOs due to infection fears, but political decisions on which businesses remained open changed consumer behavior, with commerce-driven to "essential" and online companies. SAHOs helped limit COVID-19's spread but caused economic damage as reflected in high unemployment.

Majorities of Americans supported mitigation, including state laws requiring mask-wearing. They endorsed social distancing, business restrictions, public gathering limits, a national strategy for reopening businesses and schools, a two-week national SAHO, and a ban on interstate travel (Mann 2020). However, Republicans expressed less concern than Democrats about COVID-19's severity, the consequences of economic reopening, and the need to wear masks and social distance. They also believed the president and the federal government were managing the pandemic effectively (Newport 2020; Ritter 2020). Nevertheless, only 23 percent of Americans approved of the federal government's pandemic management by August 2020, compared to 44 percent for the states' and 48 percent for local governments' management (Associated Press-NORC 2020).

24.3.2 Management of fiscal impact and response

The federal government has provided the bulk of pandemic fiscal stimuli. By large bipartisan margins, Congress enacted and Trump signed five COVID-19 relief bills from 6 March to 5 June. The Coronavirus Aid, Relief, and Economic Security (CARES) Act was the centerpiece, providing $2.2 trillion in the largest stimulus in US history. CARES boosted the economy through direct payments to citizens, enhanced unemployment benefits, and funds for businesses. Adults in households earning less than $99,000 per year received $1,200 each and $500 per child. Businesses were encouraged to retain workers through a $350 billion Paycheck Protection Program that provided forgivable loans to smaller businesses.

CARES used a major intergovernmental program, Unemployment Compensation (UC), to help the jobless. The federal government sets parameters for UC, but states determine eligibility and benefits. CARES added $600 per week to state benefits (which average $320) and extended the benefits for up to 39 weeks (Adamczyk 2020; US Department of Labor 2019). However, despite the considerable increase in unemployed people, which overwhelmed state unemployment offices, no money was allocated to help states pay their share of UC. As of September, 20 states had borrowed more than $31.3 billion from the federal government to cover their UC payments (Henderson 2020). The Federal Reserve (the US equivalent of a central bank) has accounted for about $7 trillion in stimulus action to shore up banks and credit markets. It extended more than $2.3 trillion in direct aid, including $500 billion to keep credit flowing to state and local governments.

States might face a $555 billion revenue shortfall through FY 2022 (Center for Budget 2020), although FY 2021 losses will range from about 1 percent in Idaho to perhaps 30 percent in New Mexico (National Conference 2020). Cities could experience a 13 percent revenue drop (McFarland and Pagano 2020). Revenue declines will likely be largest in Democratic jurisdictions, partly because of their stricter SAHOs. As of 7 December, Congress had provided state and local governments $277 billion (Committee 2020).

States and the federal government have managed the economy dualistically. States shut down large swaths of the economy and reopened and closed down again at their own speeds. The federal government compensated with aid and stimulus spending. The aid conformed to past practices and did not increase centralization.

However, after 5 June, Democrats (who controlled the US House) and Republicans (who controlled the US Senate) deadlocked on additional spending despite pleas from the Federal Reserve and others. The House passed a $3 trillion bill rejected by the Senate. The bipartisan National Governors Association requested $500 billion more aid for state relief (National Governors 2020); the US Conference of Mayors requested $250 billion more in direct aid to localities (Durr 2020). Democrats support more state-local aid. Most Republicans reject aid for state and local governments because they believe such aid would mainly benefit Democratic jurisdictions experiencing revenue losses due to their prolonged SAHOs and pre-COVID-19 overspending. President Trump called Democratic states and cities "poorly run" (Bowden 2020), and the Senate's Republican Majority Leader Mitch McConnell suggested states seek bankruptcy rather than federal aid. While rejecting additional aid to state and local governments, Republicans supported funding for unemployment payments, small businesses, virus mitigation programs, and aid to education. Partisan disagreements over state-local aid, as well as Republicans' desire for COVID-19 liability protections for businesses operating during the pandemic, remained the primary obstacles to passing another comprehensive COVID-19 relief bill.

However, after intense negotiations following the presidential election of 3 November, Congress passed another COVID-19 measure – the $915 billion Consolidated Appropriations/Response & Relief Act – on 21 December, which Trump signed on 27 December after having threatened to veto it. The act did not provide direct general aid to state and local governments or provide COVID-19 liability protection for businesses, but it did provide considerable specific aid, such as $151 billion for unemployment compensation, $54 billion for elementary and secondary schools, $22 billion for COVID-19 testing, tracing, and other mitigation, and $28 billion for transportation.

24.3.3 Intergovernmental relations

Executive federalism has been contentious, but federal and state agencies' bureaucratic relations continued to be largely cooperative, except when the Trump administration interfered with some federal agencies' functioning. The United States has no umbrella intergovernmental institutions. Intergovernmental relations occur politically through informal party, associational, and customary channels and bureaucratically through hundreds of federal-state-local agency fora specific to policy areas (e.g., public health). The CDC has long-standing and highly institutionalized communication channels with state and local public-health agencies.

President Trump pushed states to lead the COVID-19 response. He made little effort to formulate a unified federal-government plan and a cooperative federal-state-local plan of action. The president criticized governors and mayors, mostly

Democrats, who refused to align their SAHO policies with his preferences. After retreating from an extraordinary claim that he had total authority to reopen state economies, Trump called recalcitrant governors "mutineers" (Arsova 2020) and tweeted such blasts as LIBERATE MINNESOTA (Trump 2020) in efforts to force governors to relax their SAHOs. Trump frequently contradicted public health officials, refused to wear a mask, held large campaign rallies without social distancing, and touted unproven drugs to combat COVID-19. In many states, governors and their secretaries of health became the main COVID-19 communicators. New York Democratic Governor Andrew Cuomo's daily press conferences gained national attention because the major media paired coverage of Trump's news conferences with Cuomo's briefings.

Interstate relations have been both competitive and cooperative. The lack of a national policy on acquiring and distributing many medical supplies induced competition for several months. States bid against each other in global markets for personal protective equipment, masks, and ventilators largely because Trump pitted them against each other when he admonished governors on 16 March to "try getting" medical supplies themselves (Sheth 2020) and claimed on 19 March that the federal government was not "a shipping clerk" (Forgey 2020). Michigan Democratic Governor Gretchen Whitmer's staff dubbed the resulting interstate competition "The Hunger Games" (Mahler 2020, p. 26). Prices spiked, and some state officials feared the federal government or other states would commandeer their incoming supplies during transit (Bender and Ballhaus 2020). By mid-April, the administration, believing it had done enough, executed a "state authority handoff" (Tankersley 2020). Production of medical protective gear began to reach demand in early summer, but some shortages returned as cases spiked again (Mulvihill and Fassett 2020). Although Trump lacked constitutional authority to close or open states' economies, he did not use his commanding media position to foster coherent, national leadership. Neither the president nor governors closed state borders, but many states required a 14-day quarantine for people entering their state from other states.

Similarly, following approval of the COVID-19 vaccines in December, the Trump administration agreed to distribute the vaccines to the states but left it up to the states to decide whether to follow CDC recommendations on how to prioritize vaccinations. However, the administration's inability to make reliable deliveries made it impossible for states to schedule vaccinations with predictability.

Some states developed working relationships. Governors organized regional agreements in the West (among three states), Northeast (seven states), and Midwest (seven states) to cooperate on reopening their economies and purchase medical supplies collaboratively. Seven other geographically dispersed states joined a pact to buy rapid tests in an effort to show companies there was demand for a quick roll-out of tests (Hogan 2020). States also shared medical equipment, and some waived licensing rules for out-of-state health personnel. Some local governments collaborated regionally to enforce COVID-19 restrictions, develop consistent business-closure policies, and formulate testing policies (Mallinson 2020).

Many states experienced state-local conflicts. State governments controlled by Republicans often sought to preempt SAHO policies instituted by Democratic county officials and city mayors. Republican county and city officials often resisted COVID-19 policies instituted by Democratically controlled state governments. Some elected county sheriffs refused to enforce state mask mandates and other rules.

24.3.4 Roles of state and local governments

State and local governments continued delivering most services and switched to remote working and online public meetings fairly quickly in March and April. States implemented different SAHOs and reopening strategies, but regardless of their individual strategies, governors, county officials, and city mayors exercised emergency executive powers with little interference. Many lawsuits were filed, and some state legislatures objected to gubernatorial actions, but with little success. By December 2020, there were only four notably successful legal challenges: the Wisconsin Supreme Court ruled that a gubernatorial extension of the state's SAHO violated the state's constitution, the Michigan Supreme Court struck down the governor's SAHO and mask mandate, a US district court struck down the Pennsylvania governor's pandemic restrictions as violating the US Constitution (though the case remained on appeal as of this writing), and the US Supreme Court blocked New York's governor from enforcing an attendance limit on worship services.

Partisanship was prominent in states' COVID-19 policies, as illustrated in Figure 24.1. Democratic governors and local executives instituted earlier and more stringent SAHOs and reopened their economies more slowly than Republicans. Only 73 percent of the 26 Republican governors issued a SAHO. All Republican governors initiated reopening by 18 May, while states with Democratic governors waited until 9 June. There were also partisan divisions over mask-wearing mandates. All Democratic governors required masks by 1 August, while only 46 percent of Republican governors issued mask mandates by September.

Two factors influenced gubernatorial behavior. First, high population-density states, particularly in the Northeast, which typically had Democratic governors, were hit harder during the pandemic's early stages. However, New York's governor preempted the New York City mayor's authority to order a SAHO. This preemption delayed a statewide SAHO for five days in March and made New York City a COVID-19 super-spreader nationwide, substantially increasing the number

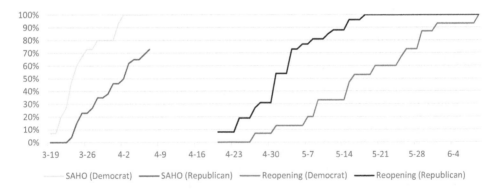

Figure 24.1 Dates of SAHOs and Reopenings by Gubernatorial Party in the United States of America.

Sources: Mervosh, S., Lu, D. and Swales, V., 2020. See Which States and Cities Have Told Residents to Stay at Home. *New York Times*, April 20. Available from: https://www.nytimes.com/interactive/2020/us/coronavirus-stay-at-home-order.html [Accessed 29 July 2020].

Lee, J. C., Mervosh, S., Avila, Y., Harvey B., Matthews, A. L., 2020. See How All 50 States Are Reopening (and Closing Again). *New York Times*. Available from: https://www.nytimes.com/interactive/2020/us/states-reopen-map-coronavirus.html [Accessed 29 July 2020].

of US cases and deaths. Many states with Republican governors with more rural residents and lower population densities saw fewer COVID-19 cases. Second, many public officials throughout the federal system adopted a partisan framing of COVID-19. Democratic officials generally focused on curbing COVID-19 transmission through strict SAHOs and slow re-openings; Republicans emphasized SAHOs' economic costs and citizens' rights to comply voluntarily with public health measures.

States also varied by how governors exercised their authority. New York's Democratic governor centralized the pandemic response in his office, causing contentious relations with New York City's Democratic mayor. Numerous other states, many with Republican governors, placed loose restrictions on personal and business behavior, while preempting local governments from creating stricter standards. Maryland's Republican Governor Larry Hogan created statewide policies but worked collaboratively with local officials who wanted to reopen their economies more slowly than other areas in the state (Davidson and Haddow 2020). Governors who sought to maintain tight control did so mainly by threatening to withhold state and federal funds from counties or cities pushing to reopen in violation of their orders and revoke licenses and permits from businesses violating their orders.

Localities have been at the forefront of service provision for COVID-19's economic victims. Concern about community spread led places like New York City to house homeless people in hotels to keep them socially distanced. Many municipalities partnered with businesses and non-profits to provide meals to the poor and unemployed, and many school districts continued giving free meals to low-income children when schools closed and switched to remote learning. Localities also helped citizens connect to the Internet and avoid utility disruptions and housing evictions. Many provided assistance to small businesses hurt by SAHOs (National League of Cities n.d.). As of September, 45 states and 56 percent of big cities had implemented housing-eviction moratoriums; 40 percent of big cities and 54 percent of states provided rent relief; 66 percent of states and 19 percent of large cities enacted a foreclosure moratorium; 33 percent of big cities and 58 percent of states offered mortgage relief; and 30 percent of states and 37 percent of large cities provided some property-tax relief (Einstein, Palmer and Fox 2020). Michigan enacted a "Pay to Stay" law allowing local governments to lower delinquent-tax amounts, thus making it easier for owners to stay in their homes. Connecticut enacted a law allowing local governments to reduce interest rates on delinquent taxes; a few states allowed localities to delay or waive late payment penalties (Collins 2020). Elementary and secondary school closures were mandated or recommended in 48 states during spring 2020. However, most states provided flexibility to school districts and local health authorities to decide how to balance in-person and online instruction in the fall. As of mid-September, 73 percent of the 100 largest school districts were online only. Four states required their schools return to some form of in-person instruction as did four states again in 2021. As of 27 January 2021, nine of the country's 20 largest school districts were teaching only online, eight were fully in person, and three combined online and in-person instruction.

Overall, the United States managed COVID-19's third wave very poorly. During and after his re-election campaign, Trump virtually ignored the pandemic. States responded diversely, although, again, Democratic governors reimposed mild to severe SAHOs and mask mandates, while Republican governors took slower and less stringent action. Even while, for example, COVID-19 cases and deaths soared in South Dakota in November to the point where the state had the nation's sixth highest death rate by 31 January 2021, its Republican governor justified her refusal to issue a mask-wearing mandate as a vindication of personal freedom.

24.4 Transformations in COVID-19 and federalism

There has been no transformation in the practice of US federalism. There was an acute failure of cooperative federalism, which would have delivered a better pandemic response, but President-elect Joseph Biden will likely seek to institute a more cooperative federalist approach. System resilience was reflected in the ability of states to respond unilaterally with sweeping authority that closed much of the nation's economy. The imposition of statewide SAHOs was unprecedented in US history. It appears that SAHOs were blunt instruments, however, and that more targeted responses might prevail in the future.

Two potential developments might accelerate centralization. First, Democrats captured the White House and Congress in the 2020 elections. They will likely increase federal authority over pandemic responses. Because Americans expect the federal government to play a large role in responding to crises such as COVID-19, centralization will be aided by widespread public disapproval of ex-President Trump's and the federal government's COVID-19 management. Second, federal and state courts may curb states' SAHO authority on civil liberties grounds. This is emerging as a major litigation objective of various religious groups and civil libertarians.

However, increased centralization will likely intensify partisan polarization that could generate even more intergovernmental conflict during another pandemic. Polarization between Democratic and Republican elites and citizens has been the overwhelmingly predominant factor in the US federal system's poor response to COVID-19. Scholars have long noted the importance of parties in shaping federalism (Detterbeck, Renzsch and Kincaid 2015), and the US pandemic case starkly highlights this finding. Bipartisan cooperation is a necessary, if not sufficient, condition for cooperative federalism; consequently, the persistence of partisan polarization will hobble the ability of the federal system to respond more effectively to future domestic crises, including another pandemic.

Bibliography

Adamczyk, A., 2020. This is the Average Unemployment Insurance Payment in Every U.S. State Without the Extra $600 in Federal Aid. *CNBC*, July 23. Available from: https://www.cnbc.com/2020/07/23/average-unemployment-insurance-payment-in-each-us-state.html

Arsova, P., 2020. Trump Calls Governors "Mutineers" for Creating Their Own Plans to Reopen the Economy. *LaCorte News*, 14 April. Available from: https://www.lacortenews.com/n/trump-claims-total-authority-to-reopen-economy

Associated Press-NORC Center for Public Affairs Research, 2020. *The August 2020 AP-NORC Center Poll.* Available from: https://apnorc.org/wp-content/uploads/2020/08/August-Topline-trump-1.pdf

Bender, M.C. and Ballhaus, R. B., 2020. How Trump Sowed Covid Supply Chaos: 'Try Getting It Yourselves'. *Wall Street Journal*, August 31. Available from: https://www.wsj.com/articles/how-trump-sowed-covid-supply-chaos-try-getting-it-yourselves-11598893051?mod=trending_now_pos3

Bowden, E., 2020. Trump Dismisses Bailouts for 'Poorly Run' States Led by Democrats. *New York Post*, April 27. Available from: https://nypost.com/2020/04/27/trump-derides-coronavirus-bailouts-for-poorly-run-democratic-states/

Brandtner, C., Bettencourt, L.M.A., Berman, M.G. and Stier, A.J., 10 August 2020. *Creatures of the State? Metropolitan Counties Compensated for State Inaction in Initial U.S. Response to Covid-19 Pandemic.* Mansueto Institute for Urban Innovation Research Paper, University of Chicago. Available from: http://dx.doi.org/10.2139/ssrn.3670927

Center for Budget and Policy Priorities, 2020. Needed: Federal Aid to Reverse Deep Public-Sector Job Cuts, Including in Education. *CBPP*, September 10. Available from: https://www.cbpp.org/blog/needed-federal-aid-to-reverse-deep-public-sector-job-cuts-including-in-education

Collins, C., 2020. *Property Tax Trends 2019 and 2020.* Cambridge: Lincoln Institute of Land Policy. Available from: https://www.lincolninst.edu/sites/default/files/pubfiles/property_tax_trends_report_2019-2020.pdf

Committee for a Responsible Federal Budget, 2020. "Update: COVID-Related State and Local Aid Will Total $280 Billion." 15 October. Available from: http://www.crfb.org/blogs/update-covid-related-state-local-aid-will-total-280-billion

Conway, D., 2019. Percentage of People with Public Health Insurance Up in 11 States, Down in Two. *Census.gov*, November 7. Available from: https://www.census.gov/library/stories/2019/11/state-by-state-health-insurance-coverage-2018.html

Davidson, N.M. and Haddow, K., 2020. State Preemption and Local Responses in the Pandemic. *American Constitution Society Expert Forum*, June 22. Available from: https://www.acslaw.org/expertforum/state-preemption-and-local-responses-in-the-pandemic/

Detterbeck, K., Wolfgang, R. and Kincaid, J., eds., 2015. *Political Parties and Civil Society in Federal Countries.* Don Mills: Oxford University Press.

Durr, S., 2020. Mayors to President Trump: Cities Need Direct Financial Assistance Now. *United States Conference of Mayors*, August 5. Available from: https://www.usmayors.org/2020/08/05/mayors-to-president-trump-cities-need-direct-financial-assistance-now/

Education Week, 2020. Map: Where Are Schools Closed? *Education Week*, September 18. Available from: https://www.edweek.org/ew/section/multimedia/map-covid-19-schools-open-closed.html

Einstein, K. L., Maxwell, P. and Fox, S., 2020. *COVID-19 Housing Policy.* Initiative on Cities, Boston University. Available from: https://www.bu.edu/ioc/files/2020/10/BU-COVID19-Housing-Policy-Report_Final-Oct-2020.pdf

Forgey, Q., 2020. 'We're Not a Shipping Clerk': Trump Tells Governors to Step up Efforts to Get Medical Supplies. *Politico*, 19 March. Available from: https://www.politico.com/news/2020/03/19/trump-governors-coronavirus-medical-supplies-137658

Henderson, T., 2020. 20 State Borrow from Feds to Pay Unemployment Benefits. *Stateline*, September 21. Available from: https://www.pewtrusts.org/en/research-and-analysis/blogs/stateline/2020/09/21/20-states-borrow-from-feds-to-pay-unemployment-benefits

Hogan, L., 2020. Governors of Maryland, Louisiana, Massachusetts, Michigan, Ohio and Virginia Announce Major Bipartisan Interstate Compact for Three Million Rapid Antigen Tests. *Maryland.gov*, August 4. Available from: https://governor.maryland.gov/2020/08/04/governors-of-maryland-louisiana-massachusetts-michigan-ohio-and-virginia-announce-major-bipartisan-interstate-compact-for-three-million-rapid-antigen-tests/

Kaiser Family Foundation, n.d. *Hospital Ownership by Type.* Available from: https://www.kff.org/other/state-indicator/hospitals-by-ownership/?currentTimeframe=0&sortModel=%7B%22colId%22:%22Location%22,%22sort%22:%22asc%22%7D [Accessed 1 September 2020].

Mallinson, D.J., 2020. Cooperation and Conflict in State and Local Innovation During COVID-19. *American Review of Public Administration*, 50 (6–7), 543–550. Mahler, J., 2020. In the Whirlwind. *New York Times Magazine*, 28 June, 20–29, 57.

Mann, B., 2020. Despite Mask Wars, Americans Support Aggressive Measures to Stop COVID-19, Poll Finds. *NPR Morning Edition*, August 4. Available from: https://www.npr.org/2020/08/04/898522180/despite-mask-wars-americans-support-aggressive-measures-to-stop-covid-19-poll-fi

McFarland, C. and Michael, A.P., 2020. *City Fiscal Conditions 2020*. Washington, DC: National League of Cities. Available from: https://www.nlc.org/resource/city-fiscal-conditions-2020

Mulvihill, G. and Fassett, C., 2020. Protective Gear for Medical Workers Begins to Run Low Again. *Associated Press*, July 7. Available from: https://apnews.com/481d933b0caa6f5fc61f466c86d4777b

National Conference of State Legislatures, 2020. Coronavirus (COVID-19): Revised State Revenue Projections. *NCSL*, September 10. Available from: https://www.ncsl.org/research/fiscal-policy/coronavirus-covid-19-state-budget-updates-and-revenue-projections637208306.aspx

National Governors Association, 2020. National Governors Association Outlines Need for 'Additional and Immediate' Fiscal Assistance to States. *National Governors Association*, April 11. Available from: https://www.nga.org/news/press-releases/national-governors-association-outlines-need-for-additional-and-immediate-fiscal-assistance-to-states/

National League of Cities, n.d. *COVID-19: Local Action Tracker*. Available from: https://covid19.nlc.org/resources/covid-19-local-action-tracker/

Newport, F., 2020. The Partisan Gap in Views of the Coronavirus. *Gallup*, May 15. Available from: https://news.gallup.com/opinion/polling-matters/311087/partisan-gap-views-coronavirus.aspx

Ritter, Z., 2020. Republicans Still Skeptical of COVID-19 Lethality. *Gallup*, May 26. Available from: https://news.gallup.com/poll/311408/republicans-skeptical-covid-lethality.aspx

Sheth, S., 2020. 'Try Getting It Yourselves': Trump Told Governors They're Responsible for Getting Their Own Medical Equipment to Treat Coronavirus Patients. *Business Insider*, 16 March. Available from: https://www.businessinsider.com/coronavirus-trump-told-governors-get-medical-equipment-on-their-own-2020-3

Tankersley, J., 2020. No Virus Deaths by Mid-May? White House Economists Say They Didn't Forecast Early End to Fatalities. *New York Times*, May 6. Available from: https://www.nytimes.com/2020/05/06/business/coronavirus-white-house-economists.html

Trump, D.J., 2020. Tweet. 27 April. Available from: https://twitter.com/realDonaldTrump/status/1251168994066944003?ref_src=twsrc%5Etfw%7Ctwcamp%5Etweetembed%7Ctwterm%5E1251168994066944003%7Ctwgr%5Eshare_3&ref_url=https%3A%2F%2Fwww.businessinsider.com%2Ftrump-tweets-to-liberate-michigan-minnesota-as-protesters-violate-orders-2020-4

U.S. Centers for Disease Control and Prevention, 2021. *Trends in Number of COVID-19 Cases and Deaths in the US Reported to CDC, by State/Territory*. Available from: https://covid.cdc.gov/covid-data-tracker/#trends_dailytrendscases

U.S. Department of Labor, May 2019. *Unemployment Compensation: Federal-State Partnership*. Available from: https://oui.doleta.gov/unemploy/pdf/partnership.pdf

Weber, L., Ungar, L., Smith, M. R., Recht, H. and Barry-Jester, A. M., 2020. Hollowed-Out Public Health System Faces More Cuts Amid Virus. *Kaiser Health News*, August 24. Available from: https://khn.org/news/us-public-health-system-underfunded-under-threat-faces-more-cuts-amid-covid-pandemic/

Wile, M., 2020. Congress Appropriates at Least $1.05 Billion to States, Territories, Tribes to Combat COVID-19. *National Conference of State Legislatures*, March 6. Available from: https://www.ncsl.org/blog/2020/03/06/congress-appropriates-at-least-105-billion-to-states-territories-tribes-to-combat-covid-19.aspx

25 The common response to COVID-19

The EU on the road toward de-crisisification?

Cristina Ares Castro-Conde

25.1 Introduction

The European Union (EU) is a unique federal arrangement. Since its establishment as a fully fledged political system by the Treaty of Maastricht in the early 1990s, it combines functional, intergovernmental, and federal features. These features vary and fluctuate across policy areas and over time. The shifting mixture of rationales for the EU – problem-solving and political – has characterized the entire process of European integration since its very inception as the European Coal and Steel Community in 1951. In the EU, political interests are based on a combination of national interests and the EU general interest.

Within the European Union, the distribution of powers is between the Member States and the supranational bodies of the EU. These supranational bodies are limited by two factors.

Firstly, EU institutions can only execute those competences explicitly transferred to them by the Member States in "the Treaties".[1]

There are three main types of EU competences:

1   **Exclusive competences**: trade, competition in the single market, and monetary issues for the euro area member countries, among others.
2   **Shared competences**: areas shared with the Member States – the most frequent type; as the economic union beyond monetary policy, economic, social, and territorial cohesion, and research.
3   **Supporting competences**: areas where the federal government supports Member States financially or administratively, i.e., health, education, and tourism.

Secondly, the principle of subsidiarity must be respected regarding powers that are not the exclusive competence of the EU. Subsidiarity in federalism means that decisions should be handled by the least centralized competent authority. The EU handles these matters under Article 5(3) of the Treaty of the European Union (TEU) and Protocol (No. 2).

Article 5(3) shows this clearly:

> under the principle of subsidiarity, in areas which do not fall within its exclusive competence, the Union shall act only if and in so far as the objectives of the proposed action cannot be sufficiently achieved by the Member States, either at central level or at regional and local level, but can rather, by reason of the scale or effects of the proposed action, be better achieved at Union level.

DOI: 10.4324/9781003251217-25

However, the EU fiscal capacity has been extraordinarily limited. Before the COVID-19 pandemic, the EU budget has represented 1 percent of the Gross National Income of all the EU Member States. Instead of constituting a tool to stimulate the economy, the common budget has been an instrument to back national public investments in infrastructures and knowledge that aims to foster a smarter allocation of national resources and better planning in most EU countries. The result has been that the application of the idea of solidarity, not just between richer and poorer social groups, but also between more and less capable Member States has been unworkable.

Yet fiscal solidarity will continue to be in need when the strategy of recovery will reach the end. Moreover,

> even in this emergency, with the creation of the Next Generation EU, the European budget has been temporarily expanded to only a little less than 2 percent of the EU GDP. In the US, by contrast, the federal budget is 21 percent of the US GDP.
>
> (Stiglitz 2020, p. 19)

Despite all this, EU bodies, above all the European Commission, have been affected by two factors: the "centralization of power induced by von der Leyen's strong

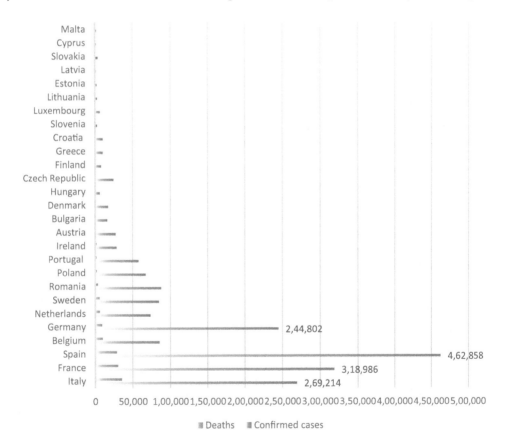

Figure 25.1 Confirmed Cases and Deaths Due to COVID-19 in the European Union*.
*EU27 confirmed cases: 1.924.458; EU27 deaths: 140.053 (On September 1, 2020).
Source: Author's own work with data issued by the Johns Hopkins University (Coronavirus Resource Center).

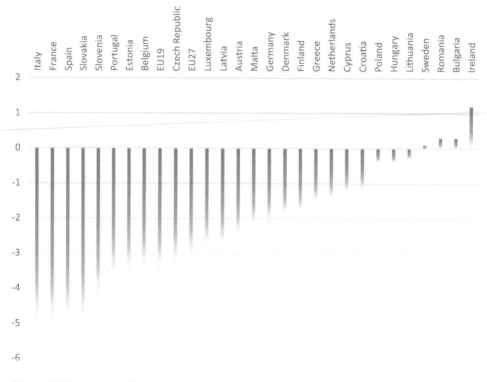

Figure 25.2 Economic Costs of COVID-19 in the European Union*.
* GDP growth in the first quarter of 2020: EU27, –3.2; EU19 (euro area member countries), –3.6.
Source: Author's own work with data issued by Eurostat.

presidential approach to crisis management" (Russack and Fenner 2020, p. 11) and the powers of the European Central Bank. Because of these factors, the EU has achieved success in responding to the COVID-19 pandemic, the main human and economic costs of which in the EU federal system are summarized in Figures 25.1 and 25.2. The reaction has demonstrated the capacity of the supranational institutions to learn from their own mistakes made during the "polycrises" of the 2010s, and it might point to a steady de-crisisification of EU policymaking.[2]

Moreover, it is worth highlighting that in response to the COVID-19 pandemic, "unlike during the economic and financial crisis, the community method was not replaced by intergovernmental action. Where formal decision-making was applied, the regular decision-making channels were used. Instead of circumventing, processes were accelerated" (Russak and Fenner 2020, p. 2).

Besides, due to their significance, this analysis emphasizes some EU pitfalls for crisis management, in comparison with other federal systems. This examination goes beyond the scope of the crisis coordination arrangements initiated by the Dutch Presidency of the Council in 2005. The Dutch Presidency included procedures for abbreviated decision-making, a crisis support team of experts, and financial resources for risk prevention (Rhinard 2019, pp. 619–620).

The "multilevel politics trap" (Zeitlin, Nicoli and Laffan 2019) must be mentioned. Mainstream country leaders still today tend to avoid uncertainty in bargaining on

Table 25.1 Key Statistics on COVID-19 in the European Union as of 10 January 2021

Cumulative Cases	Cumulative Cases per 100,000 Population	Cumulative Deaths	Cumulative Deaths per 100,000 Population	Case Fatality Percentage
17,292,252	3,892.5	373,777	84.1	2.2

Source: European Economic Forecast, Autumn 2020. Retrieved from: https://ec.europa.eu/info/sites/default/files/economy-finance/ip136_en_2.pdf

the supranational level to avoid national contestation from their Eurosceptic rivals. This adds a complicating factor into the "prisoner's dilemma" game that mainstream country leaders are forced into playing. Consequently, crucial policy decisions on sensitive areas or Treaty reform are postponed.

The gap that might emerge between the expectations of EU citizens and the delivery capacity of the supranational institutions at times of crisis may cause dissatisfaction with EU membership in several countries. There is also the fact of occasionally growing support for Eurosceptic parties and discourses to deal with as well. This is related to the fact that, in the EU, democratic legitimacy continues to rest to a great extent on a performance criterion. This is sometimes called "output legitimacy" or the ability to govern effectively. These days there is still a danger of country leaders ignoring "input legitimacy" which is "focused on citizens' attitudes toward and engagement in a political community along with the responsiveness of governments to citizens' political demands and concerns" (Schmidt 2015, p. 16) (Table 25.1).

25.2 Some enduring EU pitfalls for crisis management

In moving forward, the EU remains particularly unsuited to crisis management, for the following four reasons:

1 EU bodies can only act within competences transferred to them by the Member States.
2 EU bodies' policy solutions must fit within the EU budget.
3 EU bodies share power and have overlapping executive attributes with Member States.
4 There are many sources of EU leadership both supranational and national.

The EU is the sole organization of regional integration with autonomous supranational institutions. Regarding the legislative branch, the European Parliament – the only EU body whose members are directly elected (since 1979) – is like a house of representatives or house of commons, and the Council of the EU represents the Member States through their governments and is similar to a Senate. The European Parliament has been enormously empowered over time, especially by the last reform of "the Treaties" or the Lisbon Treaty (2009). However, the European Parliament continues to be weaker than the Council of the EU, on fiscal issues, among other relevant themes.

The Treaty of Lisbon put both chambers on an equal footing in terms of the annual budget of the EU. However, everything the EU undertakes must fit the multiannual financial framework (MFF) or the EU mid-term budgetary planning. The Lisbon Treaty did grant the European Parliament a veto right over the MFF, under a special legislative procedure called "consent." The same rationale, but under a more favorable formula for the Council, is applicable to reforming the EU budget revenues (the so-called "own resources system"), for which the procedure is also a special one referred to as "consultation." Hence, regarding EU revenues, the European Parliament holds a limited right to delay eventual changes prior to the Council's say. Indeed, for both the MFF and the own resources system, national governments have preserved their individual veto rights because all EU Council decisions must be unanimous.

Today, the basic structure of the EU legislative branch is straightforward, with an increasing balance between its two chambers, the European Parliament, and the Council of the EU. A third major EU body, the European Commission performs certain legislative functions as well, in terms of "delegated acts" at the implementation stage, under comitology (the scrutiny of its committees). However, this only works when the Commission has previously been granted these implementing powers in the text of a law passed by the legislators and is always subject to limits and the scrutiny of both chambers.[3]

Also, there is a fourth EU body that shares executive powers, the European Central Bank. That means the EU federal system divides its executive powers among the following bodies:

1   *European Council* (consisting of the 27 leaders of the Member States)
2   European Commission
3   European Central Bank
4   *Council of the European Union* (the second house of the European Union: It must approve legislation and consists of government ministers of each of the 27 Member States)

In addition, there is a consensus-based style of decision-making that characterizes the whole supranational setting. Such a complex system limits the visibility of "the opposition" on the EU level and poses a challenge for citizen control.

The EU has not suffered from a lack of leadership over time. But there are too many doors that can be opened, and behind each, you will find a potential leader. There

Table 25.2 Some Pitfalls of the European Union in Crisis Management

- **The nature of EU competences:** Supranational institutions cannot take actions beyond those competences transferred to them by the Member States in the Treaties, and the principle of subsidiarity has been applied strictly.
- **The reduced common fiscal capacity:** Until now, the total amount of own resources allocated to the Union could not exceed 1.20 percent of the sum of all the Member States' Gross National Income (GNI). The latest increase of the own resources ceiling to 2.00 percent of GNI is temporary. It will be decreased to 1.40 percent of GNI when the recovery fund for Europe comes to an end. Moreover, EU Member States have retained their individual veto rights over EU revenues.
- **Power-sharing on the EU level:** The European Commission, the European Central Bank, the EU Council, and the European Council share EU executive attributes with partial overlaps.
- **Numerous (hypothetical) sources of leadership:** Leaders include all presidents of the EU institutions, the German Chancellor, the French President, different groups of Member States, the leaders of the political groups in the European Parliament, among others.

Source: Author's own work and official data issued by the European Commission

are different presidents of EU bodies who have power in this system. These are the presidents of the European Commission, the European Central Bank, the European Council, the Council of the European Union (rotating among the Member States once every six months), among others. There are also the national leaders of France and Germany, as the EU's frontrunner Member States (Table 25.2).

25.3 What has been new in the EU response to the COVID-19 pandemic?

Compared to the past ten years of improvisations (Van Middelaar 2019), along with some other federal systems in spring 2020, the EU reacted quickly. The EU massively delivered as much support as possible for citizens and member countries.

There are three major differences in the EU response to the COVID-19 pandemic in comparison to its management of the Great Recession:

1   the speed of EU decision-making.
2   the separation of Germany from the group of Member States that is called "frugal four" (Austria, Denmark, the Netherlands, Sweden).
3   the return of the "ever closer union" formula in the EU-27 following the Brexit, as one of the options on the table at disposal to make progress (Table 25.3).

Moreover, in response to the COVID-19 pandemic, the institutions that make up the EU executive and legislative branches acted in a more harmonized manner than usual. In fact, the measures approved were connected to the working plan and the priorities for the current institutional cycle 2019–2024 that had been negotiated after the 2019 European election by the Commission, the European Parliament, and the European Council.

The genuine "game changer was the Franco-German proposal to distribute grants of € 500 billion to Member States in need" (Ladi and Tsarouhas 2020, p. 1049). A few days after this proposal, the Commission presented the Recovery plan 'Next Generation EU' with a budget of € 750 billion. The sequence of the intergovernmental and the supranational pushes was crucial. Certainly,

> the Franco-German proposal, followed by the Commission proposal, represents an instance of activism by policy entrepreneurs who sought to use the window of opportunity offered by the crisis. In doing so, they engaged in double loop learning, introducing a new organizational and normative dimension to economic governance.
>
> (Ladi and Tsarouhas 2020, p. 1051)

The EU behaved differently than it did during the former Euro area crisis. The Franco-German tandem bargained together from an early moment this time.

They did so partly because the German Chancellor Angela Merkel rapidly understood two things:

1   The concerns of her own automotive sector that "clamored for an Italian rescue to shore up their supply chains in Northern Italy as much as their sales across Europe" (Schmidt 2020, p. 1148).

Table 25.3 Core Economic Responses of the European Union to the COVID-19 Pandemic

---

EU budget

- **Immediate amendments to the EU 2020 budget:** €3.1 billion for medical supplies, testing kits, field hospitals, patient transfers for treatment in other Member States and repatriation of EU citizens; further amendments have been proposed by the European Commission (an additional €11.5 billion in 2020 to EU countries for repair and recovery).
- **Rapid redirection of cohesion funds:**
  - Coronavirus Response Investment Initiative, to support healthcare systems, medium-sized enterprises (SMEs) and labor markets, €37 billion.
  - Up to €28 billion of the 2014–2020 MFF not yet allocated to projects made available for the crisis response.
  - Up to €800 million from the EU Solidarity Fund for the hardest-hit Member States, by extending the scope of this instrument to public health crises.
  - Coronavirus Response Investment Initiative Plus (additional flexibility in the use of structural funds).
- **Three safety nets (€540 billion):**
  - **For workers:** temporary support to mitigate unemployment risks in an emergency (SURE) – loans to Member States of up to € 100 billion.
  - **For businesses:** €200 billion for a pan-European guarantee fund put in place by the European Investment Bank – loans for companies with a focus on small and medium-sized enterprises.
  - **For Member States:** Pandemic Crisis Support set up by the European Stability Mechanism – loans to euro area countries up to 2 percent of their GDP and a total of €240 billion.
- **Multiannual financial framework (MFF) for the years 2021–2027 and the EU's coronavirus recovery plan:**
  - **EU MFF 2021–2027** (€1,074.3 billion)
  - **Recovery plan "Next Generation EU"** (€750 billion)

Monetary policy
Pandemic emergency purchase program launched by the European Central Bank, €1,850 billion.

Competition policy and Economic union beyond monetary policy
Maximum flexibility in the application of EU rules on state aid measures and in general national public finances and fiscal policies to accommodate exceptional spending in order to support companies and citizens.

Source: Official data issued by the Council

2   The economic effects of the pandemic in Southern Europe could put at risk the stability of the Eurozone. Consequently, it was possible for France to break certain enduring German taboos, such as, allowing the European Commission to raise more financial resources on the markets as well as hugely extending EU common spending and grants.

Another element that facilitated the separation of Germany from the "frugal four" was the German Presidency of the Council from 1 July to 31 December 2020. This institutional position, which was conducted under the motto "Together for Europe's recovery," urged Germany to play the bridge-builder or honest broker role as well as to take more responsibility for the fate of the entire Union. Ultimately, Angela Merkel wanted to close her period as Chancellor prior to the 2021 German general election in the most determined way. And many would repeat the phrase "who but Angela Merkel's Germany, the EU's biggest economic power, could steer the EU through these rough seas?" (Koenig and Nguyen 2020, p. 1).

However, the ocean had too many sidewinds. Although all Member States wanted to compromise on two major issues – the still pending of approval MFF 2021–2017 and the new Recovery plan "Next Generation EU" – they all had different expectations.

In particular, the common negotiation position of the "frugal four" (Austria, Denmark, the Netherlands, Sweden) acted as a destabilizer during weeks due to its harsh opposition to some red lines drawn by other groups of countries. The red-liners included Southern Europe, or the Visegrad Group (Czech Republic, Hungary, Poland, Slovakia). In addition, the "frugal four" put too much emphasis on the digital agenda and new green issues, in detriment of the most traditional EU policies (i.e., the Common Agricultural Policy and cohesion policy). They also pushed for rule of law conditionality for states to receive recovery funds. Furthermore, the "frugal four" plus Finland felt uncomfortable about joint debt and new EU's own resources, and they preferred loans over grants to support recovery.

A clear example of the relevance of the honest broker role played by Germany during its last Presidency of the Council was the deal reached with Hungary and Poland on the rule of law conditionality regulation. Without any change on the agreement, the EU let the European Court of Justice rule on the mechanism before the Commission can use it.

Brexit was the third key novelty. The absence of the UK has diminished in practice the leeway of the "frugal four," and more particularly, Denmark's and Sweden's, countries that are not members of the Euro area. Without a doubt, Brexit has reduced the structural significance of the gap between Member States who are in the Euro area and those who are out.

The idea of flexible integration or country variations in EU membership was historically accepted as the last recourse for two problems:

1   Stubborn policy differences;
2   A means of formalizing relations with European countries outside the EU, such as Norway, Switzerland, or Turkey.

The elephant in the room had been the problem of accommodating British policy demands over time. Once the elephant had departed, things changed. The European Commission in 2017 had opened up the possibility of converting flexible integration into a generally acceptable alternative to the idea of "more Europe" for all EU countries. This suggestion was supported by France.

What is "more Europe"? It is the heart of the European integration process – instead of just the brain – as the Treaties never stopped to recognize. It can be read in the original functional (problem-solving) sense of more integration to complete and maintain the single market in good condition, but also according to the federal agenda. This interpretation means a greater concern about solidarity on the EU level, along with an enhanced role for the European Parliament, regional and local governments, and EU citizens.[4]

Besides, the achievement of some new advances toward a more federal Europe seems feasible today not just because of COVID-19 and Brexit but also due to the evolution of public opinion data. This took place after the end of the Great Recession. A more federal Europe emerged after the late maturing of some institutional changes introduced by the Lisbon Treaty – in particular, the empowerment of both the European and national Parliaments. The sum of all these dynamics is good news from a federal perspective when a conference on the future of Europe is about to be launched.

25.4 What must be improved in the EU to cope with crisis management?

Today "the decision-making machinery of the EU is multi-layered and has proven to be not only solid and resilient but also equipped to make speedy decisions and to modernize its way of working" (Russack and Fenner 2020, p. 13). However, horizontal coordination on the national level remains an Achilles' heel of the EU political system.

Bringing together EU countries about defining their spheres of power posed serious challenges in the first weeks of the pandemic. In those days,

> the EU looked uncoordinated with the disorganized adoption of lockdowns. The absence of exports of medical equipment from EU countries to Italy gave the impression that protectionism dominated the reaction of EU countries. The re-introduction of internal border controls and the suspension of the freedom of movement by 17 member states, with a complete lack of coordination was not a positive sign for European integration either.
>
> (Wolff and Ladi, 2020, p. 1027)

Since the Member States retain the power to decide on health, education, tourism, and other areas that are key during the pandemic, while the EU's role is just a supporting one on these domains, the reputation of the whole EU suffered.

In the health sector,

> when Covid-19 hit, the EU had two main governance frameworks through which it could organize its immediate response to the public health crisis. The first was the health security framework set up by the 2013 Decision on Serious Cross Border Threats to Health (herein the Health Threats Decision), which established a set of structures for emergency planning, preparedness, and response. The second was the Civil Protection Mechanism (CPM), which facilitates cooperation between Member States in the event of a disaster. Both performed as intended and expected in the first phase of the crisis but, reflecting the EU's limited health-related powers, their capacity and reach was inevitable insufficient.
>
> (Brooks and Geyer 2020, p. 1058)

In response to this, EU bodies decided to assume more responsibilities. Although transferring powers to them over these matters seemed unfeasible, there was quite a bit of support in most countries to empower EU institutions in relation to health. Some national data, however, indicated reluctance (see Figure 25.3).

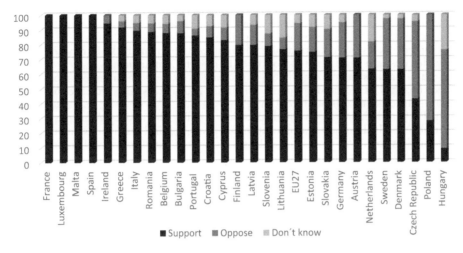

Figure 25.3 EU Member States that Support a Common European Public Health Policy.
Source: Author's own work, with data provided by the European Council on Foreign Relations.
Available from: https://ecfr.eu/special/eucoalitionexplorer/coronavirus_special/ [Accessed 1 April 2021].

Under the scope of the EU's legal basis for health, internally, the European Commission made the utmost effort to act coordinately. For instance, the European Commission began

> by creating the Covid-19 Clearing House for medical equipment within the Secretariat-General. The Clearing House, established by the Commission on the mandate of the European Council, serves to monitor and coordinate developments in Europe's supply chain of personal protective equipment (PPE), medical devices and medicines.
>
> (Russak and Fenner 2020, p. 11)

Furthermore, the Commission demonstrated great ambition with several new initiatives, which included the resourceful EU4Health Programme that will stay on the post-COVID-19 EU health agenda. This initiative will reinforce the European Centre for Disease Prevention and Control and the European Medicines Agency, make medicines accessible, deal with cross-border health threats, and support health systems. The approaching Conference on the Future of Europe will also incorporate a discussion on the future of health.

To gain capacity of response in future health emergencies, the EU bodies must put an end to Member States dependency from third countries concerning goods and services that are essential for the functioning of their public health systems. For a start, common stocks must be generated, and joint supply chains spread. Every effort should be made to strengthen medical research along with cyber security and technology development both on the national and the EU levels.

In addition, regarding communication measures on the EU level, one available solution for preserving the image of the supranational institutions would be better

Table 25.4 Possible Steps to Cope with Crisis Management in the European Union

• EU institutions should improve coordination among their communication policies. They might delegate a single spokesperson for all press conferences.
• EU bodies must stop competing with one another. In particular, the European Council should constrain itself a bit in favor of the European Commission.
• Parliamentarians and citizens should participate more. Federalism implies more politics and enhanced participation of parliamentarians and citizens. This step goes beyond transparency standards on the EU level.
• The EU must hold more political discussions on policy alternatives. All mainstream Members of the European Parliament should foster political discussions on policy alternatives about the areas affected by the COVID-19 pandemic as well as any other theme on the EU's policy portfolio.

Source: Author's own work

coordination among the communication policies of the different EU bodies. A single EU spokesperson on COVID-19 might be named. This person could systematically be the president of the European Commission.

Likewise, from a federal perspective, the EU must cultivate the democratic standards of supranational decision-making on the input side. The European Parliament should increase the visibility of the policy alternatives that are accessible to respond to the threats posed by the pandemic. This response should be geared to the general interest of the Union instead of national interests. In contrast, the prominence that the European Council acquired regarding the EU response to COVID-19 at least in spring 2020 is problematic from a federal point of view. Policy solutions were mostly framed according to individual Member States' interests, along with intergovernmental alliances. The old-style strategy of self-empowering by the European Parliament did not help much promote the interests of the EU as defined from diverse ideological positions (Table 25.4).

Notes

1 The expression "the Treaties" refers to the Treaty on the EU (TEU) and the Treaty establishing the European Community, the name of which was changed to the 'Treaty on the Functioning of the EU' (TFEU) in December 2009, following the entry into force of the Treaty of Lisbon.
2 The expression "de-crisisification of EU policy-making" is a word game that refers to a well-known article entitled "The Crisisification of Policy-making in the EU" (Rhinard 2019).
3 The term "comitology" refers to the procedures through which the European Commission, with the participation of national representatives, exercises the implementing powers eventually conferred on it by the European Parliament and the Council of the EU, following Article 291 TFUE. This article states that:

> (1). Member States shall adopt all measures of national law necessary to implement legally binding Union acts. (2). Where uniform conditions for implementing legally binding Union acts are needed, those acts shall confer implementing powers on the Commission, or, in duly justified specific cases and in the cases provided for in Articles 24 and 26 of the TEU, on the Council. (3). For the purposes of paragraph 2, the European Parliament and the Council, acting by means of regulations in accordance with the ordinary legislative procedure, shall lay down in advance the rules and general principles concerning mechanisms for control by Member States of the Commission''s

exercise of implementing powers. (4). The word 'implementing' shall be inserted in the title of implementing acts.

4 Article 1 TEU states that "this Treaty marks a new stage in the process of creating an ever-closer union among the peoples of Europe in which decisions are taken as openly as possible and as closely as possible to the citizen."

Bibliography

Brooks, E. and Geyer, R., 2020. The Development of EU Health Policy and the Covid-19 Pandemic: Trends and Implications. *Journal of European Integration*, 42 (8), 1057–1076. doi: 10.1080/07036337.2020.1853718.

European Commission, 2017. White Paper on the Future of Europe. Reflections and scenarios for the EU27 by 2025 [COM(2017)2025 of 1 March].

European Commission Website, 2021. *EU Budget Own Resources*. Available from: https://ec.europa.eu/info/strategy/eu-budget/long-term-eu-budget/2014-2020/revenue/own-resources_en#own_res [Accessed 18 February 2021].

European Council on Foreign Relations, 2020. Coronavirus Special. EU Expert Survey on European Cooperation during the Coronavirus Crisis (from 4 to 25 May 2020). Available from: https://www.ecfr.eu/eucoalitionexplorer/coronavirus [Accessed 5 April 2021].

Koenig, N. and Nguyen, T., 2020. *Five Takeaways from the German "Corona Presidency."* Policy Brief, Jacques Delors Centre/Hertie School, 15 December. Available from: https://www.delorscentre.eu/en/publications/detail/publication/five-takeaways-from-the-german-corona-presidency [Accessed 5 April 2021].

Ladi, S. and Tsarouhas, D., 2020. EU Economic Governance and Covid-19: Policy Learning and Window of Opportunity. *Journal of European Integration*, 42 (8), 1041–1056. doi: 10.1080/07036337.2020.1852231.

Rhinard, M., 2019. The Crisisification of Policy-Making in the European Union. *Journal of Common Market Studies*, 57 (3): 616–633. doi: 10.1111/jcms.12838.

Russack, S. and Fenner, D., 2020. Crisis Decision-Making. How Covid-19 Has Changed the Working Methods of the EU Institutions. CEPS Policy Insights, Number 17/July.

Schmidt, V.A., 2015. *The Eurozone's Crisis of Democratic Legitimacy: Can the EU Rebuild Public Trust and Support for European Economic Integration?* European Economy Discussion Papers, Number 15/September. Directorate-General for Economic and Financial Affairs of the European Commission. doi: 10.2765/5015 (online).

Schmidt, V.A., 2020. Theorizing Institutional Change and Governance in European Responses to the Covid-19 Pandemic. *Journal of European Integration*, 42 (8), 1177–1193. doi: 10.1080/07036337.2020.1853121.

Stiglitz, J.E., 2020. *Recovering from the Pandemic: An Appraisal of Lessons Learned*. FEPS COVID RESPONSE PAPERS, Number 10/October.

Van Middelaar, L., 2019. *Alarums and Excursions: Improvising Politics on the European Stage*. Newcastle upon Tyne: Agenda Publishing.

Wolff, S. and Ladi, S., 2020. European Union Responses to the Covid-19 Pandemic: Adaptability in Times of Permanent Emergency. *Journal of European Integration*, 42 (8), 1025–1040. doi: 10.1080/07036337.2020.1853120.

Zeitlin, J., Nicoli, F. and Laffan, B., 2019. Introduction: The European Union beyond the Polycrisis? Integration and Politicization in an Age of Shifting Cleavages. *Journal of European Public Policy*, 26 (7), 963–976. doi: 10.1080/13501763.2019.1619803.

26 The relative performance of federal and non-federal countries during the pandemic

David Cameron

26.1 Introduction

The story of COVID-19 can be divided into two broad, overlapping phases. The first phase covers the period from the initial outbreak of the pandemic at the beginning of 2020 until about January 2021. That is the time when – without a preventive vaccine – the world struggled to contain its spread and to provide health care to those who fell ill. The second phase of the story starts in early 2021, when effective vaccines began to be manufactured and administered to national populations. Assessing the performance of a country in the first phase focuses on how well the infection was contained and how many people lost their lives to the disease. Assessing performance in the second phase will continue to involve assessing infection-containment and death-reduction measures, but will in addition entail an evaluation of how effectively vaccinations were administered to a country's population.[1] This chapter restricts itself to examining performance in the first phase.

How well have federations performed in comparison with non-federal countries? Is there any evidence to suggest that federations have handled the coronavirus crisis better or worse, or differently from unitary states? It is this matter that I propose to discuss in this chapter.

A pandemic is an acid test of the relationship between citizens and their governments, particularly in democracies. It can be compared to the total mobilization of civil society that was mounted in the United Kingdom, the United States, Canada and elsewhere during the Second World War, when governments made it clear that victory could only be achieved if every citizen played an active role in the war effort. In the COVID-19 pandemic, it was manifestly true that citizens who did not wear masks, maintain social distance, and avoid travel were putting themselves and society in mortal danger. Rarely has the link between individual behavior and collective well-being been more directly drawn. Governments at all levels attempted to strike the right balance between education, exhortation, peer pressure, and coercion for optimal response to the crisis.

In this chapter, we will be scrutinizing how the pandemic was managed, not how the economy was supported or how the balance was struck between the two. Balancing the conflicting pressures of public health and the economy is an inescapable part of the responsibility of all governments coping with the pandemic, but that is not as such the focus of this chapter. How effective have the public health and medical responses to the virus been? That is the question. Clearly, the economic pressures may have led governments to close down too late or open up too soon. If those policy

DOI: 10.4324/9781003251217-26

choices have affected the performance of governments and populations in managing the pandemic, that will be reflected in the health outcomes, but the economy as such does not fall within the purview of this chapter.

26.2 COVID-19 in OECD countries

For purposes of economy of effort, and to achieve at least to some degree an apples-to-apples comparison, the chapter will concentrate on Organisation for Economic Co-operation and Development (OECD) member countries. Member states are understood to adhere to two fundamental principles: they are expected to be democratic societies committed to the rule of law and the protection of human rights; and they are meant to have open, transparent, free-market economies. In some cases – such as Turkey, which is an OECD member listed as 'not free' in the 2020 Freedom House index – these commitments appear today to be more aspirational than actual, but nevertheless OECD countries do collectively constitute a grouping of states generally exhibiting these characteristics.[2] In addition, OECD members are typically wealthier countries with more fully articulated economies and societies.[3] Restricting our detailed analysis to this group reduces somewhat the range of variables one would otherwise have to consider and makes for a more manageable analytical exercise.

Nine of the 35 OECD members we are considering here[4] are federations: Australia, Austria, Belgium, Canada, Germany, Mexico, Spain, Switzerland, and the United States of America. This offers a good range of federations of different types – with parliamentary and congressional systems, monarchical and republican forms, large and relatively small populations, and national and multinational social composition.

To assess the pandemic performance of the countries we are studying, we will use two rough and ready indicators.

- Number of COVID-19 cases per million population
- Number of COVID-19 deaths per million population

These two ratios offer at best a very rough guide to relative performance. The first, in particular, needs to be treated with great caution, given that an accurate assessment of the number of cases occurring in a country depends to a substantial degree on testing, as well as the nature of the system of testing and the extent of its use. Moreover, record-keeping and reporting capacity vary widely from one country to another (Hasell, Mathieu and Beltekian 2020). While there may be some data complexities associated with reporting on COVID-19 deaths per million, we assume those data are generally more reliable and comparable, and we will give priority to this indicator, using it to provide a rough ranking of country-by-country performance.

Table 26.1 reports the pandemic performance of OECD countries as of January 2021 against these two indicators. The primary ranking in the right-hand column indicates their rates of COVID-19 deaths per million of population. In the middle column, reporting on the number of cases per million of population, we indicate in brackets the relative ranking of the countries according to that indicator. OECD countries that are federal are noted by capital letters.

The first thing to note is that the nine federations (of the 35 OECD countries listed here) are arrayed up and down the scale from the top to the bottom. Australia is one

Table 26.1 COVID-19 Case and Death Rates in OECD Countries as of January 2021

Countries (Federal Countries in Capital Letters)	Cases per Million (Rank Order Indicated in Bracketed Number)	Deaths per Million (Rank Order Indicated in Bracketed Number)
New Zealand	474 (1)	5 (1)
South Korea	1,473 (3)	26 (2)
AUSTRALIA	1,129 (2)	36 (3)
Japan	2,899 (4)	39 (4)
Norway	11,267 (6)	102 (5)
Finland	7,685 (5)	114 (6)
Estonia	30,693 (12)	267 (7)
Turkey	28,808 (11)	295 (8)
Denmark	33,609 (14)	328 (9)
Israel	69,020 (31)	469 (10)
CANADA	19,926 (9)	492 (11)
Greece	14,581 (8)	520 (12)
Latvia	32,344 (13)	553 (13)
Ireland	37,983 (17)	570 (14)
GERMANY	25,635 (10)	612 (15)
Slovakia	43,313 (21)	697 (16)
Netherlands	55,380 (26)	764 (17)
AUSTRIA	44,936 (22)	821 (18)
Poland	38,985 (18)	910 (19)
Lithuania	64,881 (30)	916 (20)
Chile	36,572 (15)	934 (21)
Portugal	62,392 (29)	943 (22)
Colombia	39,610 (19)	997 (23)
SWITZERLAND	58,845 (27)	1046 (24)
France	46,640 (23)	1060 (25)
Sweden	54,179 (25A)	1062 (26)
MEXICO	13,675 (7)	1132 (27)
SPAIN	54,179 (25B)	1169 (28)
Hungary	37, 222 (16)	1199 (29)
UNITED STATES	76,243 (33)	1244 (30)
Italy	40,800 (20)	1396 (31)
Czech Republic	87,554 (34)	1403 (32)
United Kingdom	53, 729 (24)	1412 (33)
Slovenia	75,919 (32)	1573 (34)
BELGIUM	59, 582 (28)	1796 (35)

Source for case rates as of 24 January 2021: KFF COVID-19 Coronavirus Data Table by Country. Available from: https://www.kff.org/coronavirus-covid-19/fact-sheet/coronavirus-tracker/?utm_source=web&utm_medium=trending&utm_campaign=covid-19; KFF's data sources are: Johns Hopkins University's Coronavirus Resource Center's COVID-19 map; WHO's Coronavirus Disease (COVID-19) situation reports. As we pointed out in footnote 4, we have excluded OECD countries with less than a million population (Iceland and Luxembourg). Source for death rates as of January 22, 2021: Statista; Statista's sources: Johns Hopkins University (CSSE); World Bank; Insee. The numbers are rounded. Available from: https://www.statista.com/statistics/1104709/coronavirus-deaths-worldwide-per-million-inhabitants/ [Accessed 6 April 2021].

of the OECD's best performers, coming in third in deaths per million and second in cases per million. On the other hand, the federation of Belgium is at the bottom in 35th and final place for deaths per million, with the United States not far behind in position 30. The other six OECD federations are scattered between with no clear pattern, except perhaps for a very slight skewing toward the lower end of the ranking.

As for the performance of non-federal OECD countries, there is a similar spread. Four of the top five performers are non-federal (New Zealand, South Korea, Japan, and Norway). Equally, four of the five poorest performers are non-federal (Slovenia, United Kingdom, Czech Republic, and Italy).[5] Given that 26 of the 35 countries on the list are non-federal, it is perhaps not surprising to find them well represented at both the top and bottom of the ranking as well as in between.

26.3 The best and the worst

We will now examine in more detail those countries which find themselves either at the top of the list or the bottom.

We will begin by examining some of the poorest performers at the bottom of our list in Table 26.1. As we have noted, the country with the highest rate of deaths per million is a federation, the Kingdom of Belgium. It exemplifies to a high degree the link between governance and pandemic performance, although one would have to acknowledge as well that it is not aided by geography. Belgium is embedded in Europe, sharing a border with the Netherlands, Germany, Luxembourg, and France; its largest city, Brussels, is the de facto capital of the European Union, making it a destination for people from all over the continent.

With a society starkly divided between the French-speaking Walloons and the Dutch-speaking Flemish (plus a small German-speaking minority), the country began as a unitary state, but has been federalizing through a series of constitutional reforms that began in 1970. These alterations in the constitutional makeup of the country have not expressed a coherent design, but have been a series of decentralizing ad hoc arrangements reflecting the political and partisan pressures of the day (Bursens, Popelier and Meier 2021). The result has been a unique and highly complex federation composed of two imperfectly overlapping sets of units: three linguistically defined communities (Dutch, French, and German-speaking); and three territorially defined regions (Flanders, Wallonia, and the Brussels region). There are two distinct party systems, one for each major language community. When the pandemic struck, Belgium had been living under a caretaker government for a year, which was then hastily upgraded to full governing status in response to the crisis.

Theoretically, one might have expected that a small (11.5 million population), prosperous country with a highly developed health and social service sector would perform well in combating the coronavirus. However, Belgium did not do well, and the chief reason why seems to be lie primarily in its governance model.[6] The recurrent difficulty the country has had in forming an effective federal government suggests an institutional deficiency, and the confused scattering of jurisdictional responsibilities has made decisive action difficult. For this system to work well, an unusually high degree of coordination and a considerable capacity for intergovernmental collaboration would be necessary, and these have been notably lacking during the crisis. In addition, competition between parties representing different communities undermined the potential for coherent action and blunted or confused the pandemic policy response. Beneath the Belgian governance model lies a deeply divided society, which has driven the transformation of the country from a unitary to a federal regime. That being said, there are other federal states with deep ethnocultural differentiation that have fared better. Canada, in 11th place in deaths per million, and Switzerland in 24th position provide examples of that. Belgium's institutional structure, then – itself the expression of a deeply divided society – appears to lie at the heart of its difficulties.

The United States of America is sixth from the bottom in the OECD rankings and put in the second poorest showing among federal countries. As a rich and powerful country with a federal system offering a significant leadership and coordination role to the federal government, one might have expected the United States to be one of the highest performing federations on the list. It scored first in the Global Health Security Index in its capacity to respond to pandemics. That it did not perform as expected is chiefly the result of an abysmal failure of leadership at the national level and a partisan divide that is as evident throughout the American public-health system as it is elsewhere in US governance and society.

Former President Trump questioned and actively cast doubt on the seriousness of COVID-19 and the need to take public-health measures to combat it; as a result, the states were left to their own devices to a much greater extent than would otherwise have been the case.[7] Trump downplayed the coronavirus, contradicted his senior public-health officials, encouraged the early re-opening of the economy, and asserted that the states have the primary responsibility to combat COVID-19 and to secure the personal protective equipment (PPE) they need. His abdication of national leadership fostered a confused national response to the crisis, which encouraged a patchwork of state policies and approaches, and contributed substantially to the poor performance of the United States in combating the disease (Camacho and Glickman 2020).

It might be said that Trump inadvertently activated American federalism by his conduct. After all, while US analysts and commentators tend to pay little attention to federalism in comparison with their counterparts in other federal countries, the US states in reality had and have an indispensable constitutional role to play in confronting a public-health crisis. State governors were responsible for many of the things that really mattered in the pandemic – like whether shops would remain open, masks had to be worn, or beaches were off limits. As the virus raged across the country, it revealed just how crucial the sub-national units in the US federation are in shaping a coherent and effective pandemic response. But it brought home another point as well: that the absence of leadership from Washington undermined not only the fashioning of an effective federal response to the virus, but the effectiveness of state-level action as well. The President is the national tone-setter; his denials licensed many citizens and some political leaders across the country to contest the science and reject the public-health advice. And Washington's abdication of its national coordination role fostered at times mutually destructive behavior among the states, manifest for example, in the desperate competition for public-health supplies. The lesson from this experience is that federalism *does* matter in a public-health crisis, but that the states cannot do their job effectively if Washington does not play its part.

The often-toxic partisan division amplified the incoherence of the nation's response. There was conflict and disagreement about the size of aid packages, support for state and local governments, locking down and opening up, and mask wearing. Federal-state and state-local quarrels often reflected the partisan composition of the senior government actors (Kincaid and Leckrone 2021). These conflicts offered opportunities for skeptical Americans to contest the seriousness of the virus and for some to turn the refusal to wear masks into a partisan badge of liberty. The fragmented, partly public, partly private US health care system added to the mix. At the time of writing – March 2021 – the United States leads the world in the total number of cases and deaths from the coronavirus (Johns Hopkins University Coronavirus Resource Center 2021). On the evidence, this overall approach has proven to be a highly ineffective way of managing the pandemic.

What of poorly performing unitary countries? At or near the bottom of our list are Slovenia, the United Kingdom, the Czech Republic, and Italy. Given their size and significant position in Europe, we will focus our attention in this chapter on the United Kingdom and Italy. The Czech Republic will also be discussed very briefly.

Italy was the first country in Europe to face a major outbreak of the coronavirus. Thus, other countries in the region had the opportunity to learn from Italy's early COVID-19 experience. Thirty-fifth in the Global Health Index of pandemic preparedness, Italy did not start from a strong institutional position. Outbreaks in Italy were concentrated regionally (in the Lombardy, Emilia-Romagna, and Veneto regions in northern Italy), which placed acute strain on the local health institutions. Italy's population is the most elderly in Europe and, in contrast to the impact of the pandemic in some other European countries such as Germany, older Italians were the demographic most severely affected in the early phases. Italians have a relatively high rate of co-morbidities, and the median age of people dying from COVID-19 in Italy was 80 years. While Italy has a high functioning health care system, it is under-endowed with ICU beds, as compared to other countries; when people with mild symptoms were admitted to the hospitals in the early going, capacity was strained, making it a challenge to accommodate the really ill. Over-crowded hospitals then became incubators of infection leading to high infection rates for medical personnel.[8]

Italy's response to the crisis involved: the imposition of a quarantine to control the spread of the pandemic; the expansion of over-stretched medical facilities; and, as elsewhere, financial measures to support the failing economy (Nicola 2020). The relatively decentralized, 'federal country without federalism' system did not prove itself to be an effective instrument for addressing the pandemic (Palermo 2021). Italy's regions have grown more powerful in the 50 years since they were put in place, and – despite having primary responsibility for health care – the onset of the first wave of the pandemic led to a centralization of Italy's response.

The national government declared a state of emergency at the end of January 2020, setting the stage for implementing a set of regulations that applied throughout the country, whatever variation in concrete circumstances there may have been. National collaboration with regional governments was relatively limited. Contrary to the response in several explicitly federal systems, Francesco Palermo (2021) notes that the main instrument for managing intergovernmental relations in Italy, the Standing Conference Between the States and the Regions, actually met *less* frequently during this period than in normal times. As Palermo (2021) writes:

> After a first phase of extreme centralization, the regions (and to some extent the municipalities) gradually resumed their functions. The asymmetric impact of the virus and the equally asymmetric response by the territories revealed both the potential of such an asymmetric territorial governance and the weaknesses of an incomplete, quasi-federal system, especially as far as unclear division of powers and insufficient intergovernmental relations (IGR) are concerned.

When infections began dropping in spring, the regional governments began to assert themselves, which led to more differentiation and greater collaboration. However, confusion about roles did not abate, partly because a more limited national emergency regime continued, and tensions, sometimes political, between state and region re-surfaced.

Italy has a long tradition of short-lived coalition governments, and the tensions between political parties continued during the pandemic. Indeed, toward the end of January 2021, the government of the popular Prime Minister Giuseppe Conte collapsed after a minor party pulled out of the governing coalition.[9] Thus, Italy is struggling with political instability while still in the midst of the coronavirus crisis, making it more difficult for timely and effective measures to be implemented. Italy's indifferent performance, then, cannot be explained by any simple measure, but appears to be the product of a mixture of several factors, including bad luck and initial unfamiliarity with the disease, demography, the particular character of the country's health care system, and governance.

The United Kingdom entered the pandemic well positioned to address the challenges of COVID-19 effectively. Britain possessed strong public institutions and had recently elected a strong majority government in Westminster; in the National Health Service (NHS), it had an enviable public health system and came second after the United States in the Global Health Security Index for pandemic preparedness. Yet it sits third from bottom in the table, recording the worst performance among G7 countries, and the third highest number of COVID-19 deaths per million on our OECD list. Why is that?

Britain has devolved significant authority in health matters to the three 'home nations' of Scotland, Wales, and Northern Ireland, but with relatively little autonomous fiscal authority. This meant that the country, faced with the sudden shock of the pandemic, looked naturally to London for leadership. UK performance in the early going, then, was determined by decisions being taken by the UK government, rather than by the Scottish or Welsh governments or the Northern Ireland Assembly, and with relatively little intergovernmental collaboration. The UK government spoke of there being three phases or elements in the policy: containment (handwashing, contact tracing, etc.); delay (flattening the curve so as to not overwhelm the NHS and developing therapies and vaccines); and mitigation (protecting the most vulnerable, but letting the population at large gradually build up herd immunity). This strategy precluded early decisive measures to stop the spread of the virus. The strong public reaction to this approach led to the government rapidly shifting its policy to the suppression of the virus and its transmission with a series of increasingly stringent measures (Calnan 2020). Willing to follow the UK government in the beginning, the devolved governments became increasingly restive as time went on, frustrated by the policy lurches and U-turns. They began to set a more autonomous course, particularly with respect to the regulation of school closures and the easing of pandemic measures. All in all, in the judgment of one observer, while the National Health Service performed very well, "the management of COVID-19 in the UK has been a disaster" (Grace 2021). There is little to suggest that devolution is the culprit responsible for the UK's poor performance; instead, it seems to have been national political leadership and policy making that has most significantly shaped the United Kingdom's low ranking. Indeed, it might be hypothesized that greater devolution might have led to better results. Interestingly, Clive Grace in this volume has made the case that the likely result of Britain's pandemic experience will be to strengthen the push for greater devolution and 'federalisation' of the country, clearly not an outcome that the British government, already struggling with the fissiparous impact of Brexit, would welcome.

Before turning to a discussion of a number of high-performing countries, let me note the experience of the Czech Republic. We have seen that fighting the pandemic is closer to a marathon than a 100-yard dash, and that countries which perform well at one point in the process can falter at another. Both the United States and the United Kingdom delivered poor results in the first stage when the issue was controlling the spread of the virus, but have subsequently been global leaders in the administration of COVID-19 vaccines to their citizenry. As of 3 March 2021, Britain and the United States rank second and third among OECD countries for the number of vaccine doses administered per 100 people (OECD, 9 March 2021). The Czech Republic offers another example of variable performance in the long course of coping with the disease. One of the top performers in the first phase of the virus, through a series of mistakes the country now finds itself struggling desperately to gain control of runaway infections in the country. Rastislav Madar, a Czech epidemiologist, identifies three critical decisions in particular that the government got wrong. First the government – spurning the advice of its scientific advisors – refused to reinstate the mask-wearing mandate in the summer of 2020, just before the schools reopened. Second, after a surge of infections in October resulting largely from people not wearing masks, the government – not following its own guidelines – decided to reopen shops just before Christmas. And third, it failed to act quickly in response to the emergence of the British variant which became an increasingly important part of the post-Christmas rise in infections in January. The result is that, as of March 2021, the Czech infection rate is close to record levels, just as the number of global infections is starting to drop (Kattasova 2021).

I will turn now to the best performing countries. It is notable that three of the top four performers (New Zealand, Australia, and Japan) are island countries, and the fourth – South Korea – is bordered on three sides by water and in the north by a hard border with the hermit kingdom of North Korea. Does their geographical status make any difference with respect to pandemic control? If one compares these countries with others such as Belgium, Slovenia, the Czech Republic, or Hungary, which are physically embedded in a complex network of abutting states, one would have to acknowledge, I think, that the island or quasi-island status of the countries at the top of the OECD list is at least a facilitating condition in terms of managing a highly infectious virus. Physical contiguity with other nations and a porous land border make national isolation difficult. Imagine Belgium, seeking – through aggressive isolation from its neighbors – to pursue the same policy goal of zero COVID-19 outbreaks as New Zealand. That would seem difficult or impossible to achieve, not only because of Belgium's geographical situation, but because of its status as the de facto capital of the European Union. While I have suggested it is a facilitating condition, it would be a mistake to over-emphasize simple geographical location and specifically insularity. The United Kingdom, after all, is an island country as well, and, as we have seen, it is near the bottom of the list.

Population size and density have also been mentioned as relevant factors. The thought is that a small country will be able to marshal its citizens and manage its policy response more readily than a large country, and that an infectious disease will obviously find it easier to spread in a dense than in a dispersed population. But again, these are very far from being determining factors in successful pandemic control. True enough, New Zealand, the top performer, has a small and relatively dispersed population of just under 5 million with a density of 18 people per square kilometer. Australia, our highest achiever among federations, is a continent-sized island, with vast stretches of unpopulated territory. However, over 80 percent of its citizens live in urban settings, some of them fairly large: Sydney and Melbourne each have a population of just under 5 million people. The population density of Australia's two largest cities, though, is low. On the other hand, Japan, a geographically small country, has a large population of 126 million and a national population density ratio of 347 people per square kilometer. Its cities and mega-cities are highly crowded. These demographic realities, however, have not kept it from being the fourth highest OECD performer. While South Korea's population of 52 million is less than half the size of Japan's, its population density is even higher than Japan's at 510 people per square kilometer. Seoul has just under 10 million residents with a population density almost twice that of New York City. Yet South Korea is a top performer.

What then explains high performance? We will start by examining the case of New Zealand, which comes in first in having the lowest number of cases and number of deaths per million population. New Zealand has managed to stop the virus in its tracks; for months at a time, it has been completely virus-free (Baker, Kvalsvig and Verrall 2020). When an outbreak has occurred, they have managed to snuff it out. How so? It was by no means a foregone conclusion at the beginning that the country would bring the virus to its knees. At 35, New Zealand ranked lower than Italy in its preparation for a pandemic according to the Global Health Security Index, and much of the public health advice at the time was directed more at control than total elimination. However, a vigorous debate occurred at the early stages about which strategy to pursue. Prime Minister Jacinda Ardern chose elimination as the Government's policy goal. This set the strategic direction of the country from that point onward: all the decisions that followed were aimed at eliminating the virus, rather than simply trying to control it. The criterion of success was forbidding, but clear, and the strategy equally transparent – early, aggressive implementation of well-understood, evidence-based public-health measures.

The choice of that goal and its highly effective implementation won Ardern and her Labour Party a landslide re-election in the mid-pandemic elections in October 2020. A primary reason the Prime Minister and her government chose elimination was concern over the limited capacity of the country's health care system. To achieve the objective of effectively eliminating the virus, the Prime Minister understood that New Zealand had to act "hard and early" to prevent a loss of control. Once committed, in the words of Richard Parker,

> New Zealand's battle to contain the virus followed the classic pattern ordained by the science of virus transmission: stopping the influx of the virus from arriving travelers; procuring personal protective equipment to protect essential workers; testing, contact tracing, and isolating those who test positive; and, most of all, mobilizing the public to lockdown and socially distance so as to slow or break the chain of transmission.
>
> (Parker 2020)

To put it simply, there were three forces at work in New Zealand's successful prosecution of the war against the virus: first, there was excellent leadership, which had been exemplified earlier in Jacinda Ardern's surefooted handling of the Christchurch massacre in March 2019; secondly, there was a responsible and responsive citizenry, with sufficient trust in the country's leadership to accept the "hard and early" measures required; and thirdly, binding the two together, there was the acceptance by both the leaders and the lead of the authority of the science of epidemiology – the country followed the science. The full-scale, nationwide lockdown lasted for 26 days, followed by a moderated version of equivalent duration. Since that time, when there have been isolated outbreaks (most recently in Auckland in February 2021), the government has acted swiftly and aggressively to stamp them out.

Let us turn now to the best performing federation, Australia, which comes in third in the rankings after New Zealand and South Korea. Australia, it appears, is a case in which the federal organization of a large country was not only *not* an impediment to effective action, but overall proved to be beneficial in the prosecution of the attack on the coronavirus. Despite the decentralized constitutional framework of the country (with residual powers, for example, remaining with the states), there has been an inexorable centralization of power in the Commonwealth government, almost from Australia's inception in 1901.

> Controlling the three main tax bases and raising 80 percent of all the tax revenue in Australia, the Commonwealth has financial resources far in excess of its program requirements, while the states are dependent on the Commonwealth for almost half their revenue needs.
>
> (Fenna 2021)

One might have expected, therefore, that Australia's success in coping with the pandemic would be a story of the Commonwealth government aggressively swinging into action and pushing the state governments to one side. But this was not the case. Except for the care of the aged, which is a federal responsibility, the states have jurisdiction over most areas that matter during a pandemic: hospitals and most of public health, schools, the regulation of businesses, and the capacity to control their own state borders. While the Commonwealth government declared a 'human biosecurity emergency' under the 2015 *Biosecurity Act,* giving it sweeping powers (Edgar 2020), each of the States has public health emergency legislation and all but New South Wales declared their own states of emergency (Fenna 2021).

Each order of government implemented measures to control the virus. The Commonwealth Minister for Health, for example, issued several regulations "banning overseas travel, prohibiting cruise ships from entering ports, restricting access to remote, mainly Aboriginal communities and medical isolation zones, and controlling the prices of health-related goods such as disposable face masks, gloves, and hand sanitizer" (Edgar 2020). As for initiatives of the states, there was some variation in policy and timing, arising out of their differing circumstances, but one could argue that that was more of a benefit than a problem, permitting regional governments to respond to local needs and circumstances.

That the many semi-autonomous government actors did not by and large create confusion is owing primarily to the fact that Australia's intergovernmental actors and institutions stepped up to the challenge with what Alan Fenna calls 'loose coordination' (2021). In fact, as he points out, under the auspices of the Council of Australian Governments (COAG), state and federal leaders had begun more than a decade before to put in place legislation and intergovernmental agreements outlining the roles and responsibilities of the two orders of government in the event of a civil or biosecurity emergency of the sort COVID-19 presented. The primary responsibility of the states was recognized, as was the Commonwealth responsibility to offer financial and resource support as necessary. When the pandemic struck, then, there was a framework of understanding to guide the governments in their response. This framework was no doubt one of the factors leading to Australia ranking fourth in the Global Health Security Index. In addition, intergovernmental coordination at the apex was intensified, with COAG, the meeting of first ministers, effectively transformed into what was called the National Cabinet. As Fenna reports, this group began to meet weekly, supported by the Australian Health Protection Principals Committee whose members were the chief medical officers from the Commonwealth and state governments. The National Cabinet seems to have operated in an unusually collegial fashion, exchanging information, seeking consensus, and offering guidelines to all the participants.[10]

One area in which consensus broke down was the question of when to re-open state economies and societies that had been locked down. The Commonwealth government, faced with backstopping the enormous costs of the pandemic, was anxious to re-open as soon as possible, whereas the states, who were managing the impact of the pandemic on the ground, were reluctant to open early. Despite Commonwealth efforts, the states generally held their ground, and the resultant strategy privileged prudence and pandemic control over economic recovery, which contributed to the country's high performance in suppressing the virus.

All in all, the Australian federal system played a critical role in the management of the pandemic and in Australia's success. It allowed for the Commonwealth government to play its part in controlling the external borders of the country and giving financial and other support to the states, as well as leading the ongoing coordination function. The states managed the public health care system on the ground and generally took the lead in lockdowns, as well as in the regulation of schools and businesses. Several states also imposed their own border controls. Shared Commonwealth and state leadership proved to be very popular with the public.

Australian federalism rose to the challenge. Given that the federal government lacks operational boots on the ground, it is difficult to imagine that aggressive, unilateral action by the federal government, of the sort seen in some other formally decentralized systems, would have served the country anywhere near as well. Far from decentralized government being an impediment to high performance, in a large country with diverse conditions and dispersed populations, it appears to have contributed positively to Australia's high achievement.

26.4 Concluding thoughts on comparative performance

This brief review indicates that there is no structural impediment to high performance on the part of federal countries. As is the case with their non-federal cousins, federal countries can be found all across the performance scale, with some at or near the very top.

There appear to be some factors common to high-performing countries, whether they are federal or unitary. A decent national public-health and medical-care system is a common denominator. Also associated with high performance is broad public acceptance, shared by the political leadership, of the reality of the virus and the need to accept and act on the scientific understanding of the disease.[11] Happily, COVID-skeptics in most countries are in relatively short supply. Regulations and guidance, well explained and grounded in public-health science, tend to receive broad public acceptance. Public communication – honest, consistent, and evidence-based – builds trust and acceptance in democratic societies which inevitably depend on voluntary acquiescence more than on coercive regulation. But enforcement as a last resort helps to sustain public belief in the shared obligations of all members of society.

Our brief survey suggests that high performance in both federal and non-federal states will be heavily influenced by how well these states are governed. Effective leadership, both political and expert, appears to be critical in shaping a successful national response to the pandemic.[12] Both Belgium and Italy have been plagued by unstable government, although in the former case the federal system the Belgians have designed for themselves has exacerbated the complications, whereas in the latter governance weakness was only one contributing factor among several. The United States, in the first year of the pandemic, was badly led at the national level and driven throughout by fierce partisanship. The United Kingdom had a strong majority government and a highly regarded National Health Service; however, a willful national political leadership, uninterested in collaborating with its regional partners, led the country astray.

New Zealand and Australia, on the other hand, were very well led, but in very different ways, ways which disclose the difference between what one might call unitary and federal leadership styles. New Zealand's Prime Minister, Jacinda Ardern, did not have to bargain with autonomous regional political actors to set the country on its path. She did begin the pandemic, though, heading a coalition government, which is typical of New Zealand with its mixed member proportional electoral system, and so she had to retain the confidence of her government partners. However, part way through the pandemic, as a result of the election of 17 October 2020, her party won an absolute majority (50.01 percent of the popular vote and 65 of 120 seats), leaving her government no longer reliant on the support of other parties in Parliament. The Prime Minister of New Zealand is unequivocally the leader of the nation and the focal point of the country's politics. In terms of political offices, there is no competition. Her leadership challenge, then, was to retain the confidence of Parliament and the trust of the New Zealand people.

In Australia, however, as in most other federations, the nature of leadership and its location, particularly in the midst of a public-health crisis, are very different. Australia has constitutionally divided authority, with powerful regional politicians invested with substantial authority to act.[13] Indeed, the states, as we have seen, are primarily responsible for the institutions and the regulations required to combat COVID-19. This sets a very different context for leadership, and in fact changes its quality decisively. To begin with, leadership is to be found in two constitutionally grounded locations, in Canberra and the state capitals. In normal federal politics, the risk of sterile competition is considerable. Intergovernmental relations often invite blame-shifting and buck-passing. The Prime Minister of the country cannot force his will on the state premiers. Particularly in a crisis, there is a premium on a collaborative or collegial style of leadership, which is in fact what Australian Prime Minister Scott Morrison has provided. To a degree, normal conflictual politics were set aside in the light of the pandemic, and the National Cabinet, chaired by Morrison, operated in a collegial fashion. The states retained their autonomy and their broad scope of responsibility to manage the pandemic, while the Commonwealth government addressed the matters for which it was responsible and played a lead coordinating role. This suspension of normal politics and heightened collaboration was also apparent in other federations, such as Germany and Canada, although certainly not in all.

Good government and strong political leadership appear to be indispensable ingredients in successful pandemic performance, whatever the form of government. Achieving these qualities in a federation, though, is a more complex undertaking than it is in a unitary state.

The principle of distributed authority is expressed throughout a federation – in its constitutional and legislative structure, in its public administration, and in its citizenry and the electoral systems by which the people's representatives are chosen. A kind of federal diplomacy largely unknown in unitary systems is part of good federal practice, both administratively and politically. And citizens are members of both a provincial and a national community. They have loyalties and democratic representatives at both levels whose respective responsibilities are often not clear or not well understood. It is a world in which good government in a public-health crisis is inevitably a collegial endeavor among autonomous actors.

All that being said, I would conclude that the constitutional form of a democratic country, be it federal or non-federal, does not determine pandemic-management outcomes, but it establishes the frame within which those outcomes are determined. The pursuit of high achievement in federal and non-federal states requires different leadership styles, accountability structures, public administration practices, and citizen expectations. New Zealand performed outstandingly well, partly because it clearly set a demanding but achievable goal for itself – total victory over the virus – and pursued it zealously within a clearly defined, coherent authority structure. Australia, for its part, did a remarkable job in severely constraining the virus in a more complex constitutional and political environment in which success was determined by the collaborative performance of multiple autonomous actors. While factors such as geography and history played a noticeable role, perhaps what mattered most in confronting the coronavirus were two considerations: the quality of leadership at all levels and in all professional spheres, which established a bond of trust between the leaders and the led; and good governance, which permitted effective organization, timely interventions, and the application of the required resources of the state to combating the disease.

Please note: *This chapter was previously published by the Forum of Federations as Occasional Paper #50: http://www.forumfed.org/wp-content/uploads/2021/04/ OPS50_Relative_Performance_During_the_Pandemic1.pdf*

Notes

1 We can see already (March 5, 2021) that poor performance in the first phase is no predictor of performance in the second. The United Kingdom and the United States both did poorly in the first phase but are among the global leaders in administering the vaccine in the second phase.
2 OECD members Colombia, Hungary, and Mexico are listed as 'partly free' in the 2020 Freedom House index. The other 33 members are rated as 'free'.
3 They are all, for example, in the upper half of the nominal GDP per capita range.
4 We have excluded two OECD countries with populations less than a million from the list: Iceland and Luxembourg.
5 Despite the fact that the United Kingdom appears in this volume, albeit as a system of devolved government with 'federalised' arrangements, we will treat it in this chapter as a non-federal country, which indeed it is.

6 It is worth noting, though, that on the Global Health Security Index Belgium came in seventh place among the nine OECD federations in terms of pandemic preparedness.

7 But see Gordon, Huberfield and Jones (2020). They argue that: 'In this pandemic, US public health federalism assures that the coronavirus response depends on zip code. A global pandemic has no respect for geographic boundaries, laying bare the weaknesses of federalism in the face of a crisis." As Kumanan et al. (2008) point out, the United States, along with Canada and Australia, do confront "the challenge that authority over several of the core capacity requirements (is) primarily located at the state or province level" (p. 217).

8 The information in this paragraph is drawn chiefly from Boccia, Ricciardi and Ioannidis (2020, pp. 927–928).

9 A non-partisan technocrat, Mario Draghi, replaced the outgoing Prime Minister, Giuseppe Conte, in February 2021.

10 As with many other countries, long-term care of the elderly was an area where coordination appears to have faltered with unfortunate results. In Australia's case, the nexus between aged care, which fell under Commonwealth responsibility, and hospitals, which were the domain of the states, was at the center of the problem.

11 This might seem so obvious as to not need mentioning, but unfortunately, we have seen several cases of denialism, some in developed countries (the United States) and some in developing countries (Brazil and Tanzania). South Africa experienced an earlier case of medical denialism when former South African President Thabo Mbeki resisted the scientific evidence and medical treatment of HIV/AIDS.

12 Combating the spread of a highly infectious virus poses a distinctive challenge for political and expert leadership, because, unlike most policy fields, pandemic management requires an active commitment on the part of citizens to alter their conduct and daily practices – quarantining, wearing masks, social distancing, and the like.

13 In some federations, this regional authority has been deployed with some success to create 'bubbles' shielding sub-national units from the spread of the virus affecting other parts of the country. For several months, the Atlantic provinces of Canada established an 'Atlantic Bubble' with border controls and quarantine provisions. During this period, life went on in these provinces in a manner rather similar to life in New Zealand once that country had eliminated the virus.

Bibliography

Baker, M.G., Kvalsvig, A. and Verrall, A.J., 2020. New Zealand's COVID-19 Elimination Strategy. *The Medical Journal of Australia*, 213 (5), 198–200. Available from: https://doi.org/10.5694/mja2.50735 [Accessed 7 April 2021].

Boccia, S., Ricciardi, W. and Ioannidis, J.P.A., 2020. What Other Countries Can Learn from Italy During the COVID-19 Pandemic. *JAMA Internal Medicine*, 180 (7), 927–928. Available from: https://jamanetwork.com/journals/jamainternalmedicine/fullarticle/2764369 [Accessed 7 April 2021].

Bursens, P., Popelier, P. and Meier, P., 2021. Belgium's Response to COVID-19: How to Manage a Pandemic in a Competitive Federal System? *In*: Chattopadhyay, R., Knüpling, F., Chebenova, D., Gonzalez, P. and Whittington, L., eds. *Federalism and the Response to COVID-19: A Comparative Analysis*, Chapter 5. Canada: Routledge.

Calnan, M., 2020. England's Response to the Coronavirus Pandemic – Now Updated [online]. *Cambridge Core Blog*, 6 August 2020. Available from: https://www.cambridge.org/core/blog/2020/04/06/englands-response-to-the-coronavirus-pandemic/ [Accessed 7 April 2021].

Camacho, A.E. and Glickman, R.L., 2020. The Trump Administration's Pandemic Response is Structured to Fail. *The Regulatory Review*, University of Pennsylvania Law School, 19 May 2020. Available from: https://www.theregreview.org/2020/05/19/camacho-glicksman-trump-administration-pandemic-response-structured-fail/ [Accessed 7 April 2021].

Edgar, A., 2020. Disrupting Administrative Law in a Public Health Crisis [online]. The Regulatory Review, 24 April 2020. Available from: https://www.theregreview.org/2020/04/24/edgar-disrupting-administrative-law-public-health-crisis/ [Accessed 6 May 2021].

Fenna, A., 2021. Australian Federalism and the COVID-19 Crisis. *In*: Chattopadhyay, R., Knüpling, F., Chebenova, D., Gonzalez, P. and Whittington, L., eds. *Federalism and the Response to COVID-19: A Comparative Analysis* Chapter 3. Canada: Routledge.

Gordon, S.H., Huberfield, N. and Jones, D.K., 2020. What Federalism Means for the US Response to Coronavirus Disease 2019. Available from: https://jamanetwork.com/channels/health-forum/fullarticle/2766033 [Accessed 7 April 2021].

Grace, C., 2021. Perfect Storm: The Pandemic, Brexit, and Devolved Government in the UK. *In*: Chattopadhyay, R., Knüpling, F., Chebenova, D., Gonzalez, P. and Whittington, L., eds. *Federalism and the Response to COVID-19: A Comparative Analysis*, Chapter 23. Canada: Routledge.

Hasell, J., Mathieu, E., Beltekian, D., et al. 2020. A Cross-Country Database of COVID-19 Testing. *Scientific Data*, 7, 345. Available from: https://doi.org/10.1038/s41597-020-00688-8 [Accessed 7 April 2021].

Johns Hopkins University Coronavirus Resource Center, 2021. COVID-19 Dashboard by the Center for Systems Science and Engineering (CSSE) at Hopkins University [dataset]. 24 March. Available from: https://coronavirus.jhu.edu/map.html [Accessed 6 April 2021].

Kattasova, I., 2021. How the Czech Republic Slipped into a Covid Disaster, One Misstep at a Time [online]. *CNN*, 1 March 2021. Available from: https://www.cnn.com/2021/02/28/europe/czech-republic-coronavirus-disaster-intl/index.html [Accessed 6 May 2021].

Kincaid, J. and Leckrone, W.J., 2021. COVID-19 and American Federalism: First-Wave Responses. *In*: Chattopadhyay, R., Knüpling, F., Chebenova, D., Gonzalez, P. and Whittington, L., eds. *Federalism and the Response to COVID-19: A Comparative Analysis*, Chapter 24. Canada: Routledge.

Kumanan, W., McDougal, C., Fidler, D.P. and Lazar, H., 2008. Strategies for Implementing the New International Health Regulations in Federal Countries. *Bulletin of the World Health Organization*, 86 (3), 4.

Mammone, A., 2021. "Italy's Political Crisis is an Opportunity for the Far Right," *Al Jazeera*, 9 February 2021. Available from: https://www.aljazeera.com/opinions/2021/2/9/italys-political-crisis-is-an-opportunity-for-the-far-right [Accessed 7 April 2021].

Nicola, F.G., 2020. Exporting the Italian Model to Fight COVID-19 [online]. *The Regulatory Review*, University of Pennsylvania Law School, 23 April 2020. Available from: https://www.theregreview.org/2020/04/23/nicola-exporting-italian-model-fight-covid-19/ [Accessed 7 April 2021].

OECD, 9 March 2021. Daily Rollout of COVID-19 Vaccinations [online]. Available from: https://www.oecd.org/coronavirus/en/data-insights/ieo-2021-03-more-jabs-more-jobs [Accessed on 7 June 2021].

Palermo, F., 2021. The Impact of the Pandemic on the Italian Regional System: Centralizing or Decentralizing Effects? *In*: Chattopadhyay, R., Knüpling, F., Chebenova, D., Gonzalez, P. and Whittington, L., eds. *Federalism and the Response to COVID-19: A Comparative Analysis*, Chapter 12. Canada: Routledge.

Parker, R.W., 2020. Lessons from New Zealand's COVID-19 Success [online]. *The Regulatory Review*, 9 June 2020. Available from: https://www.theregreview.org/2020/06/09/parker-lessons-new-zealand-covid-19-success/ [Accessed 7 April 2021].

27 Comparative summary

Rupak Chattopadhyay and Felix Knüpling

27.1 The pandemic in 2020 and federalism: 24 case studies

As the world entered 2021, over 90 million people had reportedly been infected with COVID-19 around the globe, resulting in an estimated 2 million deaths. Half of these fatalities occurred in just seven countries across four continents: five federal nations (United States, India, Brazil, Russia, Germany) and three devolved unitary countries with strong devolved and decentralized governance features (Italy, Spain, and the United Kingdom).[1] This distribution underscores both the global footprint of the crisis and the extent to which some of the world's largest economies and most developed countries have been impacted by it. Even in countries where there were no extensive lockdowns during periods of rising infections, there has been significant economic disruption.

It has become increasingly clear that all countries (federal and unitary) were taken by surprise by the proliferation of the virus over the course of 2020. Consequently, in the vast majority of cases, governments struggled to formulate coherent public health and public policy responses to COVID-19. At the time of writing, the pandemic is ongoing, but it is fair to say that over the course of 2020 several lessons were learnt. This applies not just to the clinical aspects of the pandemic, but also to public policy.

Indeed, the chapters in this volume demonstrate that as the pandemic has dragged on, constituent unit governments have played an increasingly important role, even in countries where federal governments dominated decision-making. By their very nature, federations are more complex than unitary states. In unitary states, where national governments are assigned all powers, there is a single point of decision-making. In federal states, with devolved constitutional powers, decision nodes exist at two (and sometimes three) levels. Countries are federations either because they are big, or diverse (or both), or because of historical factors. No two federations are alike because their institutional arrangements were developed in response to specific historical, social, and political realities (Watts 2008). But the pandemic has highlighted the importance of intergovernmental coordination in the management of the crisis across almost all case studies in the volume. As we will see below, the effectiveness of intergovernmental cooperation has varied greatly across cases based on the robustness of the mechanisms for interaction.

COVID-19 is more than just a public-health crisis. Not only have governments been required to contain the spread of COVID-19 infections, but they have had to balance containment with preventing their economies from plunging into a death spiral, as well as coping with the social aspects of the pandemic. The economic dislocation caused by the crisis has had a massive impact on lives and livelihoods everywhere. This has required governments to step in with enormous income support programs.

DOI: 10.4324/9781003251217-27

Further, the economic disruption also had a disastrous impact on public finances everywhere and governments had to rapidly pivot in the direction of Keynesian fiscal policy aimed at providing both income support and stimulus to raise aggregate demand (Gravelle and Marples 2021). The experience of the last year has demonstrated that no one order of government can cope with a crisis of this magnitude on its own.

In this chapter, we offer a summary of observations based on the cases studies covering the 2020 calendar year. First, we identify trends in how countries differed in their response to the challenges posed by the COVID-19 pandemic. Second, we summarize how COVID-19 has affected the practice of federalism in our case studies. Third, we identify areas for further research. In recognition of the fact that the pandemic is ongoing at the time of writing, our observations are preliminary and limited to the first year of the pandemic.

27.2 Three trends

In this volume, we examined experiences from 23 federal and devolved countries as well as one supranational entity, the European Union. The cases cover both established and emerging federations from the Global North and South and countries with varied institutional structures, including presidential and parliamentary systems of government. Some federal countries have a rather clear division of competences between orders of government (often referred to as "dual federations"), while others are marked by a high degree of overlapping powers (known as "integrated federalism") (Watts 2008). Other cases, such as Italy, Spain, South Africa, United Kingdom, and the European Union, are multilevel government systems that display features of both federal and unitary systems (Anderson 2008).

In most federal countries, health care is one of the policy areas usually assigned to sub-national governments. The exact nature of this assignment is shaped by the differing needs and expectations of citizens as to how a health system should be managed (Majeed, Watts and Brown 2005). Even where health care is a concurrent power, sub-national governments (constituent units and local governments) are critical players on the frontlines of pandemic management in areas such as provision of clinical services, enforcement of public health measures, and lockdowns. Federal governments have important regulatory oversight of pharmaceuticals, the ability to close international borders and, most importantly, the fiscal tools required to respond to the health and economic impacts of the pandemic (Marchildon and Bossert 2018). Given the acute shortages of personal protective equipment (PPE) and life-saving supplies during the COVID-19 crisis, federal authorities have played an important role in coordinating the procurement and allocation of scarce resources. More recently, federal governments (and, in the case of the EU, a supranational entity) have taken the lead in certifying and securing vaccine supplies from national and global suppliers.

In the majority of cases, governments attempted to control the spread of the virus by imposing lockdowns. But not all countries implemented lockdowns of the same scale or severity. The debate in several countries revolved around the economic costs of imposing restrictions on commercial activities. This difference in responses is to be expected given the heterogeneity of the countries covered in this book, as well as the political imperatives and economic as well as social concerns that confronted decision makers in each country. Indeed, after the first wave, many countries began to gradually reopen their economies to make up for lost output, or at least to forestall further economic damage. Some countries in 2020 had to deal with a second wave (Australia, Austria, Belgium, Canada Germany, Nigeria, Pakistan, Russia, South Africa, Spain, Switzerland, United Kingdom, European Union), or even a third wave (Italy).[2] The table below shows that during 2020, there was considerable variation across countries in outcomes.

In summarizing the cases in the volume, three broad patterns of responses can be identified:

- National Government Dominated Response: Ethiopia, Italy, Kenya, Malaysia, Nepal, Nigeria, Pakistan, Russia, Spain, South Africa, United Kingdom.
- Strong Collaboration and Coordination between Orders of Government: Argentina, Australia, Austria, Canada, Germany, India, Switzerland.
- Weak Collaboration between Orders of Government: Belgium, Bosnia and Herzegovina, Brazil, Mexico, United States, the European Union.

27.2.1 *National government dominated response*

This category covers a very heterogeneous group of countries. Some are not constitutionally federal (Italy, Kenya, Spain, South Africa, United Kingdom), even though they may have multilevel institutional arrangements that allow them to function like federal systems. In the other cases (Ethiopia, Malaysia, Nepal, Nigeria, Pakistan, Russia) there are federal systems which are highly centralized either because the constituent units have poor administrative competence, or their fiscal capacity is constrained, or both. Consequently, in all these countries, federal governments dominated the response to COVID-19. In some cases, constituent units were not consulted on the measures to respond to the pandemic, while in others the constituent units were too weak to push back against national/federal policies.

Following the first COVID-19 cases in **Ethiopia**, both the federal and state governments took measures to prevent a wider outbreak of infections. Under Article 51(3) of the 1995 Constitution, public health falls under concurrent competences of the federal and state governments. Hence, federal agencies such as the Ministry of Health imposed checks and restrictions on international travel, and Ethiopian Airlines was forced to gradually suspend all international flights, save for cargo flights. The federal government closed all federal offices and asked all non-essential federal employees to work from home. At the same time, the states and some local governments placed restrictions on public movement. Bahr Dar, the capital of Amhara state, imposed a two-week lockdown on 31 March 2020. Several cities, such as Adama and Assela in Oromia, also suspended all public transportation. Tigray state was the first and the only state to invoke a state power to impose a state of emergency. Deterioration of relations between the federal government and Tigray eventually led to armed confrontation and a humanitarian crisis. Zemelak Ayele notes that in the absence of formally established intergovernmental relations fora in Ethiopia, coordination between the states and federation was initially ad hoc. With the exception of Tigray, intra-party relations offered an informal communication channel between state and federal leadership which facilitated discussion of policy measures. A federal state of emergency was proclaimed in April 2020 and expired in August 2020. State and federal authorities were faced with difficult choices between keeping the economy closed to protect public health and protecting livelihoods in a very poor country. The Federal

Ministry of Health emerged as the major locus for policy coordination during the middle of 2020 and, together with the Ministry of Peace and National Disaster and Risk Management Commission (NDRMC), formulated nationwide policies to combat COVID-19. Despite this top-down approach, authorities at the *woreda* and city level, who are responsible for providing primary health care, were important conduits for managing the pandemic.

In **Italy**, a "federal country without federalism," as Francesco Palermo writes, the national government declared a "state of emergency" in the early stages of the pandemic.[3] Thus, the national government took charge in responding to COVID-19. Although the regions, Italy's constituent units, were consulted prior to the adoption of national regulations designed to address the challenges created by the pandemic, they could not oppose measures taken by the national government. There was some flexibility for regional governments to adopt their own regulations, although only within the framework of national legislation or in the event they wished to introduce stricter rules than the national measures. Accordingly, in the early phases of the pandemic, the governance response produced a strong centralization of powers, moving authority from the regions to the center. When in May 2020 the government eased the lockdown, the role of the regions grew in relation to the lifting of national regulations, thus triggering a process of shifting responsibilities back to the regions. Indeed, a few regions began to adopt their own laws to cope with the pandemic. The process of easing the lockdown and opening the economy was primarily governed by a plethora of executive orders and regulations issued by both regional and local governments. This led to confusion because there was no coordination between the regional governments in the creation of these regulations. It also triggered conflict between the national government and various regions with regard to the constitutionality of certain measures, as there was no clarity about the distribution of emergency powers.

Rose Osoro and Victor Odanga note in their chapter that centralized decision-making was also a feature of **Kenya's** response to the pandemic. Kenya, like Italy, is not a classical federal country but instead a formally unitary country exhibiting strong decentralized or devolved features. Health, for example, is a fully devolved function. While health policy and standard setting is in the hands of the national government, the counties – Kenya's constituent units – bear the constitutional responsibility for health functions. In this context, the national government established a national coordination committee which strictly centralized the overall response process, leaving county governments to implement the national directives. Further, the committee partially drew on and re-established administrative structures which existed before the promulgation of Kenya's current 2010 constitution. This essentially set up parallel national government structures to ensure control of the response process by the center. Even though Kenya, as the authors explain, has an elaborated system of intergovernmental cooperation both vertically (through the Senate) and horizontally (through the Council of Governors), in terms of policy making, those institutions did not play a significant role during the initial phase of the pandemic. While later intergovernmental relations between the two orders of government strengthened in terms of coordination of processes and communication, the greatest missing link was the (under)resourcing of county governments. The great vertical fiscal imbalance and the underfunding of counties proved a great challenge for Kenya's counties in their efforts to implement policies to combat COVID-19.

Malaysia, as Tricia Yeoh notes, may be considered a highly centralized federal system. It was therefore not surprising that the country's federal government employed a top-down approach in attempting to manage the pandemic. In 2020, Malaysia experienced three waves of infections, with the hardest hitting the country at the end of the year. At the outbreak of the pandemic, the federal government responded early, issuing national laws and strict lockdown measures such as the Movement Control Order (MCO). The MCO, which came into force on 18 March 2020, mandated that only "essential" industries would be permitted to operate. The top-down approach employed by the federal government produced conflict with Malaysia's states, particularly in circumstances in which state governments were not consulted prior to decision-making. This was especially the case when the federal government abruptly announced that restrictions on movement and the economy would be relaxed, giving only three days' notice. Nine state governments in total reacted immediately, stating they would either not follow (Kedah, Sabah, Pahang, Penang, Kelantan, and Sarawak) or not fully comply with the new rules because they felt that the easing of restrictions by the federal government was premature. Despite the centralized nature of the response to COVID-19, many states also adopted their own measures in response to the pandemic, independent of the federal government. Several states supplemented federal aid from their own meager financial resources by providing transfers and food aid for the vulnerable, or by deferring or waving bills. Many states also relied on their own resources to conduct testing and contact tracing. This seems to indicate that if sub-national governance autonomy and decentralization in the country is to be strengthened, it is most likely to occur through a bottom-up rather than a top-down approach.

After the abolition of the monarchy in 2008 and a period of civil war, **Nepal** became a federal country in 2015 with the adoption of its new constitution. The country remains in transition, with competences still being transferred to the provinces and localities. Provinces and local governments have only limited administrative capacity and depend heavily on fiscal transfers from the federal level, particularly for health infrastructure and human resources. In this context, as Puspa Raj Kadel writes, when COVID-19 hit Nepal, the federal government adopted a centralized approach providing little room for provinces to influence the pandemic response. The government established by executive order a new ad-hoc decision-making committee under the authority of the Deputy Prime Minister to respond to the crisis. In spring 2020, the federal government ordered a nation-wide lockdown including restrictions on international (initially) and domestic (subsequently) travel. While the main decisions were taken by the federal authorities, intergovernmental cooperation did occur vertically between the federal government and provinces, as well as horizontally between provincial governments, and again vertically between the provincial and local governments. This was beneficial in managing the quarantine and isolation centers and facilitated the sharing of good practice and lessons learned in controlling the spread of COVID-19. Though Nepal's federal system managed to design and implement policies to mitigate the fallout of the pandemic, the response suffered from a lack of clarity about roles and responsibilities among the three orders of government, and the poor administrative capacity at provincial and local level, in terms of both human and financial resources.

Similar to many other countries on the African continent with a relatively young population, **Nigeria** got off relatively lightly in 2020. Julius Ihonvbere notes that while the Federal government reacted quickly to the crisis, states and local governments were caught unawares. Lagos state was the only exception where the governor recognized the potential for human and economic devastation. Some state governors as in Cross River refused even to order lockdowns. In terms of responses to COVID-19, the Nigerian system operated more like a unitary rather than a federal system. The states and local governments largely sat back and waited for federal leadership. The federal government had full authority over funds, programs, and policies. As reflected by the installation of the COVID-19 Presidential Task Force (PTF), backed up by the National Monitoring Committee as well as the National Centre for Disease Control (NCDC), the federal government's management of the pandemic emphasized the structural tendency for political power to be exercised hierarchically in Nigeria. The federally initiated national and interstate shutdown was enforced by federal police and the army. As Julius Ihonvbere explains in his chapter, the generally poor government communication infrastructure between the states, regions, and local communities was only topped by that of the barely existing interstate and intercommunal communication. Widespread acceptance of conspiracy theories surrounding COVID-19, stigma concerning patients who had recovered from the disease, and a general belief in informal treatment severely impeded both testing on a voluntary basis and the federal government's efforts to raise public awareness of and provide education on the virus. The local governments' indifference to crisis response in any shape or form, and their tendency to take action in a lethargic manner only when the state government demanded, further entrenched centralization already evident in Nigeria.

In **Pakistan**, as Sameen A. Mohsin Ali writes, the initial months of government response to COVID-19 were characterized by inaction and the downplaying of the health crisis by federal authorities, especially by Pakistan's Prime Minister Imran Khan. Guided by the National Institute of Health's National Action Plan, and with support from the Ministry of National Health, the provincial governments stepped up to create task forces. These bodies in turn planned and coordinated the enforcement of varying degrees of lockdown, the establishment of economic relief packages, the building of testing capacity, and the launch of information campaigns and designation of facilities for treatment. Local communities remained out of the policy loop and disorganized in their efforts as a result. Sidelining the vacillating federal executive and working with the provincial governments, Pakistan's military leadership, an autonomous actor in its own right, stepped in, pursuing a full lockdown strategy as of April 2020 in accordance with the provinces' Chief Ministers. This move prompted the federal government back into action, as it tasked the newly created National Coordination Committee, backed by the National Command and Operations Centre and including the Inter Services Intelligence, with the responsibility to deal with the pandemic. Intergovernmental relations and coordination between the federal government and the provinces, as well as between the provinces themselves, was entrusted to the National Disaster Management Authority. Interprovincial sparring over response measures and controversial Supreme Court rulings impeded effective civilian control and oversight of the crisis management measures. According to the author, the newly centralized management, with its adopted 'Smart Lockdown Strategy,' produced promising results.

Following reforms undertaken in the mid-2000s that altered the governance dynamics of the country, **Russia**'s response to the pandemic played out against the background of an already centralized federal system, writes Nataliya Golovanova.

Growing regional debt, in addition to the consequences of the 2008 financial crisis, intensified the power imbalance in the relationship between the federal government and the 85 constituent units in favor of the former. The crisis took a major toll on the country and some reports at the end of the year suggest that the real casualty figures are significantly higher than originally reported.[4] The federal government determined how much power was delegated to the federated entities to tackle the pandemic during both waves of COVID-19 the country experienced in 2020. Austerity measures enacted by the Russian Federation, in the form of 'Optimization Programs,' required prior approval by the federal government of regions' stringently planned processes for the provision of health care. The federal government established the Coordination Council in March 2020 to guide communication between all orders of government in pursuing the Russian Federation's "Priority Plan:" supporting the public with goods; securing economic relief for businesses; and filling gaps in regional budgets. Fearing an abrupt halt to federal funding, regional governments were eager to remain at the federal government's heel. Though the federated units had the legal powers to enforce measures in response to COVID-19, the April 2020 Presidential Decree by the federal government – which emphasized that the implementation of such measures was an independent decision on the part of the governors – pressured the heads of the constituent units to interpret the legislation as an order rather than an option. Since the decree made governors personally responsible for managing the outbreak, some quit while others resorted to excessive measures such as banning people from walking the streets of Moscow.

Contrary to its origin as a unitary state with a long-standing centralist tradition, **Spain** has since the 1980s developed its own territorially based model of federalism, explains Mario Kölling. The belated and slow reactions of the state and its 17 constituent units, the Autonomous Communities (ACs), during the COVID-19 crisis have laid bare the structural shortcomings of this model. Vertical intergovernmental coordination instruments and joint decision-making bodies were insufficient to respond to the pandemic appropriately, and horizontal intergovernmental coordination is virtually non-existent. When the pandemic hit Spain, most ACs turned to and accepted the central government's authority in managing the crisis when Prime Minister Sanchez declared the first national state of alarm. The central government also took over decision-making in the National Health Service (NHS) and in the course of the first wave of the outbreak – during which the national state of alarm was extended six times – only gradually ceded the power to deal with the pandemic back to the ACs. Inter-regional coordination on pandemic control got off to a slow start and was initially conducted through the Inter-Territorial Council for the NHS and other sectoral conferences. However, the Conference of Presidents – which brought together all the heads of government – met during the state of alarm on a weekly basis. During the second wave, which started in autumn 2020, the ACs demanded a new nationwide state of alarm in order to obtain the legal power to impose more severe social restrictions. The second state of alarm was implemented in a more decentralized manner, primarily managed by the ACs.

As Nico Steytler and Jaap de Visser argue, **South Africa**'s constitutional, financial, and political reality makes the country a "unitary state with federal features." Not surprisingly, the tendency for events to produce centralizing governance reflexes is prevalent in South Africa, particularly in times of crisis. Accordingly, in March 2020, the national government declared a national state of disaster, allowing it to issue country-wide regulations. South Africa's constituent units, the nine provinces, are almost entirely dependent for their operations on fiscal transfers from the national government, and the COVID-19 response further enhanced the already dominant role of the national government. The centralized reaction to the crisis is reflected in the administration of the economic response to the pandemic; less than 10 percent of the social and economic relief package was channeled through the provinces. The relevance of provinces (and local governments) only came to the fore in the government's "risk adjusted strategy," which theoretically enabled differentiation across provinces depending on the infection rate. Indeed, the infection rates differed vastly between provinces. However, this differentiated strategy to respond to the pandemic was never implemented and, thus, the potential benefits of multilevel government to produce tailor-made responses was not exploited. Although key policy areas in the response to the crisis such as health, disaster management, education, and social welfare are concurrent responsibilities, actions were decidedly centralized with little cooperation and coordination between orders of government. Instead of relying on existing institutions for intergovernmental relations, the national government established new structures and concentrated power in an informal cabinet committee, the National Coronavirus Command Centre, which had no provincial or local government representation.

In 2019, the World Health Organization (WHO) ranked the **United Kingdom** as the second-best prepared country to respond to a pandemic. However, as Clive Grace notes, policy errors on the part of the national government led to huge health consequences and economic damage. The response to COVID-19 was led primarily by the Government of the United Kingdom. Despite their powers in key areas of domestic policy and service delivery, the devolved governments of Scotland and Wales, and the Northern Ireland Assembly, had very limited influence in shaping policy. Collaboration between the national government and those in the devolved nations and local governments was very limited. The key coordinating mechanism for national emergencies in the United Kingdom is referred to as COBRA (**Cabinet Office Briefing Rooms**). The devolved nations had access to COBRA and did play some part in the pandemic response. The delayed measures that the UK government took to deal with the pandemic, however, rendered the situation so critical that the devolved governments had no scope for crafting tailored policy. Their influence increased once governments began to discuss how to ease lockdowns. For example, the Welsh Government declared that it was working in collaboration with the United Kingdom's other governments to take an aligned approach where it was beneficial to do so, coordinated by the UK government through meetings of COBRA. However, the power to impose a lockdown in Wales rested ultimately with the Welsh Government, which determined how it should be implemented in line with its responsibility for health and social care in the country. The author concludes that overall the response to the pandemic reflected the fundamentally centralist character of the UK government, associated with its political culture and history and the sheer weight and dominance of England.

27.2.2 *Strong collaboration between orders of government*

In a number of countries both federal as well as constituent unit governments recognized the urgency and necessity of working together to deal with the crisis. In these cases, the federal government played an important role as facilitator and coordinator for marshalling scarce resources to deal with the immediate health emergency and subsequent socioeconomic fallout of the pandemic. This is not to suggest that federal and sub-national authorities agreed on all policy issues all of the time, but rather that they remained engaged with each other in managing and seeking solutions to the crisis. In Argentina, Australia, Austria, and India, governments (federal and constituent units) disagreements between national and constituent units did sometimes end up in court. Countries in this category, on the whole, had better outcomes (see Table 27.1).

In **Argentina**, at the very start of the crisis, the President consulted with governors to define the duration and scope of early social distancing measures. Ultimately, these types of decisions were delegated to the provinces. The federal authorities also worked with the provinces to build up the diagnostic capabilities of the sub-national units and establish criteria for distributing scarce medical equipment and supplies among them. The federal government and the province of Córdoba worked with the country's main producer of ventilators to ensure that these vital pieces of equipment would not be exported. The Federal Council for Healthcare, which was created in 1981 to facilitate coordination between federal and provincial health ministries, emerged as the main forum for decision-making during the year. Also evident was considerable horizontal cooperation among provinces, including among those ruled by opposing parties. For example, the governments of the City and the Province of Buenos Aires established a special board to coordinate a range of public health measures, while another province – Córdoba – made spare medical resources (emergency doctors) available to other provinces. Certainly, there were also numerous disagreements, such as when a dozen provinces unilaterally closed their borders, and one expelled foreign citizens from their province. Despite its poor financial state, early on the federal government implemented a series of economic measures – representing approximately 5 percent of GDP – to backstop the economy and support the provinces. Matías Bianchi notes in his chapter that given the structure of Argentine federalism, where provinces have extensive responsibilities but weak finances, collaboration was essential in the first phase of the fight against COVID-19.

Australian dualism is reflected in the fact that while the Commonwealth (federal government) is provided sweeping regulatory powers under the emergency *Biosecurity Act 2015*, the States have primary responsibility for public hospitals, the government school systems, and the police and emergency services agencies. Consequently, the Commonwealth continued to acknowledge that primary responsibility for the management of communicable disease emergencies lay with the constituent units (states and territories). Not surprisingly, during the early stages of the outbreak, the two orders of government worked cooperatively to contain its spread. While the Commonwealth closed the country's borders to international travel, four of the six States closed their domestic borders. The States simultaneously invoked measures to limit gatherings, close restaurants, and restrict other services. Australia's intergovernmental arrangements, especially COAG, had laid the basis for coordinated action where needed. Hence, its transition into a "National Cabinet" comprised of the Prime Minister and State Premiers was seamless. However, as Alan Fenna explains, the Commonwealth's insistence on minimizing fiscal and economic damage and the States' preoccupation with minimizing infection did provide points of disagreement. The author further notes that, aside from in some specific operational areas such as aged care, close coordination was not necessary. The Commonwealth's acceptance of the national principles that recognize the sovereignty of States and Territories to implement policies according to local circumstances made for a largely harmonious

Table 27.1 COVID-19 Outcomes in Different Countries as of 10 January 2021

Country	Cumulative Cases	Cumulative Cases per 100,000 Population	Cumulative Deaths	Cumulative Deaths per 100,000 Population	Case Fatality Percentage
Argentina	1,703,352	3,768.8	44,273	98.0	2.6
Australia	28,582	112.1	909	3.6	3.2
Austria	378,110	4,198.2	6,614	73.4	1.7
Belgium	664,261	5,731.5	20,069	173.2	3.0
Bosnia and Herzegovina	115,379	3,516.8	4,305	131.2	3.7
Brazil	8,013,708	3,770.1	201,460	94.8	2.5
Canada	644,348	1,707.2	16,707	44.3	2.6
Ethiopia	127,792	111.2	1,985	1.7	1.6
Germany	1,908,527	2,277.9	40,343	48.2	2.1
India	10,450,284	757.3	150,999	10.9	1.4
Italy	2,257,866	3,734.4	78,394	129.7	3.5
Kenya	98,184	182.6	1,704	3.2	1.7
Malaysia	133,559	412.7	542	1.7	0.4
Mexico	1,507,931	1,169.5	132,069	102.4	8.8
Nepal	264,521	907.9	1,912	6.6	0.7
Nigeria	97,478	47.3	1,342	0.7	1.4
Pakistan	499,517	226.1	10,598	4.8	2.1
Russia	3,401,954	2,331.2	61,837	42.4	1.8
South Africa	1,214,176	2,047.2	32,824	55.3	2.7
Spain	2,025,560	4,332.3	51,690	110.6	2.6
Switzerland	475,604	5,495.4	7,545	87.2	1.6
United Kingdom	3,017,413	4,444.8	80,868	119.1	2.7
Untied States	21,761,186	6,574.3	365,886	110.5	1.7
European Union	17,292,252	3,892.5	373,777	84.1	2.2

Source: Cases and death rates as reported by the Johns Hopkins University Coronavirus Resource Center 19 January 2021
World Health Organization Weekly epidemiological update – 12 January 2021. Geneva: WHO, 2021. Available from https://www.who.int/publications/m/item/weekly-epidemiological-update

working relationship. This is particularly relevant given Australia's political and physical geography, which due to its size and sparse population lends itself to the kind of decentralized response federalism permits. The important issue is that both orders of government recognized the threat from COVID-19 and remained committed to tackling the crisis effectively.

Under **Austria's** constitution, the country is organized as an integrated federation underpinned by cooperative federalism. This implies that jurisdiction on health matters is shared between the Federation and the nine *Länder* (States). The Federation has the competence to pass and execute laws concerning public health, including pandemic prevention, except in the area of the organization of hospitals and municipal sanitation. Peter Bussjäger and Mathias Eller point out that in practice the federation relies on the *Länder* to administer federal laws, making the system highly interdependent. When the Federation used its powers to impose severe restrictions in Austria during the first wave of the pandemic, it did so with the concurrence of the states. Daily video conferences between Federal and the *Land* administrations helped coordinate policy and relief measures. As a result of this interaction, Austria was able to customize its response to deal with the needs of specific regions. For example, Tyrol, the worst affected *Land* at the start of the crisis, was able to enact more stringent regulations than those implemented by the Federal Government. The *Länder* relied on their district administrations to administer a range of public health measures. As elsewhere, there were tensions in the working relationship between the orders of government, particularly around the severity and scale of the restrictions. In Vienna for example, the city opened its parks to the public, while those owned by the Federal Government remained closed. Indeed, over the summer, the Constitutional Court struck down some severe restrictions imposed around the country. This prompted the establishment of the new "traffic light-system," from the beginning of September 2020. This new virus control mechanism was developed with the participation of the *Länder* as a way to develop regionally differentiated policy responses. In the face of a new wave in September, *Länder* found themselves inadequately resourced. Consequently, they had to call on the federal military to help enforce COVID-19 regulations. Despite Austria's very centralized federal structure, the important role of the *Land* authorities in executing regulations was at the heart of the country's COVID-19 response.

André Lecours, Daniel Beland and Jennifer Wallner note in their chapter that **Canada** is one of the world's most decentralized federations. Provinces have constitutional responsibility over public health and thus were on the frontline in managing the crisis. Crucially, this included overseeing the health care system and long-term care homes; regulating lockdown measures; and controlling movement into and on their territory. As constitutionally mandated, the federal government regulated international travel and the border with the United States. It also oversaw vaccine development and procurement efforts. The federal government played an important role in providing human and financial resources to support provincial efforts. First, at the request of the Québec and Ontario governments, it deployed members of the Armed Forces in the provinces' long-term care homes. Second, it put in place a very comprehensive fiscal response focused on mitigating the economic impact of the pandemic, including income support, unemployment support, and wage subsidies. Provinces were generally receptive to these temporary programs, even if they were sometimes given little forewarning before their announcement and implementation. Some provincial governments put in place their own complementary assistance programs. The existence of a dense network of federal–provincial relations (especially at the bureaucratic level) facilitated much intergovernmental collaboration. The collapse of sub-national finances in Canada raised the specter of centralization as the federal government stepped in to backstop the provinces. However, this concern largely dissipated as the provinces doubled-down to demand unconditional increases in federal transfers for health care (Béland and Marier 2020). Like Australia, Canada is a continental sized country with a sparse and diverse population. Given the differentiated impact of the pandemic across and within provinces, federalism was an important tool for Canada to find customized solutions.

Cooperation and coordination is the defining feature of **Germany's** integrated system, note Sabine Kropp and Johanna Schnabel. Consequently, the 16 states (*Länder*) and federal government reacted swiftly to the COVID-19 crisis in unison. While responsibility for infectious disease is vested with the *Länder* as part of their emergency management responsibilities, "measures to combat human and animal diseases which pose a danger to the public or are communicable" are concurrent powers (Article 74 of the Constitution). The German constitution allows the federal government to pass legislation regulating the response to an epidemic or pandemic, which it did by adopting the *Protection against Infection Act* 2001. At the very start of the pandemic, the worst affected *Länder* enacted unilateral restrictions. However, the federal government quickly followed suit in order to coordinate the response to the COVID-19 outbreak. The chancellor and the premiers met on a weekly basis to coordinate the introduction of measures such as: social distancing; a ban on mass gatherings; and the closure of bars, restaurants, shops, and theatres. Germany's dense network of intergovernmental relations proved resilient through the various phases of the pandemic. During the first phase, *Länder* were more willing to follow federal recommendations in determining the scale and severity of restrictions. After the first phase, there was greater initiative on the part of the *Länder* with respect to reopening the economy. The federal government came to accept that this differentiated response was more useful provided the *Länder* activated restrictions if infection rates increased above a certain threshold at the district level. Furthermore, sectoral intergovernmental fora, such as those of education ministers, allowed the *Länder* to horizontally coordinate regional approaches to a resumption in public life. Germany's coordinated approach and robust health care system ensured that the country's hospitals were never overwhelmed by the pandemic during 2020.

As in other dualist federations, in **India** no single jurisdiction had the constitutional competence or operational capability to deal with the pandemic on its own, as Rekha Saxena and Rounak Pathak explain. In India, health care is assigned to state governments. However, under the *Epidemic Diseases Act* 1897 and the *Disaster Management Act* 2005, the federal (Union) government is mandated to play a coordinating and supporting role. While the state of Karnataka was the first to invoke public health measures against COVID-19, Union support quickly followed as the states of Haryana, Maharashtra, Delhi, and Goa began to implement their own virus controls. Following the 'notification of the disaster', the Union government imposed a nationwide lockdown in late March 2020. While the states were unhappy about a lack of adequate discussion on this matter, the frequent video consultations between the Prime Minister and his state counterparts following the lockdowns saw an unprecedented level of intergovernmental interaction by the first ministers. As a result of these consultations, state governments obtained greater leeway in managing their own affairs. The states in turn relied heavily on their municipal and district administrations to test and isolate affected populations, allowing for graduated resumptions of economic activity across the country. However, the Union government continued to play an important role. Intergovernmental relations during this period were not free of conflict and the Supreme Court was called to settle some disputes. On the whole, the Union government's financial backstopping of state finances has raised the prospect of greater fiscal and policy centralization in the near term. The Union government did come under criticism for not offering the states a larger fiscal package. A better-than-expected economic recovery, with record GST collections in January 2021, may help states.[5] However, as the authors note, even the Prime Minister is on record admitting that without the coordination and cooperation between various levels of the government, containment would not have been possible.

Switzerland is a decentralized federation with the constituent units (*cantons*) possessing wide-ranging legislative and fiscal powers. However, the system also affords a degree of integration, as the *cantons* are also responsible for implementing the majority of federal laws.Prior to the pandemic, Switzerland had enacted a new "Epidemics Act" (EpidA) in early 2016. This new law, Sean Mueller, Rahel Freiburghaus, and Adrian Vatter note, was motivated by the SARS outbreak and a desire to address new challenges posed by global mobility. The EpidA distinguishes between "normal," "special," and "extraordinary" situations, which in turn has implications for how tasks are divided between the federal government and the 26 *cantons*. Under "extraordinary situations" decision-making becomes highly centralized. The Federal Council, the highest executive authority in the country, unilaterally determines whether an existing situation is deemed to be either 'special' or 'extraordinary.' The Federal Council declared that Switzerland was in a 'special situation' on 28 March 2020. Two weeks later, the same body upgraded it to an 'extraordinary situation,' allowing the Federal Council to establish measures necessary to control the spread of the virus for any part of the country, or the whole country. As the pandemic unfolded, the Federal Council consulted with the *Conference of Cantonal Directors for Health* (GDK), which has statutory representation in the coordinating body of the EpidA, as well as the *Conference of Cantonal Governments* (KdK), which was represented in the Federal Council's main "crisis unit" (*"Krisenstab des Bundesrats Corona"*). Despite the centralized but consultative approach to decision-making, it was the *cantons* which were (and continue to be) responsible for implementing rules and restrictions. The authors also note that the federal government worked closely with the *Cantons* to support affected businesses, coordinating with the Swiss National Bank and commercial banks to provide income support, including interest-free loans.

27.2.3 Weak collaboration between orders of government

The cases in this category are characterized by uncoordinated responses vertically and horizontally between jurisdictions in these countries. In each of these cases, federal and constituent unit governments were often at odds over policy. In some cases, states/provinces competed with each other to secure supplies and equipment to deal with the pandemic. This impeded the development and implementation of a national response to the crisis. As shown in Table 27.1, cases in this category had uniformly poor outcomes when measured by deaths per 100,000 people.

A formerly unitary country, **Belgium** began to federalize beginning in 1970 and has since evolved, through various stages of constitutional reform, into a highly competitive federal system, as Peter Bursens, Patricia Popelier, and Petra Meier write. The complexity of Belgium's federalism is reflected in the country's overlapping constituent units. These consist of linguistic communities based on the country's three official languages, as well as three geographic regions. The composition of Belgium is a historic product of largely economic interests, with communities and regions having exclusive but also interdependent competences. In the first place, federalization in Belgium was never intended to promote intergovernmental cooperation – either vertically or horizontally – but instead designed to respond to demands from the constituent units for greater autonomy. The complex nature of Belgium's version of federalism is echoed in the policy domain of emergency management. Responsibilities are scattered across different government levels, creating a real patchwork and making collaboration between the various levels a challenge. In the first phase of the pandemic, this system prevented – at least initially – a coordinated government response, which was also partially attributable to the fact that the country had a caretaker government. As it became clear that the response to COVID-19 would require comprehensive and coordinated decision-making, the crisis proved to be the catalyst for the installation of a federal government with full powers to handle the pandemic. A so-called *federal phase* of crisis management was announced on 13 March 2020, implying that all decisions to fight COVID-19 were to be taken by a crisis management committee composed of the federal and regional governments as well as language communities. The competitive nature of Belgian federalism, the authors argue, with its duplication of functions, led to contradictory policies at different orders of government. As the pandemic continued, challenges in coordination and collaboration among government levels persisted, rendering the response to the pandemic partially ineffective.

As Nina Sajic argues, **Bosnia and Herzegovina** is a deeply divided, polarized, and fragmented country without a common vision. The country is marked by: the political rivalry between the country's two constituent units, the Federation of Bosnia & Hercegovina (FB&H) and the Republika Srpska (SR); tensions between those advocating for more centralization and those demanding more autonomy; and a lack of trust between key political actors at the federal and constituent unit levels. When the pandemic reached the country in March 2020 and a national emergency was declared at the federal level, it triggered the federated units into action. The more centralized SR reacted first by enforcing lockdown measures, coordinated by the ad hoc Emergency Situation committee headed by the SR Prime Minister. Throughout the crisis and its fluctuating severity, this committee managed most of the restriction and relief measures enacted. In the FB&H however, overriding policy power to respond to the crisis is decentralized and vested in the ten constituting *Cantons*. The government of the FB&H enacted an overarching "Corona Law," but its interpretation, enforcement, and the extent of the measures implemented varied widely between the various *Cantons*. Intergovernmental relations in terms of horizontal coordination were virtually non-existent between the FB&H and the SR. Delays in the enforcement of restrictions as well as in the easing of controls prompted heated discussions between the two entities on several occasions.

The COVID-19 pandemic was confirmed to have spread to **Brazil** on 25 February 2020. Since health is a shared competence between all three orders of government, governors and mayors in the most affected states were the first to adopt measures to limit infections. State and federal executives differed on how the crisis should be handled. The federal government, concerned about the fragile state of Brazil's economic recovery, took time to evaluate the national threat from COVID-19 and minimize economic damage. As Eduardo Henrique Corrêa da S.P. Néris and Rodrigo Ribeiro Bedritichuk write in their chapter, the federal government passed legislation specifying what kind of measures authorities could adopt concerning virus control and preventive health policies. As the pandemic progressed in Brazil, the federal government enacted social programs to relieve unemployment and supported sub-national units with extra financial transfers. The federal government also created the "Crisis Committee" to manage the outbreak. To facilitate intergovernmental communication and coordination, the Special Secretariat for Federative Affairs (SEAF) instituted bi-weekly meetings with the Crisis Committees of the states. However, these councils and committees proved to be rather ineffective, which led to each level of government pursuing its own policies to manage the crisis. This triggered both conflict and con-fusion over whose regulations had precedence – the states' or the federations'. Con-sequently, many cases were presented to the Brazilian Supreme Court, and its rulings ultimately determined a top-down approach would be taken to pandemic manage-ment. Restrictions enacted at a higher level of government could not be challenged in degree of severity by a lower-level government. The first part of Brazil's response to COVID-19 was thus characterized by an uncoordinated and inefficient approach. It was only in the latter part of the response that institutions such as SEAF became engaged in trying to shape a more coordinated response. Bringing in the municipal governments was crucial since they are both constitutionally significant but also have wide-ranging responsibility for the delivery of services.

Mexico was among the countries very severely impacted by the COVID-19 pan-demic in 2020, as measured by mortality. Competence for public health policy is shared between all three orders of government and the existing health care system is deeply fragmented, as Laura Flamand, Monica Naime, and Juan C. Olmeda highlight in their chapter. The lack of political will at the federal level to push for a collabora-tive response obstructed a coordinated and efficient management of the crisis. Follow-ing the first two recorded deaths of COVID-19 patients in March 2020, the Mexican effort to tackle the health crisis was led individually by the state governments. While the federal government did declare the pandemic a health emergency via the National Public Health Council, this did not entail binding legislation to be enforced by the states. In addition to the declaration, the federal government reallocated financial re-sources to an emergency fund, implemented measures for the reorganization of public and private hospitals to equip them for COVID-19 patient care and, from the end of March 2020, recommended social distancing as part of a national health campaign. By this point, 10 of Mexico's 32 governors had already closed education facilities in their states. Despite their heavy financial dependence on federal transfers, the states (some with outright opposition to federal policies in mind) extended closures to cul-tural venues and businesses, introduced restrictions on public gatherings, established punitive measures for failing to adhere to restrictions, and adopted their own testing procedures and economic relief programs. Disputes between the states and federal government continued to escalate with several governors calling for a revision of the 1978 fiscal pact, and in September 2020, nine governors left the National Conference of Governors.

The **United States** ranked first on the 2019 Global Health Security Index. Yet by all accounts the country performed very poorly in responding to the COVID-19 pandemic in 2020, as John Kincaid and J. Wesley Leckrone describe. While the federal government, including the US Centers for Disease Control and Prevention (CDC), began screening for COVID-19 as early as January 2020 and barred entry of foreign nationals traveling from China, President Trump pushed states to lead the COVID-19 response. Under the dualist structure of American federalism, health care is predominantly a state responsibility and the president made no effort to cen-tralize executive decision-making authority. His administration also failed to for-mulate a cooperative federal-state-local plan of action. In the absence of apex-level intergovernmental institutions, coordination relied largely on sector-specific bureaucratic channels, including the CDC and its state and local public-health counterparts. Consequently, state governors and their secretaries of health became the main COVID-19 communicators. The lack of a national policy on acquiring and distributing medical supplies induced competition for several months. States bid against each other in global markets for personal protective equipment, masks, and ventilators. Ultimately, states developed working relationships, where some governors concluded regional agreements on coordinating the reopening of their economies and purchasing arrangements for medical supplies. As large urban areas were hit badly by the pandemic, municipalities were at the forefront of providing services to affected populations as well as giving support to marginalized groups. Partisan polarization around the seriousness of COVID-19 and necessary relief measures made the situation worse. This is reflected by the country's high number of COVID-19 casualties in 2020.

The **European Union** is not a conventional federation but an international organization exhibiting federal features (Kincaid 1999). In her chapter, Christina Ares explains that the decision-making authority of the EU is limited because EU institutions can only execute those competences explicitly transferred to them by the Member States. The EU nonetheless responded reasonably quickly and on a broad policy front to the COVID-19 crisis, although at the beginning of the pandemic it failed to effectively coordinate national policies among its Member States. While the EU only plays a supportive role in public health policy, it was able to compensate by exercising its political influence in the areas of monetary and economic policy. It enforced immediate amendments to the EU 2020 budget and the Multiannual Financial Framework (MFF) of 2014–2020, redirected financial resources from the cohesion fund to the Coronavirus Response Investment Initiative (CRII) and CRIIPlus, and made loans available to Member States via the temporary support for unemployment emergency (SURE), the European Investment Bank, and the European Stability Mechanism. Most significant, however, was the announcement of EU's ambitious COVID-19 Recovery Plan, which amounts to €2,364.3 billion euros. Discussions conducted at the level of the Member States were vital to the successful bridging of differing stances on the nature of spending, the size of the funds made available for tackling the pandemic, and the form in which state aid is to be given – loans or grants. Particularly important were the talks at which the German and French governments sought to find common ground. Horizontal communication between the legislative and executive branches within the EU, as well as between the Member States themselves, however, remains an issue. Connecting the approval of COVID-19 response measures to the working plan and the priorities for the current institutional cycle 2019–2024 of the Commission proved a step in the right direction in this regard.

27.3 Common threads

While the broad categorization of responses above highlights the differences in the ways in which the countries tackled the crisis, and the political and institutional arrangements that shaped the approach, we can nevertheless also establish broad commonalities between the different case studies. Identifying these common threads enables us to draw preliminary conclusions about the impact that COVID-19 has had on the practice of federalism globally.

27.3.1 *Adequacy of legislative and regulatory arrangements*

Writing during the first half of 2020, Francesco Palermo (2020) noted that few federal countries declared the state of emergency, such as Australia, Ethiopia, and Mexico. Spain declared a 'state of alarm' and South Africa declared a 'state of disaster'. In the United States, President Trump issued this first five-state disaster declaration in its history. In his analysis, Palermo writes that during the first part of 2020, pandemic management in a large number of federations like Argentina, Austria, Belgium, Brazil, Canada, Germany, Switzerland, India, Malaysia, Pakistan, and Russia was still being undertaken within the framework of ordinary public health and disaster management. However, by the end of the year, more and more countries found it necessary to proclaim states of emergency to deal with the pandemic. Such that by the end of 2020, only four countries – India, Malaysia, Pakistan, and the United Kingdom – had not invoked emergency measures. In countries such as Canada, Germany, Kenya, and Russia no national states of emergency were proclaimed but constituent units did proclaim local emergencies (Table 27.2).

Despite the proclamation of national emergencies in a vast majority of cases, in most countries, constituent units did not cede additional powers to national governments even if there were varying degrees of centralization in some spheres of decision-making. In 16 of 24 cases, constituent units did not cede any power to the federal government (See Table 27.3). It should be noted that in some of these countries like Malaysia and South Africa constituent units were already relatively weak to begin with (Majeed, Watts and Brown 2005). In five cases, significant powers were ceded (even if temporarily). For example, constituent units in Belgium allowed federal authorities to decide on the operation and organization of schools and cultural institutions, while the declaration of the 'extraordinary situation' according to Switzerland's epidemic act allowed the federal government to strip the constituent units of their competences. In practice, the Cantons were integrated into the decision-making process and in the implementation of these decisions.

In Spain, the Autonomous Communities gave up authority over Internal Affairs, Transport, Urban Matters, and Health for a three-month period. In Italy,

Table 27.2 States of Emergency Proclamations by Level of Government

Country	National	Sub-national	None	Country	National	Sub-national	None
Argentina	X			Malaysia			X
Australia	X			Mexico	X		
Austria	X			Nepal	X		
Bosnia	X			Nigeria	X		
Belgium	X			Pakistan			X
Brazil	X			Russia		X	
Canada		X		S.Africa[6]	X		
Ethiopia	X			Spain	X		
Germany		X		Switzerland	X		
India			X	UK			X
Italy	X			USA	X		
Kenya		X		Euro Union	X		

the state of emergency enabled the national government to seize the powers of the regions in all spheres deemed necessary, but in practice, this was limited to policies around the opening/closing economic activities and on movement and transport. The Nigerian case is unique where in accordance with the 'Quarantine Act,' states can only make regulations where the president fails to do so. This has allowed the federal government to undertake pandemic management measures as if Nigeria were a unitary state.[7] In three countries, relatively limited powers were ceded to upper tier governments. In Austria, the *Länder* allowed the federal government to make procurements on their behalf, while in Kenya, the national government took over record-keeping of COVID-19 matters and resource mobilization, and in the case of the EU, Member States relied on it to oversee vaccine development and distribution.

27.3.2 Increased Apex-level Intergovernmental Relations (IGR)

It is well established in the literature that the development of IGR and coordination processes between different orders of government in federal systems can facilitate more effective and efficient policymaking and service delivery (Chattopadhyay and Whittington 2019; Poirier, Saunders and Kincaid 2015). Indeed, vertical and horizontal forms of coordination can facilitate the development of innovative policy action that would not otherwise be possible. In early 2020, a report by the World Health Organization reinforced this view when it concluded that coordination among the national and sub-national governments is the "first step of an effective response" (WHO 2020).

In the context of the public health and humanitarian crisis engendered by COVID-19, no single order of government had either the policy competence or the human, technical, or financial resources to deal with it alone. Therefore, both vertical and horizontal coordination became necessary. Tackling COVID-19 required all orders of government to do more than exchange data and information. Decisions on

Table 27.3 Powers Ceded by Constituent Units

No Powers Ceded	Extensive Powers Ceded	Limited Powers Ceded
1 Argentina	1 Belgium	1 Austria
2 Australia	2 Italy	2 Kenya
3 Bosnia	3 Nigeria	3 European Union
4 Brazil	4 Spain	
5 Canada	5 Switzerland	
6 Ethiopia		
7 Germany		
8 India		
9 Malaysia		
10 Mexico		
11 Nepal		
12 Pakistan		
13 Russia		
14 South Africa		
15 United Kingdom		
16 United States		

the scope and scale of lockdowns, as well as resumption of economic activities – while informed by science and data in most countries – were ultimately political in nature. Authors noted in 14 cases (Argentina, Australia, Austria, Belgium, Canada, Ethiopia, Germany, India, Kenya, Pakistan, South Africa, Spain, Switzerland, EU) that first ministers (heads of federal and constituent unit governments) met more frequently than in previous years.

For example, in Canada, the Prime Minister or his deputy met with provincial premiers almost weekly since the start of the COVID crisis. In comparison, this group had met only 16 times between 1993 and 2017. In Germany, the normally bi-annual meetings between the Chancellor and Minster-Presidents were convened bi-weekly at the beginning of the pandemic. Many of these countries, such as Austria, Australia, Canada, Germany, and South Africa, had well-established apex-level IGR mechanisms even before the pandemic (Poirier, Saunders and Kincaid 2015). But even countries where such mechanisms were underdeveloped, such as India and Spain, there were unprecedented levels of interaction through much of 2020. In Spain, where cooperation got off to a slow start, the Conference of Presidents ended up meeting more frequently in 2020 alone than it had in the previous 15 years. In India, the meetings between the Prime Minister and State Chief Ministers happened with much greater frequency than meetings of the Interstate Council over the last 20 years. Six cases (Italy, Malaysia, Nepal, Nigeria, Russia, and United Kingdom) in which authors noted no increased interaction between first ministers were countries where pandemic policy making was highly centralized. The importance of good IGR was particularly evident in the larger federations (population > 80 million), where greater coordination between orders of government resulted in better outcomes as measured in Cumulative Cases per 100,000 and deaths per 100,000 (Table 27.4).

It should be noted that, overall, the frequency of first ministers' meetings did not guarantee a particular outcome. The Belgian case is instructive in this regard where collaboration between orders of government remained weak. The increased frequency of meetings in the majority of cases underscores that in these countries national governments and constituent units saw each other as partners in the fight against COVID-19.

Table 27.4 Outcome in Large Federations (Pop.> 80 million)

Country	Cumulative Cases per 100,000	Cumulative Deaths per 100,00
Brazil	3,770.1	94.8
Ethiopia	111.2	1.7
Germany	2,277.9	48.2
India	757.3	10.9
Mexico	1,169.5	102.4
Nigeria	47.3	0.7
Pakistan	226.1	4.8
Russia	2,331.2	42.4
United States	6,574.3	110.5
European Union	3,892.5	84.1

Source: Extracted from Table 27.1

27.3.3 Executive federalism was the dominant mode of IGR, but...

Almost everywhere, the legislative basis for responding to epidemics or disasters empowers executive authorities (Dhar Chakrabarti 2015). The importance of first minister's meetings has been discussed in the previous section. The centrality of the executive, particularly, the federal or national executive, was even more in evidence in countries such as Italy, Malaysia, and Nigeria where the national government was at the forefront of pandemic management. In countries, where there were no or very weak pre-existing intergovernmental forums, such as the United States and Brazil, the Presidents periodically consulted with State Governors, even if they disagreed on policy prescriptions. For safety reasons, in several countries, it was not possible to convene regular sittings of national and constituent unit legislatures, which effectively remained in suspended animation. It took several months before parliaments migrated to virtual or mixed sittings in all countries, ceding policy space to national and sub-national executives in the meantime. In over half the cases (Bosnia, Belgium, Brazil, Germany, Italy, Kenya, Pakistan, Spain, South Africa, Switzerland, United Kingdom) national or sub-national legislatures expressed displeasure at being sidelined. But, in the case of the presidential federations (Argentina, Brazil, Mexico, the United States), legislatures played an active role in COVID policy. For example, early on in the pandemic, the Brazilian Congress declared a state of 'public calamity,' lifting the government's obligation to comply with the primary balance target, while the United States Congress was very active in putting together four COVID relief packages in Spring 2020.

In Austria, Australia, Brazil, Ethiopia, India, Italy, Pakistan, Spain, and the United States, a range of executive actions, particularly around the imposition of COVID-19 restrictions, were challenged in court. In most cases, the courts found in favor of decisions made by executives at the federal and constituent unit levels. The exceptions were Austria and the United States, where the court struck down specific restrictions.

27.3.4 Local government emerges as an important player

Over the course of 2020, it has become clear even in very highly centralized countries that sub-national governments, particularly local governments, have an important role to play in pandemic management. In many federations, even when local and metropolitan governments are not constitutionally recognized, as the order of government closest to the people it is seen as being the most responsive to community needs. In many countries, urban local governments also have a broad mandate coupled with significant financial and human resources which allow them to deliver key public services (Steytler 2009).

With the exception of five countries (Australia, Malaysia, Nepal, Nigeria, and Pakistan), local governments have been an indispensable part of national strategies to avoid blanket lockdowns which were the norm in most countries during early 2020. The near absence of local government as a player in these cases was largely a function of their limited mandates and capacity. In most of the other case studies, local governments (urban and rural) were at the forefront to enforcing local restrictions, organizing testing and tracing, and in some cases delivering COVID relief (India, Mexico, South Africa). Indeed, federal and constituent unit governments relied on local governments in Austria, Belgium, Brazil, Canada, Germany, Mexico, India,

Italy, and Spain to be proactive in implementing more stringent measures than those mandated by higher order governments in response to local public health conditions.

27.3.5 Erosion of sub-national fiscal capacity

The impact of COVID-19 on the global and national economies is stark. Extended shutdowns and job losses have destroyed livelihoods in many parts of the world. The International Monetary Fund (IMF) in its January 2021 World Economic Output projected that most major economies would perform poorly in 2020. Table 27.5 below illustrates the dire economic situation in some of the larger federations.

With the exception of a few federations such as Belgium, Canada, Switzerland, and the United States, constituent units in general raise very little of their own source revenue (Shah and Kincaid 2007). In the vast majority of federations, constituent unit taxation powers are limited, and they remain dependent on federal transfers either in the form of shared taxes, special purpose or ad hoc grants, or fiscal equalization payments. In countries such as Austria, Australia, India, and Nigeria, the states' share of value-added taxes (VAT/GST) represent a significant source of income for the states. In Canada and the United States where states can raise income taxes, sub-national revenues tend to be more buoyant (Kitchen, McMillan and Shah 2019).

However, in 2020, decreased economic activity and loss of jobs has expectedly led to lower revenue for all orders of government, in most countries. The impact, however, of this downturn is asymmetric. While federal revenues have been impacted, the fact that federal governments have the ability to monetize debt and greater fiscal capacity makes a huge difference to their ability to weather the economic storm. State and local governments, however, are much more vulnerable to economic shocks like COVID, and this is reflected in the fiscal deficit now facing the sub-national orders. The fiscal shock has not spared either the highly fiscally decentralized (e.g., Canada) or fiscally more centralized (e.g., Australia and Austria) federations. Our cases studies noted that in most countries federal governments stepped in with support packages

Table 27.5 Estimated Change in GDP in Percentage in 2020

Country	2020	2021
United States	–3.4	5.1
EURO AREA	–7.2	4.2
Germany	–5.4	3.5
Italy	–9.2	3.0
Spain	–11.1	5.9
United Kingdom	–10.0	4.5
Canada	–5.5	3.6
India	–8.0	11.5
Russia	–3.6	3.0
Brazil	–4.5	3.6
Mexico	–8.5	4.3
Nigeria	–3.2	1.5
South Africa	–7.5	2.8

Note: For India, data and forecasts are presented on a fiscal year basis, with FY2020/2021 starting in April 2020. World Economic Output, IMF, January 2021. Available from: https://www.imf.org/en/Publications/WEO/Issues/2021/01/26/2021-world-economic-outlook-update [Accessed 5 April 2021].

for constituent units. This support took different forms, ranging from enhanced lines of credit to special purpose grants. At the time of writing, Belgium, Bosnia, and Mexico were the only case studies where the federal government had not stepped up with additional resources.

Constituent unit revenues often declined more steeply than economic output. The scale of the crisis can be illustrated through a few examples. In May 2020, projections were released which indicated that Germany was predicted to suffer a year-on-year reduction in tax revenue of about 11 percent for the *Länder* and 15 percent for the municipalities (OECD 2020). The economy was projected to contract by –5.4 percent during the same period (Table 2). In India, even as the economy contracted by –8 percent, despite federal transfers, tax revenues of the 15 largest states declined by 14 percent during the April 2020-January 2021 period (Sahu 2021). Tombe et al. (2020) estimated that Canadian provinces were likely to see a $35 billion shortfall in 2020/21, with knock-on effects on local governments. Budget documents from 2020 indicated Ontario expected to lose almost 10 percent of tax revenue in 2020, while the Canadian economy was expected to shrink by –5.5 percent (Government of Ontario 2020). At the time of writing, deferred tax collection in Austria was likely to result in a 12 percent decrease in states' revenues (OECD 2020). In the United States, Kincaid and Leckrone note in this volume, the National Governors Association requested $500 billion in aid for state relief and the US Conference of Mayors requested $250 billion more in direct aid to localities.

Predictably, in all cases, federal and national governments have announced considerable budgetary measures to help sub-national governments cope with the fiscal shocks. Federal and state governments have also provided fiscal assistance to municipalities to support their frontline work in providing basic services. These measures have taken the form of additional transfers to sub-national governments, tax deferrals, concessional loans, and income support measures. Even the EU has shown flexibility on the issue of new debt raised by Member States. Given that most transfers earmarked for COVID-19 relief have come in the form of special purpose grants, in some countries (such as the United States), political wrangling has vitiated policy making and further complicated pandemic management.

In the years to come, the primary challenge for sub-national governments, particularly local governments, will be uncertainty over which types of revenue streams are likely to recover. While it is too early to make a definitive assessment, local governments who rely on property taxes and fees appear particularly vulnerable if commercial properties remain unoccupied, or if commuters stop using public transit or parking in municipal facilities as a result of remote working becoming the norm. Given the IMF's expectation that economic output will remain below 2019 levels in most major countries at least into 2022, it is highly likely that sub-national governments will continue to suffer from fiscal constraints (OECD 2020).

27.3.6 Laboratory federalism

Various case studies corroborate the hypothesis that federalism can contribute to intergovernmental learning (Oates 1999) or 'policy transfers' based on *New State Ice Co. v. Liebmann*, 285 U.S. 262 (1932) (Dolowitz and Marsh 2000). All case studies provide evidence of policy transfers. Due to space constraints, we will illustrate this by highlighting one case from each region.

During the first phase of the pandemic, Argentina's Federal Council for Healthcare (COFESA in Spanish) provided a platform where states could work together to create tools to link their information systems to the 'DetectAr' program (aimed at identification, detection, and tracing COVID-19 cases), and the integrated database system (SISA in Spanish), allowing them to monitor and locate stocks of medicines and equipment around the country. The chapter on Canada notes that the pandemic also marked the first time one saw the concerted use of social media to communicate intergovernmental responses to a major emergency, as well as community engagement tool by individual governments. Throughout the first wave of the pandemic, apart from Ontario, other provinces periodically imposed generalized border restrictions on interprovincial travel or requirements to self-isolate if visiting from another region in the country.

In Kenya, the Council of Governors (CoG) made significant strides toward the support of the most vulnerable in select counties through partnership with development partners. These measures initially included the provision of 'dignity hygiene products' for women in the reproductive age within quarantine/isolation facilities and supported by tele-counselors for manning hotlines in three counties. This became a template for future expansion. In India, Uttar Pradesh became one of the first states to rope in local governments to provide more granular approaches to quarantine and isolating infected wards. This approach eventually allowed states to take more responsive and graduated approach to imposing restrictions based on local conditions.

In Australia, Victoria's strong quarantine measures in the early phase of the pandemic in response to errors made initially in the quarantining of overseas arrivals in the state, served as a template for others states to refine their own quarantine regulations. In another example from Australia, contact tracing methods employed in New South Wales which were considered to be effective were adopted by Victoria.

In Germany, early lockdown restrictions implemented in Bavaria, one of Germany's most severely impacted *Land*, set the tone for Germany's increased nationwide restrictions later in March 2020. Also, the City State of Berlin designed a so-called "traffic light system" consisting of three indicators: the reproductive value ("R factor"); the number of available ICU beds in the City State; and the number of new infections per 100,000 people over a period of seven days. When all three indicators hit a predefined mark, the government would respond by introducing stricter lockdown measures. This approach was later adopted by other *Länder* in the fall of 2020.

27.3.7 Increased digitalization

Most notably, the COVID crisis has pushed forward the process of the digitalization of administrative governance. This was not restricted to just federations. While this was not an issue we asked authors to explore in detail, the issue of digital delivery of public services was raised in a number of case studies. The point is particularly highlighted by Bussjäger and Eller in their chapter on Austria, but it also reflects the findings of the OECD (2020). As in other sectors, the majority of meetings of government officials or parliamentarians were held virtually in most countries in order to comply with social distancing requirements. Thus, video conferencing has become the new normal. The pandemic has also increased the need for digitalizing communications between the state and citizens, as well as between administrative units themselves. Thus, digitalization of administrative procedures has also taken place during the crisis. In countries such as Canada and India, governments have launched digital apps to track and stop the spread of the coronavirus.

It is probable that this will have an enormous impact on the way in which governments communicate both internally and externally with their citizens in the future. The push for increased digitalization of administrative service delivery as well as inter-agency communication will most likely have an impact on federal governance. This is already evident in the digitalization of education. The transition to digital schooling has been led by locally managed school districts in the Global North, but remains a challenge in the Global South. Issues of access remain to be addressed, however, even in Europe and the Americas. Figures from the OECD (2020) indicate that even in a wealthy country like Italy, almost 42 percent of the population have no access to computers or tablets at home.

The other area where digitization of service delivery has assumed importance is health care. Although digital technologies, such as those used for telemedicine, have existed for decades, they have had poor penetration into the market because of heavy regulation. As recently as 2019, a US survey showed that 38 percent of chief executive officers of US health care systems reported having no digital component in their overall strategic plan. COVID-19 has changed much in this regard, where patients increasingly prefer virtual consultations to ones in person.

Administrative systems across orders of government will have to be harmonized in order to ensure interoperability, assign clear responsibilities, and avoid duplication and inconsistencies. Such a process will warrant strong collaboration between orders of government. At the same time, digitalization requires substantial financial investment which – in the face of low fiscal capacities of many constituent units – will in all likelihood have to be carried by the federal government in most countries. The issue of access is particularly salient in countries such as Ethiopia where informational and communications technological penetration is relatively low. This, though, potentially carries the risk of a process of centralization, or at least tension between orders of government about the scope and objectives of a digitalized administrative governance system. Federal governments could aim to entice constituent units dependent on transfers toward preferred policy behavior.

27.4 Outlook

It is clear that many possible factors play a role in determining the outcome of a country's response to the COVID-19 pandemic. There are many factors which we have not – or have only peripherally – discussed in this book. We have considered the impact the pandemic had on federal and multilevel systems and, vice-versa, how federal and multilevel systems have responded to the pandemic. Regarding the constitutional form of a country, we have focused our analysis on the question of multilevel government as opposed to unitary government systems. At the same time, we have not examined questions around democracy and authoritarian rule in depth, or explicitly compared the performance of parliamentary systems with presidential systems. Other important factors influencing pandemic response derive from political leadership, how governments communicate policies to their constituencies, and what level of trust a body politic has in its leaders and scientists. Also significant, of course, is the capacity and resilience of a country's health system.

Further, there are many other important factors which lie outside the realm of politics, such as the geographic location of a country and how tightly it is integrated with other countries, its population density and the degree of urbanization, as well as demographic factors. The older a society, the more likely COVID-19 will have a lethal impact. And even the climate may play a role. There is emerging evidence that the virus spreads less effectively outside, and in indoor environments where there is effective ventilation, and thus warmer countries may have an advantage in controlling the spread of the virus.

Finally, the timeline of developments was important at the beginning of the crisis. In Europe, for example, the pandemic hit Italy first; therefore, other countries had some time to adapt and learn from the Italian experience. Thus, one could say that luck was a factor here, too.

All these factors or variables have to be taken into account or controlled for if attempting to answer the question what impact a system of governance had on the efficacy of pandemic response. It is important to emphasize that, at the time of writing, the pandemic was not over and it is likely to be some time before one can properly reflect upon events and offer a more definitive verdict on how the COVID-19 crisis affected the practice of federalism globally. Inevitably, the question arises of whether unitary countries have been more successful than federal ones. In his chapter in this book comparing the relative performance of federal versus non-federal countries within the OECD, David Cameron argues that the structure of government, federal or non-federal, does not determine pandemic-management outcomes. Indeed, what mattered most in confronting COVID were the quality of leadership at all levels and in all professional spheres, which established a bond of trust between the leaders and the led; and good governance, which permitted effective organization, timely interventions, and the application of the required resources of the state to combating the disease.

We also saw the potential challenges of federalism come to the forefront. The system of checks and balances and power sharing exhibited by federal systems of government prevents them from imposing uniform policies across the country. Indeed, as some authors argue, regulatory overlaps and coordination deficits may have hindered the pursuit of effective responses to the pandemic in 2020. Also, in some federal systems, the pandemic has enhanced conflicts between the federal and sub-national level or even between the constituent units with regard to competences and enacted measures.

There were conspicuous cases of ineffective governance by the constituent units, particularly in developing federations such as Ethiopia and Nepal, because of a lack of sub-national capacity. Sub-national governments were ineffective owing to a lack of human and financial resources necessary to fulfil their functions. Thus, decision-makers should be aware of the risk of overburdening weak and newly established governing institutions with demands that they cannot meet.

It will also be interesting to analyze the impact of the pandemic on the political discussions around federalism. The pandemic ignited debates in almost all countries around either the relevance of federalism or its effectiveness in responding to the crisis, circling around the tension between the need or desire for uniform solutions and approaches with the need or desire for regionally tailored solutions and approaches. In some countries – Ethiopia, Nigeria, and Malaysia, for example – there seem to be strong calls for further decentralization of powers to constituent units and local governments. In other federations, at times, many called for more centralization in the faces of seemingly fragmented and uncoordinated policies. Gaining a better understanding what difference federalism may have made compared to other governance systems will be important for this debate.

27.5 Concluding thoughts

This survey of 24 case studies aimed to develop an understanding of how federalism mediated responses to the COVID-19 pandemic. Furthermore, it intended to consider whether the strain of dealing with the crisis changed the character of federalism in these systems. The variety in approaches that we have seen across the cases is reflective of the diversity among federations, including in their politics and institutional structure. The pandemic and its social-economic fallout has been too overwhelming for any one sphere of government to handle by itself. Consequently, as is apparent from this survey, countries where different orders of government collaborated closely generally achieved better outcomes during 2020. A major lesson of the study of this period of pandemic is the importance of building robust mechanisms for intergovernmental coordination and cooperation. The need for vertical cooperation has proven as important as horizontal cooperation in order to manage the pandemic policy response. Indeed, the actual pattern of response is shaped by a variety of factors, such as political leadership, the state of the health care system, and political culture, which go far beyond the constitutional structures for assigning power in the given country.

Acknowledgment

For comments on an earlier drafts of the chapter, we are grateful to David Cameron, John Kincaid, and Sandeep Shastri.

Notes

1 Bing COVID tracker Updated 19 January 2021 at 10:20 AM.
2 WHO Coronavirus Disease (COVID-19) Dashboard Data: 19 January 2021, 6:44 PM CE.
3 Palermo, Francesco. (2012). Italy: A Federal Country without Federalism?. https://www. researchgate.net
4 New Data Triples Russia's Covid-19 Death Toll – The New York Times (nytimes.com).
5 "January GST Collection Highest at INR 1.2 Lakh Crore", *Financial Express*, 2 February 2021.
6 A "State of Disaster" is distinct from a "State of Emergency" that can be declared by the President section 37 of the Constitution of South Africa and in terms of the State of Emergency Act 1997. The South African Human Rights Commission, Tseliso Thipanyane, has argued that the measures introduced in fact amounts to a State of Emergency (a point echoed by others), but President Ramaphosa did not want to use that term due to its association with the days of apartheid. For more, see Labuschaigne, Melodie; Staunton, Ciara: *COVID-19: State of Disaster in South Africa, VerfBlog*, 11 April 2020, https:// verfassungsblog.de/covid-19-state-of-disaster-in-south-africa/.
7 The Law and Human Rights in Nigeria's Response to the COVID-19 Pandemic I Bill of Health (harvard.edu).

Bibliography

Anderson, G., 2008. *Federalism: An Introduction*. Toronto: Oxford University Press.
Bronskill, J., 2021. Federal Liberals Earmark $7.2 Billion for Health Care, Vaccination, Municipalities. *The Canadian Press*, 25 March. Available from: https://www.cp24.com/ news/federal-liberals-earmark-7-2-billion-for-health-care-vaccination-municipalities-1.5362599?cache=yes%3FclipId%3D89578%3FautoPlay%3Dtrue [Accessed 5 April 2021].
Cameron, D. 2021.*The Impact of COVID-19 on Federal Countries*. University of Toronto: Unpublished.

Chattopadhyay, R. and Whittington, L., 2020. *Apex-level Intergovernmental Relations in Federal Systems: Comparative Perspectives and Lessons for the Indian Context*. Ottawa: World Bank and Forum of Federations.

Dhar Chakrabarti, P.G., 2015. *Federalism and Disaster Management Forum of Federations*, Occassional Paper Number 10. Government of Ontario, 2020. Ontario's Economic and Fiscal Outlook in Brief. *2020 Ontario Budget*. Available from: https://budget.ontario.ca/2020/brief.html#section-0 [Accessed 5 April 2021].

Gravelle, J.G. and Marples, D.J., 2021. Fiscal Policy and Recovery from the COVID-19 Recession. *Congressional Research Service Report*. R46460, 1 February.

International Monetary Fund, January 2021. World Economic Outlook Update. Available from: https://www.imf.org/en/Publications/WEO/Issues/2021/01/26/2021-world-economic-outlook-update [Accessed 5 April 2021].

Kincaid, J., 1999. Confederal Federalism and Citizen Representation in the European Union. *West European Politics* 22 (2), 34–58.

Kitchen, H., McMillan, M. and Shah, A., 2019. Higher-Order Fiscal Transfers to Local Governments: An Overview of Worldwide Practices. *In*: Kitchen, H., McMillan, M. and Shah, A., eds. *Local Public Finance and Economics*. Cham: Palgrave Macmillan, 441–469.

Majeed, A., Watts, R.L. and Brown, D.M., 2005. *Distribution of Powers and Responsibilities in Federal Countries*. *Global Dialogue on Federalism*. Volume 2. Montreal: McGill-Queens University Press.

Marchildon, G.P. and Bossert, T.J., eds., 2018. *Federalism and Decentralisation in Health Care: A Decision Space Approach*. Toronto: University of Toronto Press.

OECD, 2020. *The Territorial Impact of COVID-19: Managing the Crisis across Orders of Government. OECD Policy Responses to Coronavirus (COVID-19)*. Paris: Organization for Economic Cooperation and Development.

Palermo, F. 2020. 'Is There a Space for Federalism in Times of Emergency?', *VerfBlog*, 13 May 2020. Available from: https://verfassungsblog.de/is-there-a-space-for-federalism-in-times-of-emergency/

Poirier, J. and Saunders, C., 2015. Conclusion: Comparative Experience of Intergovernmental Relations in Federal Systems. *In*: Poirier, J., Saunders, C. and Kincaid, J., eds. *Intergovernmental Relations in Federal Systems*. Toronto: Oxford University Press, 440–498.

Shah, A., 2007. ed. *The Practice of Fiscal Federalism. Comparative Perspectives*. Montreal: McGill-Queens University Press.

Steytler, N. 2009. *Local Government and Metropolitan Regions in Federal Systems. Global Dialogue on Federalism*. Volume 6. Montreal: McGill-Queens University Press.

Tombe, T., Beland, D., Lecours, A. and Paquet. M., 2020. Critical Juncture in Fiscal Federalism? Canada's Response to COVID-19. *Canadian Journal of Political Science* 53 (2), 239–243.

Watts, R.L., 2008. *Comparing Federal Systems*. Montreal: McGill Queens University Press.

WHO, 2020. Laboratory Testing Strategy Recommendations for COVID-19. Available from: https://apps.who.int/iris/bitstream/handle/10665/331509/WHO-COVID-19-lab_testing-2020.1-eng.pdf [Accessed 5 April 2021].

Postscript

Since the period of analysis in this volume ends in January 2021, it is important to provide a postscript to provide an overview of the course of the pandemic in the first half of 2021. As of June 2021, almost all country cases in the volume reported new waves of infections. Argentina, Australia, Austria, Belgium, Canada Germany, Nigeria, Pakistan, Russia, South Africa, Spain, Switzerland, United Kingdom, European Union all experienced a third wave. Countries like India and Malaysia experienced a third wave. Countries such as Brazil, Mexico, and Russia have experienced high plateaus, rather than waves.

In most federations of the Global North, vaccination rollout during the first quarter of 2021 combined with improved health interventions led to significantly improved outcomes measured by lower case fatalities (CFR) than earlier waves. Furthermore, death rates measured in number per million were also considerably lower during the waves in 2021 (Figures 27.1 and 27.2).

The presidential federations Argentina, Brazil, Mexico, and Russia outcomes measured in CFR plateaued at relatively high levels, despite declining slightly from their 2020 peaks. Only in Argentina has there been a consistent decline, while in Russia, there has been a constant increase in CFR. Argentina which did very well through the first wave suffered quite badly in the second wave in late 2020 and third wave in 2021, as measured by deaths per million. Russia's situation has consistently worsened into 2021 (Figures 27.3 and 27.4).

A look at select federations in the Global South is also instructive. In Ethiopia, India, and Malaysia, falling CFR during most of 2020 saw slight reversal in 2021, as caseloads increased in these countries. In Pakistan, CFR has remained high since the beginning of the pandemic. In South Africa, which had a devastating first wave, CFRs have continued to rise. The selection of these cases is based on availability of data. When looking at deaths per million, both India and Malaysia, which has managed to keep fatalities low during the first wave, suffered significantly during the second wave. Fatalities also climbed in Pakistan during 2021 (Figure 27.5).

The other major event of 2021 is the large-scale roll out of vaccinations for COVID. The chart below provides an overview of relative vaccination rates in the number of cases where the data is available. As has been widely reported in the press, there is a big disparity in access to vaccines between the Global North and South, and this is reflected in the data on federations (Figure 27.6).

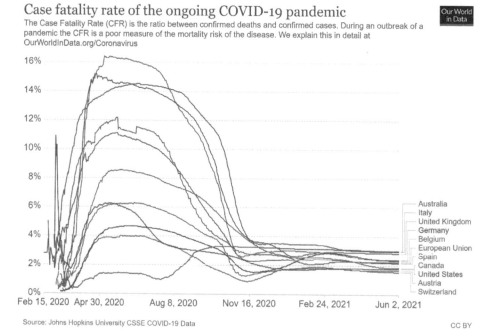

Figure 27.1 Case Fatality Rate of the Ongoing COVID-19 Pandemic.

While the analysis of the pandemic in the period after vaccines were rolled out is outside the scope of the volume, it was important to provide an update of what has happened during the period following the period under study.

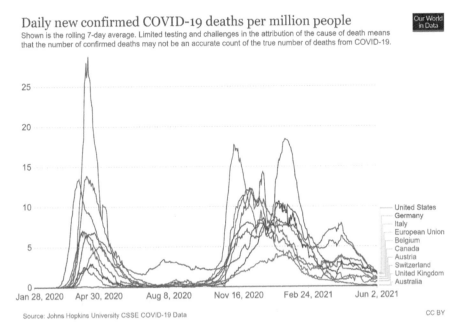

Figure 27.2 Daily New Confirmed COVID-19 Deaths per Million People.

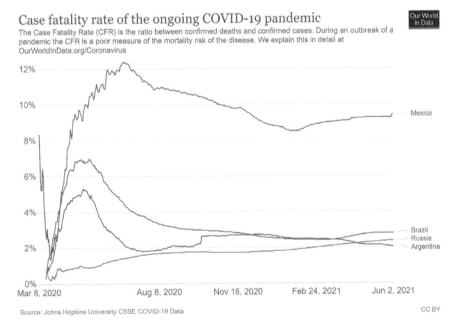

Figure 27.3 Case Fatality Rate of the Ongoing COVID-19 Pandemic.

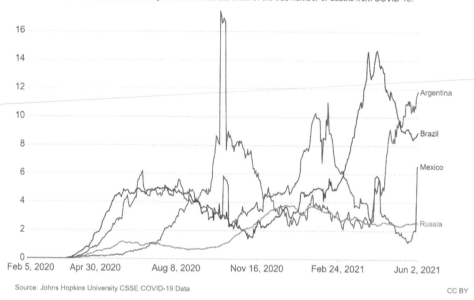

Figure 27.4 Daily New Confirmed COVID-19 Deaths per Million People.

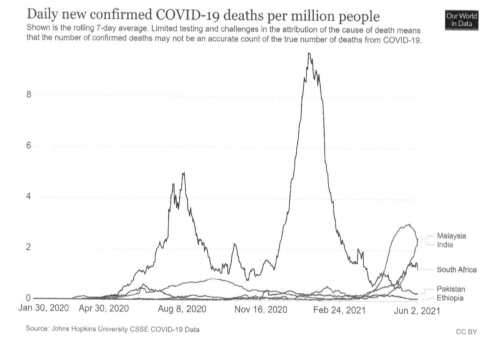

Figure 27.5 Daily New Confirmed COVID-19 Deaths per Million People.

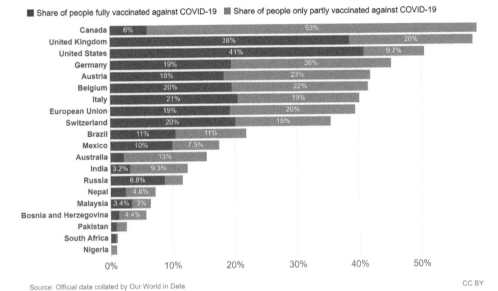

Figure 27.6 Share of People Vaccinated against COVID-19, June 2, 2021.

Index

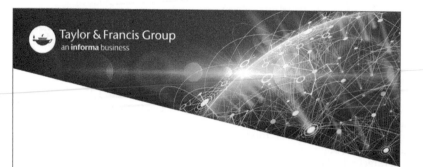